SANFORD GUIDE®

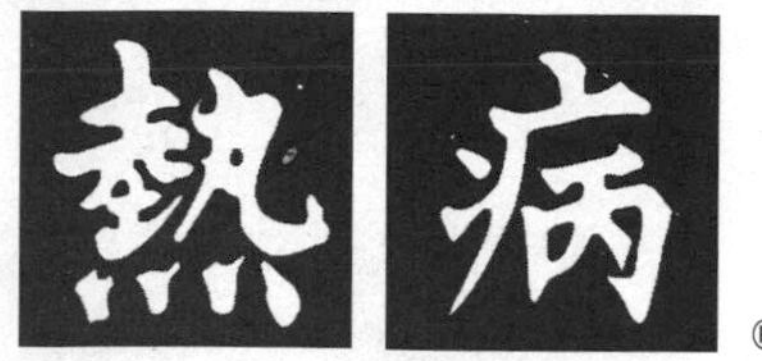

Forty-First Edition

THE SANFORD GUIDE TO ANTIMICROBIAL THERAPY 2011

David N. Gilbert, M.D.
Robert C. Moellering, Jr., M.D.
George M. Eliopoulos, M.D.
Henry F. (Chip) Chambers, M.D.
Michael S. Saag, M.D.

THE SANFORD GUIDE TO ANTIMICROBIAL THERAPY 2011
(41ST EDITION)

Editors

David N. Gilbert, M.D.
Chief of Infectious Diseases and Director, Earl A. Chiles Research Institute
Providence Portland Medical Center, Oregon

Robert C. Moellering, Jr., M.D.
Shields Warren-Mallinckrodt Professor of Medical Research, Harvard Medical School, Boston, Massachusetts

George M. Eliopoulos, M.D.
Chief, James L. Tullis Firm, Beth Israel Deaconess Hospital, Professor of Medicine, Harvard Medical School, Boston, Massachusetts

Henry F. (Chip) Chambers, M.D.
Chief of Infectious Diseases, San Francisco General Hospital, Professor of Medicine, University of California at San Francisco

Michael S. Saag, M.D.
Director, UAB Center for AIDS Research, Professor of Medicine and Director, Division of Infectious Diseases, University of Alabama, Birmingham

Contributing Editors

Douglas Black, Pharm. D.
Professor of Pharmacy, University of Washington, Seattle

David O. Freedman, M.D.
Director, Travelers Health Clinic, Professor of Medicine, University of Alabama, Birmingham

Managing Editor
Jeb C. Sanford

Emeritus
Jay P. Sanford, M.D. (1928-1996)
Merle A. Sande, M.D. (1935-2007)

The SANFORD GUIDES are updated annually and published by:

Antimicrobial Therapy, Inc.
P.O. Box 276, 11771 Lee Highway, Sperryville, VA 22740-0276 USA
Tel (+1) 540-987-9480 *Fax* (+1) 540-987-9486 *Email*: info@sanfordguide.com
www.sanfordguide.com

Acknowledgements
Thanks to Ushuaia Solutions, SA, Argentina, for assistance with the design layout of the manuscript; Royalty Press, Westville, NJ for printing and Fox Bindery, Quakertown, PA for finishing this edition of the Sanford Guide to Antimicrobial Therapy.

Note to Readers

Since 1969, the SANFORD GUIDE has been independently prepared and published. Decisions regarding the content of the SANFORD GUIDE are solely those of the editors and the publisher. We welcome your questions, comments and feedback concerning the SANFORD GUIDE. All of your feedback is reviewed and taken into account in preparing the next edition.

Every effort is made to ensure the accuracy of the content of this guide. However, current full prescribing information available in the package insert of each drug should be consulted before prescribing any product. The editors and publisher are not responsible for errors or omissions or for any consequences from application of the information in this book and make no warranty, express or implied, with respect to the currency, accuracy, or completeness of the contents of the publication. Application of this information in a particular situation remains the professional responsibility of the practitioner.

Content-related notices are published on our website at:
http://www.sanfordguide.com/notices

Printed in the United States of America
ISBN 978-1-930808-65-2
Pocket Edition (English)

QUICK PAGE GUIDE TO THE SANFORD GUIDE*

* Adapted from materials provided by Stephanie Troy, M.D., Stanford Univ. Med. Ctr.

—TABLE OF CONTENTS—

ABBREVIATIONS

3TC = lamivudine
AB,% = percent absorbed
ABC = abacavir
ABCD = amphotericin B colloidal dispersion
ABLC = ampho B lipid complex
ACIP = Advisory Committee on Immunization Practices
AD = after dialysis
ADF = adefovir
AG = aminoglycoside
AIDS = Acquired Immune Deficiency Syndrome
AM-CL = amoxicillin-clavulanate
AM-CL-ER = amoxicillin-clavulanate extended release
AMK = amikacin
Amox = amoxicillin
AMP = ampicillin
Ampho B = amphotericin B
AM-SB = ampicillin-sulbactam
AP = atovaquone proguanil
AP Pen = antipseudomonal penicillins
APAG = antipseudomonal aminoglycoside (tobra, gent, amikacin)
ARDS = acute respiratory distress syndrome
ARF = acute rheumatic fever
ASA = aspirin
ATS = American Thoracic Society
ATV = atazanavir
AUC = area under the curve
Azithro = azithromycin
bid = twice a day
BL/BLI = beta-lactam/beta-lactamase inhibitor
BW = body weight
C&S = culture & sensitivity
CAPD = continuous ambulatory peritoneal dialysis
CARB = carbapenems (DORI, ERTA, IMP, MER)
CDC = Centers for Disease Control
Cefpodox = cefpodoxime proxetil
Ceftaz = ceftazidime
Ceph= cephalosporin
CFB = ceftobiprole
CFP = cefepime
Chloro = chloramphenicol
CIP = ciprofloxacin; **CIP-ER** = CIP extended release
Clarithro = clarithromycin; **ER** = extended release
Clav = clavulanate
Clinda = clindamycin
CLO = clofazimine
Clot = clotrimazole
CMV = cytomegalovirus
CQ = chloroquine phosphate
CrCl = creatinine clearance
CRRT = continuous renal replacement therapy
CSD = cat-scratch disease
CSF = cerebrospinal fluid

CXR = chest x-ray
d4T = stavudine
Dapto = daptomycin
DBPCT = double-blind placebo-controlled trial
dc = discontinue
ddC = zalcitabine
ddI = didanosine
DIC = disseminated intravascular coagulation
div. = divided
DLV = delavirdine
Dori = doripenem
DOT = directly observed therapy
DOT group = B. distasonis, B. ovatus, B. thetaiotaomicron
Doxy = doxycycline
DR = delayed release
DRSP = drug-resistant S. pneumoniae
DS = double strength
EBV = Epstein-Barr virus
EES = erythromycin ethyl succinate
EFZ = efavirenz
ENT = entecavir
ER = extended release
ERTA = ertapenem
Erythro = erythromycin
ESBLs = extended spectrum β-lactamases
ESR = erythrocyte sedimentation rate
ESRD = endstage renal disease
ETB = ethambutol
Flu = fluconazole
Flucyt = flucytosine
FOS-APV = fosamprenavir
FQ = fluoroquinolone (CIP, Oflox, Lome, Peflox, Levo, Gati, Moxi, Gemi)
FTC = emtricitabine
G = generic
GAS = Group A Strep
Gati = gatifloxacin
GC = gonorrhea
Gemi = gemifloxacin
Gent = gentamicin
gm = gram
GNB = gram-negative bacilli
Griseo = griseofulvin
HEMO = hemodialysis
HHV = human herpesvirus
HIV = human immunodeficiency virus
HLR = high-level resistance
H/O = history of
HSCT = hematopoietic stem cell transplant
HSV = herpes simplex virus
IA = injectable agent/anti-inflammatory drugs
ICAAC = International Conference on Antimicrobial Agents & Chemotherapy

IDSA = Infectious Diseases Society of America
IDV = indinavir
IFN = interferon
IMP = imipenem-cilastatin
INH = isoniazid
Inv = investigational
IP = intraperitoneal
IT = intrathecal
Itra = itraconazole
IVDU = intravenous drug user
IVIG = intravenous immune globulin
Keto = ketoconazole
LAB = liposomal ampho B
LCM = lymphocytic choriomeningitis virus
LCR = ligase chain reaction
Levo = levofloxacin
LP/R = lopinavir/ ritonavir
M. Tbc = Mycobacterium tuberculosis
Macrolides = azithro, clarithro, dirithro, erythro, roxithro
mcg = microgram
MER = meropenem
Metro = metronidazole
mg = milligram
Mino = minocycline
Moxi = moxifloxacin
MQ = mefloquine
MSSA/MRSA = methicillin-sensitive/resistant S. aureus
NB = name brand
NF = nitrofurantoin
NAI = not FDA-approved (indication or dose)
NFR = nelfinavir
NNRTI = non-nucleoside reverse transcriptase inhibitor
NRTI = nucleoside reverse transcriptase inhibitor
NSAIDs = non-steroidal
NUS = not available in the U.S.
NVP = nevirapine
O Ceph 1,2,3 = oral cephalosporins—*see Table 10C*
Oflox = ofloxacin
P Ceph 1,2,3,4 = parenteral cephalosporins—*see Table 10C*
P Ceph 3 AP = parenteral cephalosporins with antipseudomonal activity—*see Table 10C*
PCR = polymerase chain reaction
PEP = post-exposure prophylaxis
PI = protease inhibitor
PIP = piperacillin
PIP-TZ = piperacillin-tazobactam
po = per os (by mouth)
PQ = primaquine
PRCT = Prospective randomized controlled trials
PTLD = post-transplant lymphoproliferative disease
Pts = patients

ABBREVIATIONS (2)

Pyri = pyrimethamine
PZA = pyrazinamide
qid = 4 times a day
QS = quinine sulfate
Quinu-dalfo = **Q-D** = quinupristin-dalfopristin
R = resistant
RFB = rifabutin
RFP = rifapentine
Rick = Rickettsia
RIF = rifampin
RSV = respiratory syncytial virus
RTI = respiratory tract infection
RTV = ritonavir
rx = treatment
S = potential synergy in combination with penicillin, AMP, vanco, teico

SA = Staph. aureus
SD = serum drug level after single dose
Sens = sensitive (susceptible)
SM = streptomycin
SQV = saquinavir
SS = steady state serum level
STD = sexually transmitted disease
subcut = subcutaneous
Sulb = sulbactam
Tazo = tazobactam
TBc = tuberculosis
TC-CL = ticarcillin-clavulanate
TDF = tenofovir
TEE = transesophageal echocardiography
Teico = teicoplanin
Telithro = telithromycin

Tetra = tetracycline
Ticar = ticarcillin
tid = 3 times a day
TMP-SMX = trimethoprim-sulfamethoxazole
TNF = tumor necrosis factor
Tobra = tobramycin
TPV = tipranavir
TST = tuberculin skin test
UTI = urinary tract infection
Vanco = vancomycin
VISA = vancomycin intermediately resistant S. aureus
VL = viral load
Vori = voriconazole
VZV = varicella-zoster virus
WHO = World Health Organization
ZDV = zidovudine

ABBREVIATIONS OF JOURNAL TITLES

AAC: Antimicrobial Agents & Chemotherapy
Adv PID: Advances in Pediatric Infectious Diseases
AHJ: American Heart Journal
AIDS Res Hum Retrovir: AIDS Research & Human Retroviruses
AJG: American Journal of Gastroenterology
AJM: American Journal of Medicine
AJRCCM: American Journal of Respiratory Critical Care Medicine
AJTMH: American Journal of Tropical Medicine & Hygiene
Aliment Pharmacol Ther: Alimentary Pharmacology & Therapeutics
Am J Hlth Pharm: American Journal of Health-System Pharmacy
Amer J Transpl: American Journal of Transplantation
AnEM: Annals of Emergency Medicine
AnIM: Annals of Internal Medicine
AnPharmacother: Annals of Pharmacotherapy
AnSurg: Annals of Surgery
Antivir Ther: Antiviral Therapy
ArDerm: Archives of Dermatology
ArIM: Archives of Internal Medicine
ARRD: American Review of Respiratory Disease
BMJ: British Medical Journal
BMTr: Bone Marrow Transplantation
Brit J Derm: British Journal of Dermatology
Can JID: Canadian Journal of Infectious Diseases
Canad Med J: Canadian Medical Journal
CCM: Critical Care Medicine
CCTID: Current Clinical Topics in Infectious Disease
CDBSR: Cochrane Database of Systematic Reviews
CID: Clinical Infectious Diseases
Clin Micro Inf: Clinical Microbiology and Infection
CMN: Clinical Microbiology Newsletter
Clin Micro Rev: Clinical Microbiology Reviews
CMAJ: Canadian Medical Association Journal

COID: Current Opinion in Infectious Disease
Curr Med Res Opin: Current Medical Research and Opinion
Derm Ther: Dermatologic Therapy
Dermatol Clin: Dermatologic Clinics
Dig Dis Sci: Digestive Diseases and Sciences
DMID: Diagnostic Microbiology and Infectious Disease
EID: Emerging Infectious Diseases
EJCMID: European Journal of Clin. Micro. & Infectious Diseases
Eur J Neurol: European Journal of Neurology
Exp Mol Path: Experimental & Molecular Pathology
Exp Rev Anti Infect Ther: Expert Review of Anti-Infective Therapy
Gastro: Gastroenterology
Hpt: Hepatology
ICHE: Infection Control and Hospital Epidemiology
IDC No. Amer: Infectious Disease Clinics of North America
IDCP: Infectious Diseases in Clinical Practice
IJAA: International Journal of Antimicrobial Agents
Inf Med: Infections in Medicine
J AIDS & HR: Journal of AIDS and Human Retrovirology
J All Clin Immun: Journal of Allergy and Clinical Immunology
J Am Ger Soc: Journal of the American Geriatrics Society
J Chemother: Journal of Chemotherapy
J Clin Micro: Journal of Clinical Microbiology
J Clin Virol: Journal of Clinical Virology
J Derm Treat: Journal of Dermatological Treatment
J Hpt: Journal of Hepatology
J Inf: Journal of Infection
J Med Micro: Journal of Medical Microbiology
J Micro Immunol Inf: Journal of Microbiology, Immunology, & Infection
J Ped: Journal of Pediatrics
J Viral Hep: Journal of Viral Hepatitis

JAC: Journal of Antimicrobial Chemotherapy
JACC: Journal of American College of Cardiology
JAIDS: JAIDS Journal of Acquired Immune Deficiency Syndromes
JAMA: Journal of the American Medical Association
JAVMA: Journal of the Veterinary Medicine Association
JCI: Journal of Clinical Investigation
JCM: Journal of Clinical Microbiology
JIC: Journal of Infection and Chemotherapy
JID: Journal of Infectious Diseases
JNS: Journal of Neurosurgery
JTMH: Journal of Tropical Medicine and Hygiene
Ln: Lancet
LnID: Lancet Infectious Disease
Mayo Clin Proc: Mayo Clinic Proceedings
Med Lett: Medical Letter
Med Mycol: Medical Mycology
MMWR: Morbidity & Mortality Weekly Report
NEJM: New England Journal of Medicine
Neph Dial Transpl: Nephrology Dialysis Transplantation
Ped Ann: Pediatric Annals
Peds: Pediatrics
Pharmacother: Pharmacotherapy
PIDJ: Pediatric Infectious Disease Journal
QJM: Quarterly Journal of Medicine
Scand J Inf Dis: Scandinavian Journal of Infectious Diseases
Sem Resp Inf: Seminars in Respiratory Infections
SGO: Surgery Gynecology and Obstetrics
SMJ: Southern Medical Journal
Surg Neurol: Surgical Neurology
Transpl Inf Dis: Transplant Infectious Diseases
Transpl: Transplantation
TRSM: Transactions of the Royal Society of Medicine

TABLE 1A – CLINICAL APPROACH TO INITIAL CHOICE OF ANTIMICROBIAL THERAPY*

Treatment based on presumed site or type of infection. In selected instances, treatment and prophylaxis based on identification of pathogens. Regimens should be reevaluated based on pathogen isolated, antimicrobial susceptibility determination, and individual host characteristics. *(Abbreviations on page 2)*

ANATOMIC SITE/DIAGNOSIS/ MODIFYING CIRCUMSTANCES	ETIOLOGIES (usual)	SUGGESTED REGIMENS*		ADJUNCT DIAGNOSTIC OR THERAPEUTIC MEASURES AND COMMENTS
		PRIMARY	ALTERNATIVE[§]	
ABDOMEN: *See Peritoneum, page 44; Gallbladder, page 15; and Pelvic Inflammatory Disease, page 23*				
BONE: Osteomyelitis. Microbiologic diagnosis is essential. If blood culture negative, need culture of bone. Culture of sinus tract drainage not predictive of bone culture. Review: *Ln 364:369, 2004.* For comprehensive review of antimicrobial penetration into bone, *see Clinical Pharmacokinetics 48:89, 2009.*				
Hematogenous Osteomyelitis				
Empiric therapy—Collect bone and blood cultures before empiric therapy				
Newborn (<4 mos.) *See Table 16 for dose*	S. aureus, Gm-neg. bacilli, Group B strep	**MRSA possible: Vanco+ (Ceftaz or CFP)**	**MRSA unlikely: (Nafcillin** or **oxacillin)** + **(Ceftaz or CFP)**	*Table 16 for dose.* Severe allergy or toxicity: (**Linezolid**[NAI] 10 mg/kg IV/po q8h + **aztreonam**). Could substitute **clindamycin** for linezolid.
Children (>4 mos.)—Adult: Osteo of extremity	S. aureus, Group A strep, Gm-neg. bacilli rare	**MRSA possible: Vanco**	**MRSA unlikely: Nafcillin** or **oxacillin**	Severe allergy or toxicity: **Clinda** or **TMP-SMX** or **linezolid**[NAI]. Adults: **ceftaz** 2 gm IV q8h, **CFP** 2 gm IV q12h. *Peds dosages in Table 16. See Table 10 for adverse reactions to drugs.*
		Add **Ceftaz or CFP** if Gm-neg. bacilli on Gram stain (**Adult doses below.** *Peds Doses: Table 16.*		
Adult (>21 yrs) **Vertebral osteo ± epidural abscess**; other sites *(NEJM 355:2012, 2006)*	S. aureus most common but variety other organisms. **Blood & bone cultures essential.**	**MRSA possible: Vanco** 1 gm IV q12h; if over 100 kg, 1.5 gm IV q12h	**MRSA unlikely: Nafcillin** or **oxacillin** 2 gm IV q4h	**Dx: MRI early to look for epidural abscess.** Allergy or toxicity: **TMP-SMX** 8–10 mg/kg per day div. IV q8h or **linezolid** 600 mg IV/po q12h *(AnIM 138:135, 2003)*[NAI]. *See MRSA specific therapy comment.* Epidural abscess ref.: *ArIM 164:2409, 2004.*
Specific therapy—Culture and in vitro susceptibility results known				
	MSSA	**Nafcillin** or **oxacillin** 2 gm IV q4h or **cefazolin** 2 gm IV q8h	**Vanco** 1 gm q12h IV; if over 100 kg, 1.5 gm IV q12h	**Other options if susceptible in vitro and allergy/toxicity issues:** 1) **TMP/SMX** 8-10 mg/kg/d IV div q8h. Minimal data on treatment of osteomyelitis; 2) **Clinda** 600-900 mg IV q8h – have lab check for inducible resistance especially if erythro resistant *(CID 40:280,2005)*; 3) [(**Cip** 750 mg po bid or **levo** 750 mg po q24h) + **rif** 300 mg po bid]; 4) **Daptomycin** 6 mg/kg IV q24h; –clinical failure secondary to resistance reported *(J Clin Micro 44:595;2006)*; 5) **Linezolid** 600 mg po/IV bid – anecdotal reports of efficacy *(J Chemother 17:643,2005)*, optic & peripheral neuropathy with long-term use *(Neurology 64:926, 2005)*; 6) **Fusidic acid**[NUS] 500 mg IV q8h + **rif** 300 mg po bid. *(CID 42:394, 2006)*.
	MRSA—*See Table 6, page 75; IDSA Guidelines CID 52 (Feb 1):1, 2011.*	**Vanco** 30-60 mg/kg per day in 2-3 divided doses to achieve target trough concentrations of 15-20 mcg/mL recommended for serious infections.	**Linezolid** 600 mg q12h IV/po ± **RIF** 300 mg po/IV bid	
Hemoglobinopathy: Sickle cell/thalassemia	Salmonella; other Gm-neg. bacilli	**CIP** 400 mg IV q12h	**Levo** 750 mg IV q24h	Thalassemia: transfusion and iron chelation risk factors.
Contiguous Osteomyelitis Without Vascular Insufficiency				
Empiric therapy: Get cultures!				
Foot bone osteo due to nail through tennis shoe	P. aeruginosa	**CIP** 750 mg po bid or **Levo** 750 mg po q24h	**Ceftaz** 2 gm IV q8h or **CFP** 2 gm IV q12h	*See Skin—Nail puncture, page 53.* Need debridement to remove foreign body.
Long bone, post-internal fixation of fracture	S. aureus, Gm-neg. bacilli, P. aeruginosa	**Vanco** 1 gm IV q12h + [**ceftaz** or **CFP**]. *See Comment*	**Linezolid** 600 mg IV/po bid[NAI] + (**ceftaz** or **CFP**). *See Comment*	Often necessary to remove hardware after union to achieve eradication. May need revascularization. **Regimens listed are empiric.** Adjust after culture data available. If susceptible Gm-neg. bacillus, **CIP** 750 mg po bid or **Levo** 750 mg po q24h. For other *S. aureus* options: *See Hem. Osteo. Specific Therapy, page 4).*

* **DOSAGES SUGGESTED are for adults (unless otherwise indicated) with clinically severe (often life-threatening infections). Dosages also assume normal renal function, and not severe hepatic dysfunction.**

§ **ALTERNATIVE THERAPY INCLUDES these considerations: allergy, pharmacology/pharmacokinetics, compliance, costs, local resistance profiles.**

TABLE 1A (2)

ANATOMIC SITE/DIAGNOSIS/ MODIFYING CIRCUMSTANCES	ETIOLOGIES (usual)	SUGGESTED REGIMENS*		ADJUNCT DIAGNOSTIC OR THERAPEUTIC MEASURES AND COMMENTS
		PRIMARY	ALTERNATIVE[§]	
BONE/Contiguous Osteomyelitis Without Vascular Insufficiency/Empiric therapy *(continued)*				
Osteonecrosis of the jaw	Probably rare adverse reaction to bisphosphonates	Infection may be secondary to bone necrosis and loss of overlying mucosa. Treatment: minimal surgical debridement, chlorhexidine rinses, antibiotics (e.g. PIP-TZ). *NEJM 355:2278, 2006.*		
Prosthetic joint	*See prosthetic joint, page 30*			
Spinal implant infection	S. aureus, coag-neg staphylococci, gram-neg bacilli	Onset within 30 days culture, treat & then suppress until fusion occurs	Onset after 30 days remove implant, culture & treat	For details: *CID 44:913, 2007.*
Sternum, post-op	S. aureus, S. epidermidis	**Vanco** 30-60 mg/kg per day in 2-3 divided doses to achieve target trough concentrations of 15-20 mcg/mL recommended for serious infections.	**Linezolid** 600 mg po/IV[NAI] bid	Sternal debridement for cultures & removal of necrotic bone. For *S. aureus* options: *Hem. Osteo. Specific Therapy, page 4.*
Contiguous Osteomyelitis With Vascular Insufficiency. Ref.: *CID S115–22, 2004*				
Most pts are **diabetics** with peripheral neuropathy & infected skin ulcers *(see Diabetic foot, page 14)*	Polymicrobic [Gm+ cocci (to include MRSA) (aerobic & anaerobic) and Gm-neg. bacilli (aerobic & anaerobic)]	Debride overlying ulcer & submit bone for histology & culture. Select antibiotic based on culture results & treat for 6 weeks. **No empiric therapy unless acutely ill.** If acutely ill, *see suggestions, Diabetic foot, page 14.* Revascularize if possible.		**Diagnosis of osteo:** Culture bone biopsy (gold standard). Poor concordance of culture results between swab of ulcer and bone – need bone. *(CID 42:57, 63, 2006).* Sampling by needle puncture inferior to biopsy *(CID 48:888, 2009).* Osteo more likely if ulcer >2 cm², positive probe to bone, ESR >70 & abnormal plain x-ray *(JAMA 299:806, 2008).* **Treatment:** (1) **Revascularize if possible;** (2) Culture bone; (3) Specific antimicrobial(s). Reviews: *BMJ 339:b4905, 2006; Plast Reconstr Surg 117: (7 Suppl) 2125, 2006.*
Chronic Osteomyelitis: Specific therapy By definition, implies presence of dead bone. **Need valid cultures**	S. aureus, Enterobacteriaceae, P. aeruginosa	**Empiric rx not indicated.** Base systemic rx on results of culture, sensitivity testing. If acute exacerbation of chronic osteo, rx as acute hematogenous osteo. Surgical debridement important.		**Important adjuncts:** removal of orthopedic hardware, surgical debridement, vascularized muscle flaps, distraction osteogenesis (Ilizarov) techniques. Antibiotic-impregnated cement & hyperbaric oxygen adjunctive. **NOTE: RIF + (vanco or β-lactam)** effective in animal model and in a clinical trial of S. aureus chronic osteo *(SMJ 79:947, 1986).*
BREAST: Mastitis—Obtain culture; need to know if MRSA present. Review with definitions: *Ob & Gyn Clin No Amer 29:89, 2002*				
Postpartum mastitis				
Mastitis without abscess Ref.: *JAMA 289:1609, 2003*	S. aureus; less often S. pyogenes (Gp A or B), E. coli bacteroides species, maybe Corynebacterium sp., & selected coagulase-neg. staphylococci (e.g., S. lugdunensis)	**NO MRSA: Outpatient: Dicloxacillin** 500 mg po qid or **cephalexin** 500 mg po qid. **Inpatient: Nafcillin/oxacillin** 2 gm IV q4h	**MRSA Possible: Outpatient: TMP-SMX-DS** tabs 1-2 po bid or, if susceptible, **clinda** 300 mg po qid **Inpatient: Vanco** 1 gm IV q12h; if over 100 kg, 1.5 gm IV q12h.	If no abscess, ↑ freq of nursing may hasten response; discuss age-specific risks to infant of drug exposure through breast milk with pediatrician. Corynebacterium sp. assoc. with chronic granulomatous mastitis *(CID 35:1434, 2002).* Bartonella henselae infection reported *(Ob & Gyn 95:1027, 2000).*
Mastitis with abscess				With abscess, d/c nursing. **I&D standard;** needle aspiration reported successful *(Am J Surg 182:117, 2001).* Resume breast feeding from affected breast as soon as pain allows.
Non-puerperal mastitis with abscess	S. aureus; less often Bacteroides sp., peptostreptococcus, & selected coagulase-neg. staphylococci	*See regimens for Postpartum mastitis, page 5.*		**If subareolar & odoriferous**, most likely anaerobes; need to **add metro** 500 mg IV/po tid. If not subareolar, staph. Need pretreatment aerobic/anaerobic cultures. Surgical drainage for abscess.

 NOTE: All dosage recommendations are for adults (unless otherwise indicated) and assume normal renal function.

TABLE 1A (3)

ANATOMIC SITE/DIAGNOSIS/ MODIFYING CIRCUMSTANCES	ETIOLOGIES (usual)	SUGGESTED REGIMENS* PRIMARY	ALTERNATIVE§	ADJUNCT DIAGNOSTIC OR THERAPEUTIC MEASURES AND COMMENTS
BREAST: Mastitis *(continued)*				
Breast implant infection	Acute: *S. aureus, S. pyogenes*. TSS reported. Chronic: Look for rapidly growing Mycobacteria	Acute: **Vanco** 1 gm IV q12h; if over 100 kg, 1.5 gm q12h.	Chronic: Await culture results. *See Table 12* for mycobacteria treatment.	*Lancet Infect Dis 5:94, 462, 2005.* Coag-negative staph also common *(Aesthetic Plastic Surg 31:325, 2007).*
CENTRAL NERVOUS SYSTEM				
Brain abscess				
Primary or contiguous source In 20 pts standard cultures found 22 bacterial strains; molecular methods found 72 bacterial strains *(CID 48:1169, 2009).*	Streptococci (60–70%), bacteroides (20–40%), Enterobacteriaceae (25–33%), S. aureus (10–15%), S. anginosus grp. Rare: Nocardia *(below)* Listeria *(CID 40:907, 2005). See S. aureus Comment*	**P Ceph 3** [(**cefotaxime** 2 gm IV q4h or **ceftriaxone** 2 gm IV q12h) + (**metro** 7.5 mg/kg q6h or 15 mg/kg IV q12h)] Duration of rx unclear; treat until response by neuroimaging (CT/MRI)	**Pen G** 3-4 million units IV q4h + **metro** 7.5 mg/kg q6h or 15 mg/kg IV q12h	If CT scan suggests cerebritis or abscesses <2.5 cm and pt neurologically stable and conscious, start antibiotics and observe. Otherwise, surgical drainage necessary. Experience with Pen G (HD) + metro without ceftriaxone or nafcillin/oxacillin has been good. We use ceftriaxone because of frequency of isolation of Enterobacteriaceae. **S. aureus rare without positive blood culture; if S. aureus, use vanco until susceptibility known.** Strep. anginosus group esp. prone to produce abscess.
Post-surgical, post-traumatic	S. aureus, Enterobacteriaceae	**For MSSA:** (**Nafcillin** or **oxacillin**) 2 gm IV q4h + (**ceftriaxone** or **cefotaxime**)	**For MRSA: Vanco** 1 gm IV q12h + (**ceftriaxone** or **cefotaxime**)	Adjust vanco dose to achieve trough level of 15-20 µg/mL. Aspiration of abscess usually necessary for dx & rx. If P. aeruginosa suspected, susbstitute (Cefepime or Ceftazidime) for (Ceftriaxone or Cefotaxime).
HIV-1 infected (AIDS)	Toxoplasma gondii	*See Table 13A, page 136*		
Nocardia: Haematogenous abscess Ref: *Can Med J 171:1063, 2004*	N. farcinica, N. asteroides & N. basiliensis	**TMP-SMX:** 15 mg/kg/day of TMP & 75 mg/kg/day of SMX, IV/po div in 2-4 doses + **Imipenem** 500 mg q6h IV. If multiorgan involvement some add **amikacin** 7.5 mg/kg q12h. After 3-6 wks of IV therapy, switch to po therapy. Immunocompetent pts: **TMP-SMX**, **minocycline** or **AM-CL** x 3+ months. Immunocompromised pts: Treat with 2 drugs for at least one year.	**Linezolid** 600 mg IV or po q12h + meropenem 2 gm q8h	Measure peak sulfonamide levels: target 100-150 mcg/mL 2 hrs post dose. **Linezolid** 600 mg po bid reported effective *(Ann Pharmacother 41:1694, 2007).* For in vitro susceptibility testing: Wallace (+1) 903-877-7680 or U.S. CDC (+1) 404-639-3158. In vitro resistance to TMP-SMX may be increasing *(Clin Infect Dis 51:1445, 2010),* but whether this is associated with worse outcomes is not known; TMP-SMX remains a drug of choice for CNS nocardia infection. If sulfonamide resistant or sulfa-allergic, **amikacin** plus one of: **IMP**, **MER**, **ceftriaxone** or **cefotaxime**.
Subdural empyema: In adult 60–90% are extension of sinusitis or otitis media. Rx same as primary brain abscess. Surgical emergency: must drain. Review in *LnID 7:62, 2007.*				
Encephalitis/encephalopathy *IDSA Guideline: CID 47:303, 2008. (For Herpes see Table 14A, page 150 and for rabies, Table 20B, page 198)*	In 253 pts, etiol in 52%: H. simplex (42%), VZV (15%), M. TB (15%), Listeria (10%) *(CID 49:1838, 2009).* Other: arbovirus, West Nile, rabies, Lyme, Parvo B19, CSD.	Start IV **acyclovir** while awaiting results of CSF PCR for H. simplex. For amebic encephalitis *see Table 13A.*		**Strain of bat rabies:** may not require a break in the skin to infect. Eastern equine encephalitis causes focal MRI changes in basal ganglia and thalamus *(NEJM 336:1867, 1997).* **Cat-scratch ref.:** *PIDJ 23:1161, 2004.* Ref. on **West Nile** & related viruses: *NEJM 351:370, 2004.* **Parvovirus B19** *(CID 48:1713, 2009).* Review of all etiologies: *LnID 10:835, 2010.*
Meningitis, "Aseptic": Pleocytosis of up to 100s of cells, CSF glucose normal, neg. culture for bacteria *(see Table 14A, page 145)* Ref: *CID 47:783, 2008*	Enteroviruses, HSV-2, LCM, HIV, other viruses, drugs (NSAIDs, metronidazole, carbamazepine, TMP-SMX, IVIG), rarely leptospirosis	For all but leptospirosis, IV fluids and analgesics. D/C drugs that may be etiologic. For lepto (**doxy** 100 mg IV/po q12h) or (**Pen G** 5 million units IV q6h) or (**AMP** 0.5–1 gm IV q6h). Repeat LP if suspect partially-treated bacterial meningitis. **Acyclovir** 5-10 mg/kg IV q8h sometimes given for HSV-2 meningitis (Note: this entity is distinct from HSV encephalitis where early rx is mandatory).		If available, PCR of CSF for enterovirus. HSV-2 unusual without concomitant genital herpes. For lepto, positive epidemiologic history and concomitant hepatitis, conjunctivitis, dermatitis, nephritis. For complete list of implicated drugs: *Inf Med 25:331, 2008.*

NOTE: All dosage recommendations are for adults (unless otherwise indicated) and assume normal renal function.

TABLE 1A (4)

ANATOMIC SITE/DIAGNOSIS/ MODIFYING CIRCUMSTANCES	ETIOLOGIES (usual)	SUGGESTED REGIMENS*		ADJUNCT DIAGNOSTIC OR THERAPEUTIC MEASURES AND COMMENTS
		PRIMARY	ALTERNATIVE[§]	
CENTRAL NERVOUS SYSTEM *(continued)*				
Meningitis, Bacterial, Acute: Goal is empiric therapy, then CSF exam within 30 min. If focal neurologic deficit, give empiric therapy, then head CT, then LP. *(NEJM 354:44,2006; Ln ID 10:32, 2010; IDSA Pract. Guid., CID 39:1267, 2004)* **NOTE:** In children, treatment caused CSF cultures to turn neg. in 2 hrs with meningococci & partial response with pneumococci in 4 hrs *(Peds 108:1169, 2001)*				
Empiric Therapy—CSF Gram stain is negative—immunocompetent				
Age: Preterm to <1 mo *LnID 10:32, 2010*	Group B strep 49%, E. coli 18%, listeria 7%, misc. Gm-neg. 10%, misc. Gm-pos. 10%	**AMP** 100 mg/kg IV q6h + **cefotaxime** 50 mg/kg IV q6h	**AMP** 100 mg/kg IV q6h + **gentamicin** 2.5 mg/kg IV q8h	Regimens active vs. Group B strep, most coliforms, & listeria. If premature infant with long nursery stay, S. aureus, enterococci, and resistant coliforms potential pathogens. **Optional empiric regimens: [nafcillin + (ceftazidime or cefotaxime)]. If high risk of MRSA,** use vanco + cefotaxime. Alter regimen after culture/sensitivity data available.
		Intraventricular treatment not recommended. Repeat CSF exam/culture 24–36 hr after start of therapy		
Age: 1 mo– 50 yrs ***See footnote***[1] for empiric treatment rationale. Hearing loss is most common neurologic sequela *(LnID 10:32, 2010)*.	S. pneumo, meningococci, H. influenzae now very rare, **listeria unlikely if young adult & immunocompetent** (add **ampicillin** if suspect listeria: 2 gm IV q4h)	Adult dosage: [(**Cefotaxime** 2 gm IV q4–6h OR **ceftriaxone** 2 gm IV q12h)] + (**dexamethasone**) + **vanco**[2].	(**MER** 2 gm IV q8h) (Peds: 40 mg/kg IV q8h) + IV **dexamethasone** + **vanco**[2]	**For pts with severe pen. allergy: Chloro** 12.5 mg/kg IV q6h (max. 4 gm/day) (for meningococcus) + **TMP-SMX** 5 mg/kg q6–8h (for listeria if immunocompromised) + **vanco**. Rare meningococcal isolates chloro-resistant. High chloro failure rate in pts with resistant S. pneumo. **So far, no vanco-resistant S. pneumo.** **Value of dexamethasone** documented in children with H. influenzae and adults with S. pneumo *(NEJM 357:2431 & 2441, 2007; LnID 4:139, 2004)*. Decreased inflammatory markers in adults *(CID 49:1387, 2009)*. **Give 1st dose 15–20 min. prior to, or concomitant with, 1st dose of antibiotic. Dose: 0.15 mg/kg IV q6h x 2–4 days.**
		Dexamethasone: 0.15 mg/kg IV q6h x 2–4 days. **Give with, or just before, 1st dose of antibiotic to block TNF production *(see Comment)*.**		
		See footnote[2] *for Vanco Adult dosage and*[3] *for ped. dosage*		
Age: >50 yrs or alcoholism or other **debilitating assoc diseases** or **impaired cellular immunity**	S. pneumo, listeria, Gm-neg. bacilli. Note absence of meningococcus.	(**AMP** 2 gm IV q4h) + (**ceftriaxone** 2 gm IV q12h or **cefotaxime** 2 gm IV q4–6h) + **vanco** + IV **dexamethasone**	**MER** 2 gm IV q8h + **vanco** + IV **dexamethasone**. ***For severe pen. Allergy, see Comment***	**Severe penicillin allergy: Vanco** 15 mg/kg q8h + **TMP-SMX** 5 mg/kg q6–8h pending culture results. Chloro has failed vs. pen-resistant S. pneumo.
		For vanco dose, see *footnote*[2]. Dexamethasone dose: 0.15 mg/kg IV q6h x 2–4 days; 1st dose before, or concomitant with, 1st dose of antibiotic.		
Post-neurosurgery Ventriculostomy/lumbar catheter; ventriculo-peritoneal (atrial) shunt) or Penetrating trauma w/o basilar skull fracture	S. epidermidis, S. aureus, P. acnes. Facultative and aerobic gram-neg bacilli, including: P. aeruginosa & A. baumannii (may be multi-drug resistant)	**Vanco** 15 mg/kg IV q8h (to achieve trough level of 15-20 µg/mL) + (**Cefepime** or **Ceftaz** 2 gm IV q8h)	**Vanco** 15 mg/kg IV q8h (to achieve trough level of 15-20 µg/mL) + (**MER** 2 gm IV q8h)	• If possible, remove infected shunt or catheter. • Logic for intraventricular therapy: goal is to achieve a 10-20 ratio of CSF concentration to bacterial MIC of infecting bacteria. • Use only preservative-free drug. Clamp/close catheter for 1 hr after 1st dose. • Timing of new V-P shunt *(CID 39:1267, 2004)*. • Acinetobacter meningitis *(LnID 9:245, 2009; JAC 61:908, 2008)*. • Review of nosocomial bacterial meningitis *(NEJM 362, 146, 2010)*.
		• **If severe Pen/Ceph allergy**, for possible gram-neg, substitute either: Aztreonam 2 gm IV q6-8h or CIP 400 mg IV q8-12h. • **If IV therapy inadequate, may need intraventricular therapy:** Intraventricular daily drug doses *(CID 39:1267, 2004)*: **Adult: Vanco** 10-20 mg; **Amikacin** 30 mg; **Tobra** 5-20 mg; **Gent** 4-8 mg; **Colistin** 10 mg (or 5 mg q12h), **Polymyxin B** 5 mg; **Peds: Gent** 1-2 mg; **Polymyxin B** 2 mg.		
Trauma with basilar skull fracture	S. pneumoniae, H. influenzae, S. pyogenes	**Vanco** 15 mg/kg IV q8h (to achieve trough level of 15-20 µg/mL) + (**Ceftriaxone** 2 gm IV q12h or **Cefotax** 2 gm IV q6h) + [**Dexamethasone** 0.15 mg/kg IV q6h x 2-4 d (1st dose with or before 1st antibiotic dose)]		

[1] **Rationale:** Hard to get adequate CSF concentrations of anti-infectives, hence MIC criteria for in vitro susceptibility are lower for CSF isolates *(ArIM 161:2538, 2001)*.
[2] **Vanco adult dose:** 15 mg/kg IV q8h to achieve trough level of 15-20 µg/mL.
[3] **Dosage of drugs used to treat children ≥1 mo of age: Cefotaxime** 50 mg/kg per day IV q6h; **ceftriaxone** 50 mg/kg IV q12h; **vanco** 15 mg/kg IV q6h to achieve trough level of 15-20 µg/mL.

Abbreviations on page 2. *NOTE: All dosage recommendations are for adults (unless otherwise indicated) and assume normal renal function.*

TABLE 1A (5)

ANATOMIC SITE/DIAGNOSIS/ MODIFYING CIRCUMSTANCES	ETIOLOGIES (usual)	SUGGESTED REGIMENS* PRIMARY	ALTERNATIVE[§]	ADJUNCT DIAGNOSTIC OR THERAPEUTIC MEASURES AND COMMENTS
CENTRAL NERVOUS SYSTEM/Meningitis, Bacterial, Acute *(continued)*				
Empiric Therapy—Positive CSF Gram stain				
Gram-positive diplococci	S. pneumoniae	Either (**ceftriaxone** 2 gm IV q12h or **cefotaxime** 2 gm IV q4–6h) + **vanco** 15 mg/kg IV q8h (to achieve 15-20 μg/mL trough) + timed **dexamethasone** 0.15 mg/kg q6h IV x 2–4 days.		**Alternatives: MER** 2 gm IV q8h or **Moxi** 400 mg IV q24h. **Dexamethasone** does not block penetration of vanco into CSF *(CID 44:250, 2007)*.
Gram-negative diplococci	N. meningitidis	(**Cefotaxime** 2 gm IV q4–6h or **ceftriaxone** 2 gm IV q12h)		**Alternatives: Pen G** 4 mill. units IV q4h or **AMP** 2 gm q4h or **Moxi** 400 mg IV q24h or **chloro** 1 gm IV q6h
Gram-positive bacilli or coccobacilli	Listeria monocytogenes	**AMP** 2 gm IV q4h ± **gentamicin** 2 mg/kg loading dose then 1.7 mg/kg q8h		**If pen-allergic, use TMP-SMX 5 mg/kg (TMP comp) q6–8h or MER 2 gm IV q8h**
Gram-negative bacilli	H. influenzae, coliforms, P. aeruginosa	(**Ceftazidime** or **cefepime** 2 gm IV q8h) + **gentamicin** 2 mg/kg 1st dose then 1.7 mg/kg q8h		**Alternatives: CIP** 400 mg IV q8–12h; **MER** 2 gm IV q8h
Specific Therapy—Positive culture of CSF with in vitro susceptibility results available. Interest in monitoring/reducing intracranial pressure: *CID 38:384, 2004*				
H. influenzae	β-lactamase positive	**Ceftriaxone** 2 gm IV q12h (adult), 50 mg/kg IV q12h (peds)		**Pen. allergic: Chloro** 12.5 mg/kg IV q6h (max. 4 gm/day.)
Listeria monocytogenes *(CID 43:1233, 2006)*		**AMP** 2 gm IV q4h ± **gentamicin** 2 mg/kg loading dose, then 1.7 mg/kg q8h		**Pen. allergic: TMP-SMX** 20 mg/kg per day div. q6–12h. One report of greater efficacy of AMP + TMP-SMX as compared to AMP + gentamicin *(JID 33:79, 1996)*. **Alternative: MER** 2 gm IV q8h. Success reported with **linezolid** + **RIF** *(CID 40:907, 2005)* after AMP rx for brain abscess with meningitis.
N. meningitidis	Pen MIC 0.1–1 mcg per mL	**Ceftriaxone** 2 gm IV q12h x 7 days *(see Comment)*; if β-lactam allergic, **chloro** 12.5 mg/kg (up to 1 gm) IV q6h		Rare isolates chloro-resistant *(NEJM 339:868 & 917, 1998)*. **Alternatives: MER** 2 gm IV q8h or **Moxi** 400 mg q24h.
S. pneumoniae **NOTES:** 1. Assumes dexamethasone just prior to 1st dose & x 4 days. 2. If MIC ≥1, repeat CSF exam after 24–48h. 3. Treat for 10–14 days	Pen G MIC <0.1 mcg/mL	**Pen G** 4 million units IV q4h or **AMP** 2 gm IV q4h		**Alternatives: Ceftriaxone** 2 gm IV q12h, **chloro** 1 gm IV q6h
	0.1–1 mcg/mL	**Ceftriaxone** 2 gm IV q12h or **cefotaxime** 2 gm IV q4–6h		**Alternatives: Cefepime** 2 gm IV q8h or **MER** 2 gm IV q8h
	≥2 mcg/mL	**Vanco** 15 mg/kg IV q8h (15-20 μg/mL trough target) + (**ceftriaxone** or **cefotaxime** as above)		**Alternatives: Moxi** 400 mg IV q24h
	Ceftriaxone MIC ≥1 mcg/mL	**Vanco** 15 mg/kg IV q8h (15-20 μg/mL trough target) + (**ceftriaxone** or **cefotaxime** as above)		**Alternatives: Moxi** 400 mg IV q24h If MIC to ceftriaxone >2 mcg/mL, add **RIF** 600 mg po/IV 1x/day.
E. coli, other coliforms, or P. aeruginosa	**Consultation advised**—need susceptibility results	(**Ceftazidime** or **cefepime** 2 gm IV q8h) ± **gentamicin**		**Alternatives: CIP** 400 mg IV q8–12h; **MER** 2 gm IV q8h. For intraventricular therapy: drug dosing, *see Meningitis, Post-neurosurgery, page 7*.
Prophylaxis for H. influenzae and N. meningitides				
Haemophilus influenzae type b Household and/or day care contact: residing with index case for ≥4 hrs in a day. Day care contact or same day care facility as index case for 5-7 days before onset		**Children: RIF** 20 mg/kg po (not to exceed 600 mg) q24h x 4 doses. **Adults: RIF** 600 mg q24h x 4 days		**Household:** If there is one unvaccinated contact ≤4 yr in the household, give RIF to all household contacts except pregnant women. **Child Care Facilities:** With 1 case, if attended by unvaccinated children ≤2 yr, consider prophylaxis + vaccinate susceptibles. If all contacts >2 yr: no prophylaxis. If ≥2 cases in 60 days & unvaccinated children attend, prophylaxis recommended for children & personnel *(Am Acad Ped Red Book 2006, page 313)*.

 NOTE: All dosage recommendations are for adults (unless otherwise indicated) and assume normal renal function.

TABLE 1A (6)

ANATOMIC SITE/DIAGNOSIS/ MODIFYING CIRCUMSTANCES	ETIOLOGIES (usual)	SUGGESTED REGIMENS*		ADJUNCT DIAGNOSTIC OR THERAPEUTIC MEASURES AND COMMENTS
		PRIMARY	ALTERNATIVE[§]	
CENTRAL NERVOUS SYSTEM/Meningitis, Bacterial, Acute/Prophylaxis for H. influenzae and N. meningitides *(continued)*				
Prophylaxis for Neisseria meningitidis exposure (close contact) **NOTE:** CDC reports **CIP-resistant group B meningococcus** from selected counties in N. Dakota & Minnesota. **Avoid CIP**. Use **ceftriaxone**, **RIF**, or single 500 mg dose of **azithro** *(MMWR 57:173, 2008)*.		[**Ceftriaxone** 250 mg IM x 1 dose (child <15 yr 125 mg IM x 1)] **OR** [**RIF** 600 mg po q12h x 4 doses. (Children >1 mo 10 mg/kg po q12h x 4 doses, <1 mo 5 mg/kg q12h x 4 doses)] **OR** If not CIP-resistant, **CIP** 500 mg po x 1 dose (adult)		**Spread by respiratory droplets**, not aerosols, hence close contact req. ↑ risk if close contact for at least 4 hrs during wk before illness onset (e.g., housemates, day care contacts, cellmates) or exposure to pt's nasopharyngeal secretions (e.g., kissing, mouth-to-mouth resuscitation, intubation, nasotracheal suctioning).
		Spiramycin[NUS] 500 mg po q6h x 5 days. Children 10 mg/kg po q6h x 5 days.		Primary prophylactic regimen in many European countries.
Meningitis, chronic Defined as symptoms + CSF pleocytosis for ≥4 wks	M. tbc 40%, cryptococcosis 7%, neoplastic 8%, Lyme, syphilis, Whipple's disease	Treatment depends on etiology. No urgent need for empiric therapy, but when TB suspected treatment should be expeditious.		Long list of possibilities: bacteria, parasites, fungi, viruses, neoplasms, vasculitis, and other miscellaneous etiologies—*see chapter on chronic meningitis in latest edition of Harrison's Textbook of Internal Medicine*. Whipple's: *JID 188:797 & 801, 2003*.
Meningitis, eosinophilic *LnID 8:621, 2008*	Angiostrongyliasis, gnathostomiasis, baylisascaris	Corticosteroids	Not sure antihelminthic therapy works	1/3 lack peripheral eosinophilia. Need serology to confirm diagnosis. Steroid ref.: *LnID 8:621, 2008*. Automated CSF count may not correctly identify eosinophils *(CID 48: 322, 2009)*.
Meningitis, HIV-1 infected (AIDS) *See Table 11, Sanford Guide to HIV/AIDS Therapy*	As in adults, >50 yr: also consider cryptococci, M. tuberculosis, syphilis, HIV aseptic meningitis, Listeria monocytogenes	If etiology not identified: treat as adult >50 yr + obtain CSF/serum cryptococcal antigen *(see Comments)*	For crypto rx, *see Table 11A, page 109*	C. neoformans most common etiology in AIDS patients. H. influenzae, pneumococci, Tbc, syphilis, viral, histoplasma & coccidioides also need to be considered. Obtain blood cultures. L. monocytogenes risk >60x ↑, ¾ present as meningitis *(CID 17:224, 1993)*.
EAR				
External otitis				
Chronic	Usually 2° to seborrhea	Eardrops: [(**polymyxin B** + **neomycin** + **hydrocortisone** qid) + **selenium sulfide shampoo**]		Control seborrhea with dandruff shampoo containing selenium sulfide (Selsun) or [(ketoconazole shampoo) + (medium potency steroid solution, triamcinolone 0.1%)].
Fungal	Candida species	**Fluconazole** 200 mg po x 1 dose & then 100 mg po x 3-5 days.		
"Malignant otitis externa" Risk groups: Diabetes mellitus, AIDS, chemotherapy. Ref: *Oto Clinics N Amer 41:537, 2008*	Pseudomonas aeruginosa in >90%	(**IMP** 0.5 gm IV q6h) or (**MER** 1 gm IV q8h) or [**CIP** 400 mg IV q12h (or 750 mg po q12h)] or (**ceftaz** 2 gm IV q8h) or (**CFP** 2 gm q12h) or (**PIP** 4–6 gm IV q4–6h + **tobra**) or (**TC** 3 gm IV q4h + **tobra** dose Table 10D)		CIP po for treatment of early disease. Debridement usually required. R/O osteomyelitis: CT or MRI scan. If bone involved, treat for 4–6 wks. PIP without Tazo may be hard to find: extended infusion of PIP-TZ (4 hr infusion of 3.375 gm every 8h) may improve efficacy *(CID 44:357, 2007)*.
"Swimmer's ear" *PIDJ 22:299, 2003*	Pseudomonas sp., Enterobacteriaceae, Proteus sp. (Fungi rare.) Acute infection usually 2° S. aureus	Eardrops: **Oflox 0.3% soln bid** or [(**polymyxin B** + **neomycin** + **hydrocortisone**) qid] or (**CIP** + **hydrocortisone bid**) --active vs. gm-neg bacilli. For acute disease: **dicloxacillin** 500 mg po 4x/day. If MRSA a concern, use **TMP-SMX**, **doxy** or **clinda**		Rx includes gentle cleaning. Recurrences prevented (or decreased) by drying with alcohol drops (1/3 white vinegar, 2/3 rubbing alcohol) after swimming, then antibiotic drops or 2% acetic acid solution. Ointments should not be used in ear. Do not use neomycin drops if tympanic membrane punctured.

 NOTE: All dosage recommendations are for adults (unless otherwise indicated) and assume normal renal function.

TABLE 1A (7)

ANATOMIC SITE/DIAGNOSIS/ MODIFYING CIRCUMSTANCES	ETIOLOGIES (usual)	SUGGESTED REGIMENS*		ADJUNCT DIAGNOSTIC OR THERAPEUTIC MEASURES AND COMMENTS
		PRIMARY	ALTERNATIVE[§]	
EAR *(continued)*				
Otitis media—infants, children, adults				
Acute Two PRDB trials indicate efficacy of antibiotic rx if age < 36 mos & definite AOM *(NEJM 364:105, 116 & 168, 2011)*				
Initial empiric therapy of acute otitis media (AOM) **NOTE: Treat children <2 yr old**. If >2 yr old, afebrile, no ear pain, neg./questionable exam— consider analgesic treatment without antimicrobials. Favorable results in mostly afebrile pts with waiting 48hrs before deciding on antibiotic use *(JAMA 296:1235, 1290, 2006)*	Overall detection in middle ear fluid: No pathogen 4% Virus 70% Bact. + virus 66% Bacteria only 92% Bacterial pathogens from middle ear: S. pneumo 49%, H. influenzae 29%, M. catarrhalis 28%. Ref.: *CID 43:1417 & 1423, 2006.* Children 6 mo-3 yrs, 2 episodes AOM/yr & 63% are virus positive *(CID 46:815 & 824, 2008).*	**If NO antibiotics in prior month:** **Amox** po HD[4] For dosage, *see footnote*[5]. **All doses are pediatric** **Duration of rx:** <2 yr old x 10 days; ≥2 yr x 5–7 days. Appropriate duration unclear. 5 days may be inadequate for severe disease *(NEJM 347:1169, 2002)* **For adult dosages, see *Sinusitis, pages 47–48, and Table 10***	**Received antibiotics in prior month:** **Amox** HD[4] or **AM-CL** extra-strength[4] or **cefdinir** or **cefpodoxime** or **cefprozil** or **cefuroxime axetil**	**If allergic to β-lactam drugs?** If history unclear or rash, effective oral ceph OK; avoid ceph if IgE-mediated allergy, e.g., anaphylaxis. High failure rate with **TMP-SMX** if etiology is DRSP or H. influenzae *(PIDJ 20:260, 2001)*; **azithro x 5 days or clarithro x 10 days** (both have ↓ activity vs. DRSP). **Up to 50% S. pneumo resistant to macrolides**. Rationale & data for single dose azithro, 30 mg per kg: *PIDJ 23:S102 & S108, 2004*. **Spontaneous resolution occurred in:** 90% pts infected with M. catarrhalis, 50% with H. influenzae, 10% with S. pneumoniae; overall 80% resolve within 2–14 days *(Ln 363:465, 2004)*. Risk of DRSP ↑ if age <2 yr, antibiotics last 3 mo, &/or daycare attendance. Selection of drug based on (1) effectiveness against β-lactamase producing H. influenzae & M. catarrhalis & (2) effectiveness against S. pneumo, inc. DRSP. **Cefaclor, loracarbef, & ceftibuten less active vs. resistant S. pneumo.** than other agents listed. Variable acceptance of drug taste/smell by children 4–8 yrs old. *[PIDJ 19 (Suppl.2):S174, 2000]*.
Treatment for clinical failure after 3 days	Drug-resistant S. pneumoniae main concern	**NO antibiotics in month prior to last 3 days:** **AM-CL** high dose or **cefdinir** or **cefpodoxime** or **cefprozil** or **cefuroxime axetil** or IM **ceftriaxone** x 3 days. *For dosage, see footnote*[5] **All doses are pediatric** Duration of rx as above	**Antibiotics in month prior to last 3 days:** [(IM **ceftriaxone**) or (**clindamycin**) and/or tympanocentesis] *See clindamycin Comments*	**Clindamycin** not active vs. H. influenzae or M. catarrhalis. S. pneumo resistant to macrolides are usually also resistant to clindamycin. Definition of failure: no change in ear pain, fever, bulging TM or otorrhea after 3 days of therapy. Tympanocentesis will allow culture. **Newer FQs active vs. drug-resistant S. pneumo (DRSP), but not approved for use in children** *(PIDJ 23:390, 2004)*. **Vanco is active vs. DRSP.** Ceftriaxone IM x 3 days superior to 1-day treatment vs. DRSP *(PIDJ 19:1040, 2000)*. AM-CL HD reported successful for pen-resistant S. pneumo AOM *(PIDJ 20:829, 2001)*.
After >48hrs of nasotracheal intubation	Pseudomonas sp., klebsiella, enterobacter	**Ceftazidime** or **CFP** or **IMP** or **MER** or (**Pip-Tz**) or **TC-CL** or **CIP**. *(For dosages, see Ear, Malignant otitis externa, page 9)*		With nasotracheal intubation >48 hrs, about ½ pts will have otitis media with effusion.
Prophylaxis: acute otitis media *PIDJ 22:10, 2003*	Pneumococci, H. influenzae, M. catarrhalis, Staph. aureus, Group A strep *(see Comments)*	**Sulfisoxazole** 50 mg/kg po at bedtime or **amoxicillin** 20 mg/kg po q24h	**Use of antibiotics to prevent otitis media is a major contributor to emergence of antibiotic-resistant S. pneumo!** Pneumococcal protein conjugate vaccine decreases freq. AOM & due to vaccine serotypes. Adenoidectomy at time of tympanostomy tubes ↓ need for future hospitalization for AOM *(NEJM 344:1188, 2001)*.	

[4] **Amoxicillin UD or HD** = amoxicillin usual dose or high dose; **AM-CL HD** = amoxicillin-clavulanate high dose. **Dosages in footnote[5].** Data supporting amoxicillin HD: *PIDJ 22:405, 2003*.

[5] **Drugs & peds dosage (all po unless specified) for acute otitis media: Amoxicillin UD** = 40 mg/kg per day div q12h or q8h. **Amoxicillin HD** = 90 mg/kg per day div q12h or q8h. **AM-CL HD** = 90 mg/kg per day of amox component. **Extra-strength AM-CL oral suspension** (Augmentin ES-600) available with 600 mg AM & 42.9 mg CL / 5 mL—dose: 90/6.4 mg/kg per day div bid. **Cefuroxime axetil** 30 mg/kg per day div q12h. **Ceftriaxone** 50 mg/kg IM x 3 days. **Clindamycin** 20–30 mg/kg per day div qid (may be effective vs. DRSP but no activity vs. H. influenzae).
Other drugs suitable for drug (e.g., penicillin)-sensitive S. pneumo: TMP-SMX 4 mg/kg of TMP q12h. **Erythro-sulfisoxazole** 50 mg/kg per day of erythro div q6–8h. **Clarithro** 15 mg/kg per day div q12h; **azithro** 10 mg/kg per day x 1 & then 5 mg/kg q24h on days 2–5. Other FDA-approved regimens: 10 mg/kg q24h x 3 days & 30 mg/kg x 1. **Cefprozil** 15 mg/kg q12h; **cefpodoxime proxetil** 10 mg/kg per day as single dose; **cefaclor** 40 mg/kg per day div q8h; **loracarbef** 15 mg/kg q12h. **Cefdinir** 7 mg/kg q12h or 14 mg/kg q24h.

Abbreviations on page 2. *NOTE: All dosage recommendations are for adults (unless otherwise indicated) and assume normal renal function.*

TABLE 1A (8)

ANATOMIC SITE/DIAGNOSIS/ MODIFYING CIRCUMSTANCES	ETIOLOGIES (usual)	SUGGESTED REGIMENS*		ADJUNCT DIAGNOSTIC OR THERAPEUTIC MEASURES AND COMMENTS
		PRIMARY	ALTERNATIVE[§]	
EAR *(continued)*				
Mastoiditis				
Acute				
Outpatient	Strep. pneumoniae 22%, S. pyogenes 16%, **Staph. aureus** 7%, H. influenzae 4%, P. aeruginosa 4%, others <1%	Empirically, same as Acute otitis media, above; need **vanco** or **nafcillin/oxacillin** if culture + for S. aureus.		Has become a rare entity, presumably as result of the aggressive treatment of acute otitis media. Small ↑ in incidence in Netherlands where use of antibiotics limited to children with complicated course or high risk *(PIDJ 20:140, 2001)*. ↑ incidence reported from US also *(Arch Otolaryngol Head Neck Surg 135: 638, 2009)*. Unusual causes of acute mastoiditis: nocardia *(AIDS Reader 17: 402, 2007)*, TB, actinomyces *(EarNoseThroat Journal 79: 884, 2000)*.
Hospitalized		**Cefotaxime** 1–2 gm IV q4–8h (depends on severity) or **ceftriaxone** 1 gm IV q24h		
Chronic	Often polymicrobic: anaerobes, S. aureus, Enterobacteriaceae, P. aeruginosa	Treatment for acute exacerbations or perioperatively. No treatment until surgical cultures obtained. Empiric regimens: **IMP** 0.5 gm IV q6h, **TC-CL** 3.1 gm IV q6h, **PIP-TZ** 3.375 gm IV q4–6h or 4.5 gm q8h, or 4 hr infusion of 3.375 gm q8h, **MER** 1 gm IV Q8h.		May or may not be associated with chronic otitis media with drainage via ruptured tympanic membrane. Antimicrobials given in association with surgery. Mastoidectomy indications: chronic drainage and evidence of osteomyelitis by MRI or CT, evidence of spread to CNS (epidural abscess suppurative phlebitis, brain abscess).
EYE—General Reviews: *CID 21:479, 1995; IDCP 7:447, 1998*				
Eyelid: Little reported experience with CA-MRSA *(Ophthal 113:1455, 2006)*				
Blepharitis	Etiol. unclear. Factors include Staph. aureus & Staph. epidermidis, seborrhea, rosacea, & dry eye	Lid margin care with baby shampoo & warm compresses q24h. Artificial tears if assoc. dry eye *(see Comment)*.		Usually topical ointments of no benefit. If associated rosacea, add doxy 100 mg po bid for 2 wk and then q24h.
Hordeolum (Stye)				
External (eyelash follicle)	Staph. aureus	Hot packs only. Will drain spontaneously		Infection of superficial sebaceous gland.
Internal (Meibomian glands): Can be acute, subacute or chronic.	Staph. aureus, MSSA	Oral **dicloxacillin** + hot packs		Also called acute meibomianitis. Rarely drain spontaneously; may need I&D and culture. Role of fluoroquinolone eye drops is unclear: MRSA often resistant to lower conc.; may be susceptible to higher concentration of FQ in ophthalmologic solutions of gati, levo or moxi.
	Staph. aureus, MRSA-CA	**TMP/SMX-DS**, tabs ii po bid		
	Staph. aureus, MRSA-HA	**Linezolid** 600 mg po bid possible therapy if multi-drug resistant.		
Conjunctiva: *NEJM 343:345, 2000*				
Conjunctivitis of the newborn (**ophthalmia neonatorum**): by day of onset post-delivery—all doses pediatric				
Onset 1st day	Chemical due to silver nitrate prophylaxis	None		Usual prophylaxis is erythro ointment; hence, silver nitrate irritation rare.
Onset 2–4 days	N. gonorrhoeae	**Ceftriaxone** 25–50 mg/kg IV x 1 dose *(see Comment)*, not to exceed 125 mg		Treat mother and her sexual partners. Hyperpurulent. Topical rx inadequate. **Treat neonate for concomitant Chlamydia trachomatis.**
Onset 3–10 days	Chlamydia trachomatis	**Erythro base or ethylsuccinate syrup** 12.5 mg/kg q6h x 14 days. No topical rx needed.		Diagnosis by antigen detection. Alternative: **Azithro suspension** 20 mg/kg po q24h x 3 days. Treat mother & sexual partner.
Onset 2–16 days	Herpes simplex types 1, 2	Topical anti-viral rx under direction of ophthalmologist.		Also give Acyclovir 60 mg/kg/day IV div 3 doses *(Red Book online, accessed Jan 2011)*.
Ophthalmia neonatorum prophylaxis: **erythro** 0.5% ointment x 1 or **tetra** 1% ointment[NUS] x 1 application				
Pink eye (viral conjunctivitis) Usually unilateral	Adenovirus (types 3 & 7 in children, 8, 11 & 19 in adults)	No treatment. If symptomatic, cold artificial tears may help.		Highly contagious. Onset of ocular pain and photophobia in an adult suggests associated keratitis—rare.

viations on page 2. *NOTE: All dosage recommendations are for adults (unless otherwise indicated) and assume normal renal function.*

TABLE 1A (9)

ANATOMIC SITE/DIAGNOSIS/ MODIFYING CIRCUMSTANCES	ETIOLOGIES (usual)	SUGGESTED REGIMENS*		ADJUNCT DIAGNOSTIC OR THERAPEUTIC MEASURES AND COMMENTS
		PRIMARY	ALTERNATIVE[§]	
EYE/Conjunctiva *(continued)*				
Inclusion conjunctivitis **(adult)** Usually unilateral	Chlamydia trachomatis	**Doxy** 100 mg bid po x 1–3 wk	**Erythro** 250 mg po qid x 1–3 wk	Oculogenital disease. Diagnosis by culture or antigen detection or PCR—availability varies by region and institution. Treat sexual partner.
Trachoma --a chronic bacterial keratoconjunctivitis linked to poverty	Chlamydia trachomatis	**Azithro** 20 mg/kg po single dose—78% effective in children; Adults: 1 gm po.	**Doxy** 100 mg po bid x minimum of 21 days or **tetracycline** 250 mg po qid x 14 days.	Starts in childhood and can persist for years with subsequent damage to cornea. Topical therapy of marginal benefit. Avoid doxy/tetracycline in young children. Mass treatment works *(NEJM 358:1777 & 1870, 2008; JAMA 299:778, 2008)*.
Suppurative conjunctivitis: Children and Adults				
Non-gonococcal; non-chlamydial *Med Lett 46:25, 2004; Med Lett 50:11, 2008*	Staph. aureus, S. pneumoniae, H. influenzae, et al. Outbreak due to atypical S. pneumo. *NEJM 348:1112, 2003*	Ophthalmic solution: **Gati** 0.3%, **Levo** 0.5%, or **Moxi** 0.5%. All 1–2 gtts q2h while awake 1st 2 days, then q4–8h up to 7 days.	**Polymyxin B + trimethoprim** solution 1–2 gtts q3–6h x 7–10 days. **Azithro** 1%, 1 gtt bid x 2 days, then 1 gtt daily x 5 days.	**FQs** best spectrum for empiric therapy but expensive: $40–50 for 5 mL. High concentrations ↑ likelihood of activity vs. S. aureus—even MRSA. **TMP** spectrum may include MRSA. Polymyxin B spectrum only Gm-neg. bacilli but no ophthal. prep of only **TMP**. Most S. pneumo resistant to **gent** & tobra. **Azithro** active vs. common gm+ pathogens.
Gonococcal (peds/adults)	N. gonorrhoeae	**Ceftriaxone** 25-50 mg/kg IV/IM (not to exceed 125 mg) as one dose in children; 1 gm IM/IV as one dose in adults		
Cornea (keratitis): Usually serious and often sight-threatening. Prompt ophthalmologic consultation essential! Herpes simplex most common etiology in developed countries; bacterial and fungal infections more common in underdeveloped countries.				
Viral				
H. simplex	H. simplex, types 1 & 2	**Trifluridine**, one drop q1-2h up to 9x/day until re-epithelialized, then one drop q4h up to 5x/day, for total course of 21 days.	**Vidarabine** ointment— useful in children. Use 5x/day for up to 21 days (currently listed as discontinued in U.S.).	Fluorescein staining shows topical dendritic figures. 30–50% rate of recurrence within 2 years. 400 mg acyclovir po bid ↓ recurrences, p 0.005 *(NEJM 339:300, 1998)*.
Varicella-zoster ophthalmicus	Varicella-zoster virus	**Famciclovir** 500 mg po tid or **valacyclovir** 1 gm po tid x 10 days	**Acyclovir** 800 mg po 5x/day x 10 days	Clinical diagnosis most common: dendritic figures with fluorescein staining in patient with varicella-zoster of ophthalmic branch of trigeminal nerve.
Bacterial *(Med Lett 46:25, 2004)*		**All rx listed for bacterial, fungal, & protozoan is topical**		
Acute: No comorbidity	*S. aureus, S. pneumo., S. pyogenes, Haemophilus sp.*	**Moxi:** eye gtts. 1 gtt tid x 7 days	**Gati:** eye gtts. 1-2 gtts q2h while awake x 2 days, then q4h x 3-7 days.	Prefer Moxi due to enhanced lipophilicity & penetration into aqueous humor. Survey of *Ophthal 50 (suppl 1) 1, 2005.* **Note:** despite high conc. may fail vs. MRSA.
Contact lens users	P. aeruginosa	**Tobra** or **gentamicin** (14 mg/mL) + **piperacillin** or **ticarcillin** eye drops (6–12 mg/mL) q15–60 min around clock x 24–72 hrs, then slow reduction	**CIP** 0.3% or **Levo** 0.5% drops q15–60 min around clock x 24–72 hrs	Pain, photophobia, impaired vision. Recommend alginate swab for culture and sensitivity testing.
Dry cornea, diabetes, immunosuppression	Staph. aureus, S. epidermidis, S. pneumoniae, S. pyogenes, Enterobacteriaceae, listeria	**Cefazolin** (50 mg/mL) + **gentamicin** or **tobra** (14 mg/mL) q15–60 min around clock x 24–72 hrs, then slow reduction	**Vanco** (50 mg/mL) + **ceftazidime** (50 mg/mL) q15–60 min around clock x 24–72 hrs, then slow reduction. *See Comment*	Specific therapy guided by results of alginate swab culture and sensitivity. CIP 0.3% found clinically equivalent to cefazolin + tobra; only concern was efficacy of CIP vs. S. pneumoniae *(Ophthalmology 163:1857, 1996)*.
Fungal	Aspergillus, fusarium, candida. No empiric therapy—*see Comment*	**Natamycin** (5%) drops q3–4 hrs with subsequent slow reduction	**Ampho B** (0.05–0.15%) q3–4 hrs with subsequent slow reduction	No empiric therapy. Wait for results of Gram stain or culture in Sabouraud's medium.

 NOTE: All dosage recommendations are for adults (unless otherwise indicated) and assume normal renal function.

TABLE 1A (10)

ANATOMIC SITE/DIAGNOSIS/ MODIFYING CIRCUMSTANCES	ETIOLOGIES (usual)	SUGGESTED REGIMENS*		ADJUNCT DIAGNOSTIC OR THERAPEUTIC MEASURES AND COMMENTS
		PRIMARY	ALTERNATIVE[§]	
EYE/Cornea (keratitis) *(continued)*				
Mycobacteria: Post-refractive eye surgery	*Mycobacterium chelonae*	**Gati** or **Moxi** eye drops: 1 gtt qid, probably in conjunction with other active antimicrobials		Used in conjunction with other topical and/or systemic anti-mycobacterial agents (*J Cataract Refract Surg 33:1978, 2007; Ophthalmology 113:950, 2006*).
Protozoan Soft contact lens users. Ref: *CID 35:434, 2002.*	Acanthamoeba sp.	No primary/alternative; just one suggested regimen: Topical 0.02% chlorhexidine & 0.02% polyhexamethylene biquinide (PHMB), alone or in combination. Often combined with either propamidine isethionate or hexanide *(see Comment)*. Eyedrops q waking hour for 1 wk, then slow taper		Uncommon. Trauma and soft contact lenses are risk factors. To obtain suggested drops: Leiter's Park Ave Pharmacy (800-292-6773; www.leiterrx.com). Cleaning solution outbreak: *MMWR 56: 532, 2007*. Review in *Am J Ophthamol 148:487, 2009.*
Lacrimal apparatus				
Canaliculitis	Actinomyces most common. Rarely, Arachnia, fusobacterium, nocardia, candida	Remove granules & irrigate with **pen G** (100,000 mcg/mL) **Child: AM-CL** or **cefprozil or cefuroxime** *(See dose on Table 16)*	If fungi, irrigate with **nystatin** approx. 5 mcg/mL: 1 gtt tid	Digital pressure produces exudate at punctum; Gram stain confirms diagnosis. Hot packs to punctal area qid. M. chelonae reported after use of intracanalic plugs *(Ophth Plast Reconstr Surg 24: 241, 2008)*.
Dacryocystitis (lacrimal sac)	S. pneumo, S. aureus, H. influenzae, S. pyogenes, P. aeruginosa	Often consequence of obstruction of lacrimal duct. Empiric therapy based on Gram stain of aspirate—*see Comment.*		Need ophthalmologic consultation. Surgery may be required. Can be acute or chronic. Culture to detect MRSA.
Endophthalmitis: For post-op endophthalmitis, *see CID 38:542, 2004*				
Bacterial: Haziness of vitreous key to diagnosis. Needle aspirate of both vitreous and aqueous humor for culture prior to therapy. Intravitreal administration of antimicrobials essential.				
Postocular surgery (cataracts)				
Early, acute onset (incidence 0.05%)	S. epidermidis 60%, Staph. aureus, streptococci, & enterococci each 5–10%, Gm-neg. bacilli 6%	**Immediate ophthal. consult.** If only light perception or worse, immediate vitrectomy + intravitreal vanco 1 mg & intravitreal ceftazidime 2.25 mg. No clear data on intravitreal steroid. May need to repeat intravitreal antibiotics in 2–3 days. Can usually leave lens in.		
Low grade, chronic	Propionibacterium acnes, S. epidermidis, S. aureus (rare)	May require removal of lens material. Intraocular **vanco** ± vitrectomy.		
Post filtering blebs for glaucoma	Strep. species (viridans & others), H. influenzae	Intravitreal and topical agent and consider systemic **AM-CL**, **AM-SB** or **cefprozil or cefuroxime**		
Post-penetrating trauma	Bacillus sp., S. epiderm.	Intravitreal agent as above + systemic **clinda** or **vanco**. Use topical antibiotics post-surgery (tobra & cefazolin drops).		
None, suspect hematogenous	S. pneumoniae, N. meningitidis, Staph. aureus	(**cefotaxime** 2 gm IV q4h or **ceftriaxone** 2 gm IV q24h) + **vanco** 30-60 mg/kg/day in 2-3 div doses to achieve target trough serum concentration of 15-20 mcg/mL pending cultures. Intravitreal antibiotics as with early post-operative.		
IV heroin abuse	Bacillus cereus, Candida sp.	Intravitreal agent + (systemic **clinda** or **vanco**)		
Mycotic (fungal): Broad-spectrum antibiotics, often corticosteroids, indwelling venous catheters	Candida sp., Aspergillus sp.	Intravitreal **ampho B** 0.005–0.01 mg in 0.1 mL. *Also see Table 11A, page 107 for concomitant systemic therapy. See Comment.*		With moderate/marked vitritis, options include systemic rx + vitrectomy ± intravitreal ampho B *(CID 27:1130 & 1134, 1998)*. Report of failure of ampho B lipid complex *(CID 28:1177, 1999)*.
Retinitis				
Acute retinal necrosis	Varicella zoster, Herpes simplex	IV **acyclovir** 10–12 mg/kg IV q8h x 5–7 days, then 800 mg po 5x/day x 6 wk		Strong association of VZ virus with atypical necrotizing herpetic retinopathy *(CID 24:603, 1997)*.
HIV+ (AIDS) CD4 usually <100/mm³	Cytomegalovirus	*See Table 14, page 148*		Occurs in 5–10% of AIDS patients

bbreviations on page 2. *NOTE: All dosage recommendations are for adults (unless otherwise indicated) and assume normal renal function.*

TABLE 1A (11)

ANATOMIC SITE/DIAGNOSIS/ MODIFYING CIRCUMSTANCES	ETIOLOGIES (usual)	SUGGESTED REGIMENS*		ADJUNCT DIAGNOSTIC OR THERAPEUTIC MEASURES AND COMMENTS
		PRIMARY	ALTERNATIVE[§]	
EYE/Retinitis *(continued)*				
Progressive outer retinal necrosis	VZV, H. simplex, CMV (rare)	**Acyclovir** 10-12 mg/kg IV q8h for 1-2 weeks, then (**valacyclovir** 1000 mg po tid, or **famciclovir** 500 mg po tid, or **acyclovir** 800 mg po tid). Ophthalmology consultation imperative: approaches have also included intra-vitreal injection of anti-virals (foscarnet, ganciclovir implant). In rare cases due to CMV use **ganciclovir/valganciclovir** *(see CMV retinitis, Table 14A)*.		Most patients are highly immunocompromised (HIV with low CD4 or transplantation). In contrast to Acute Retinal Necrosis, lack of intraocular inflammation or arteritis *(Surv Ophthalmol 49:131, 2004)*. May be able to stop oral antivirals when CD4 recovers with ART *(Ocul Immunol Inflammation 15:425, 2007)*.
Orbital cellulitis *(see page 51 for erysipelas, facial)*	S. pneumoniae, H. influenzae, M. catarrhalis, S. aureus, anaerobes, group A strep, occ. Gm-neg. bacilli post-trauma	**Nafcillin** 2 gm IV q4h (or if **MRSA-vanco** 30-60 mg/kg/day in 2-3 div doses to achieve target trough serum concentration of 15-20 mcg/mL) + **ceftriaxone** 2 gm IV q24h + **metro** 1 gm IV q12h		**If penicillin/ceph allergy: Vanco** + **levo** 750 mg IV once daily + **metro** IV. Problem is frequent inability to make microbiologic diagnosis. Image orbit (CT or MRI). Risk of cavernous sinus thrombosis. If vanco intolerant, another option for s. aureus is dapto 6 mg/kg IV q24h.
FOOT				
"Diabetic"—Two thirds of patients have triad of neuropathy, deformity and pressure-induced trauma. Refs.: *Ln 366:1725, 2005; NEJM 351:48, 2004; JAC 65 (suppl 3): 3, 2010.*				
Ulcer without inflammation	Colonizing skin flora	No antibacterial therapy		**General:** 1. Glucose control, eliminate pressure on ulcer 2. **Assess for peripheral vascular disease**—very common *(CID 39:437, 2004)* **Principles of empiric antibacterial therapy:** 1. Include drug predictably active vs. MRSA. If outpatient, can assume community-associated MRSA (CA-MRSA) until culture results available. 2. As culture results dominated by S. aureus & Streptococcus species, empiric drug regimens should include strep & staph. Role of enterococci uncertain. 3. Severe limb and/or life-threatening infections require initial parenteral therapy with predictable activity vs. Gm-positive cocci, coliforms & other aerobic Gm-neg. rods, & anaerobic Gm-neg. bacilli. 4. **NOTE:** The regimens listed are suggestions consistent with above principles. Other alternatives exist & may be appropriate for individual patients. 5. Is there an associated osteomyelitis? Risk increased if ulcer area >2 cm², positive probe to bone, ESR >70 and abnormal plain x-ray. Negative MRI reduces likelihood of osteomyelitis *(JAMA 299:806, 2008)*. MRI is best imaging modality *(CID 47:519 & 528, 2008)*.
Ulcer with <2 cm of superficial inflammation	*S. aureus (assume MRSA), S. agalactiae (Gp B), S. pyogenes predominate*	**Oral therapy:** (**TMP-SMX-DS** or **minocycline**) plus (**Pen VK** or selected **O Ceph 2, 3**, or **FQ**) *Dosages in footnote[6]*		
Ulcer with >2 cm of inflammation with extension to fascia. **Osteomyelitis** *See Comment.*	As above, plus coliforms possible	**Oral therapy:** (**AM-CL-ER** plus **TMP-SMX-DS**) or [(**CIP** or **Levo** or **Moxi**) plus **linezolid**] or **ERTA** OR **Parenteral therapy:** [based on prevailing susceptibilities: (**AM-SB** or **TC-CL** or **PIP-TZ** or **ERTA** or other carbapenem)] plus [**vanco** (or alternative anti-MRSA drug as below) until MRSA excluded]. See IDSA practice guidelines for additional options *(CID 39:885, 2004)*. *Dosages in footnotes[7, 8]*		

(Continued on next page)

[6] **TMP-SMX-DS** 1-2 tabs po bid, **minocycline** 100 mg po bid, **Pen VK** 500 mg po qid, (O Ceph 2, 3: **cefprozil** 500 mg po q12h, **cefuroxime axetil** 500 mg po q12h, **cefdinir** 300 mg po q12h or 600 mg po q24h, **cefpodoxime** 200 mg po q12h), **CIP** 750 mg po bid. **Levo** 750 mg po q24h.

[7] **AM-CL-ER** 2000/125 mg po bid, **TMP-SMX-DS** 1-2 tabs po bid, **CIP** 750 mg po bid, **Levo** 750 mg po q24h, **Moxi** 400 mg po q24h, **linezolid** 600 mg po bid.

Abbreviations on page 2. *NOTE: All dosage recommendations are for adults (unless otherwise indicated) and assume normal renal function.*

TABLE 1A (12)

ANATOMIC SITE/DIAGNOSIS/ MODIFYING CIRCUMSTANCES	ETIOLOGIES (usual)	SUGGESTED REGIMENS*		ADJUNCT DIAGNOSTIC OR THERAPEUTIC MEASURES AND COMMENTS
		PRIMARY	ALTERNATIVE[§]	
FOOT/Diabetic *(continued)*				
Extensive local inflammation plus systemic toxicity. Treatment modalities of limited efficacy & expensive: Neg pressure (wound vac) *(Ln 366:1704, 2005)*; growth factor (becaplermin); and hyperbaric oxygen *(CID 43:188, 193, 2006)*	As above, plus anaerobic bacteria. Role of enterococci unclear.	**Parenteral therapy:** (**Vanco** plus **β-lactam/β-lactamase inhibitor**) or (**vanco** plus [**Dori**, **IMP** or **MER**]). Other alternatives: 1. **Dapto** or **linezolid** for vanco 2. (**CIP** or **Levo** or **Moxi** or **aztreonam**) plus **metronidazole** for β-lactam/β-lactamase inhibitor *Dosages in footnote[8]* **Assess for arterial insufficiency!**		*(Continued from previous page)*
Onychomycosis: *See Table 11, page 110, fungal infections*				
Puncture wound: Nail/Toothpick	P. aeruginosa	Cleanse. Tetanus booster. Observe.		*See page 4. 1–2% evolve to osteomyelitis.* After toothpick injury *(PIDJ 23:80, 2004)*: S. aureus, Strep sp, and mixed flora.
GALLBLADDER				
Cholecystitis, cholangitis, biliary sepsis, or common duct obstruction (partial: 2nd to tumor, stones, stricture). Cholecystitis Ref: *NEJM 358:2804, 2008.*	Enterobacteriaceae 68%, enterococci 14%, bacteroides 10%, Clostridium sp. 7%, rarely candida	**PIP-TZ** or **AM-SB** or **TC-CL** or **ERTA** If life-threatening: **IMP** or **MER** or **Dori** *Dosages in footnote[8].* * Add vanco to these regimens to cover gram-positives.	**P Ceph 3** + **metro** OR **Aztreonam*** + **metro** OR **CIP*** + **metro** OR **Moxi**	In severely ill pts, antibiotic therapy complements adequate biliary drainage. 15-30% pts will require decompression: surgical, percutaneous or ERCP-placed stent. Whether empirical therapy should always cover pseudomonas & anaerobes is uncertain. Ceftriaxone associated with biliary sludge of drug (by ultrasound 50%, symptomatic 9%, *NEJM 322:1821, 1990)*; clinical relevance still unclear but has led to surgery *(MMWR 42:39, 1993)*.
GASTROINTESTINAL				
Gastroenteritis—Empiric Therapy (laboratory studies not performed or culture, microscopy, toxin results NOT AVAILABLE) (Ref.: *NEJM 350:38, 2004)*				
Premature infant with necrotizing enterocolitis	Associated with intestinal flora	Treatment and rationale as for diverticulitis/peritonitis, *page 20. See Table 16, page 187 for pediatric dosages.*		Pneumatosis intestinalis on x-ray confirms diagnosis. Bacteremia-peritonitis in 30–50%. If Staph. epidermidis isolated, add vanco (IV).
Mild diarrhea (≤3 unformed stools/day, minimal associated symptomatology)	Bacterial *(see Severe, below)*, viral (norovirus), parasitic. Viral usually causes mild to moderate disease. For traveler's diarrhea, *see page 18*	Fluids only + lactose-free diet, avoid caffeine		**Rehydration: For po fluid replacement, see *Cholera, page 17.*** **Antimotility:** Loperamide (Imodium) 4 mg po, then 2 mg after each loose stool to max. of 16 mg per day. Bismuth subsalicylate (Pepto-Bismol) 2 tablets (262 mg) po qid. Do not use if suspect hemolytic uremic syndrome. **Hemolytic uremic syndrome (HUS):** Risk in **children** infected with E. coli 0157:H7 is 8–10%. Early treatment with TMP-SMX or FQs ↑ risk of HUS *(NEJM 342:1930 & 1990, 2000)*. Controversial meta-analysis: *JAMA 288:996 & 3110, 2002.* **Norovirus**: Etiology of over 90% of non-bacterial diarrhea (± nausea/vomiting). Lasts 12-60 hrs. Hydrate. No effective antiviral. **Other potential etiologies:** Cryptosporidia—no treatment in immunocompetent host *(see Table 13A & JID 170:272, 1994)*. Cyclospora—usually chronic diarrhea, responds to TMP-SMX *(see Table 12A & AIM 123:409, 1995)*. Klebsiella oxytoca identified as cause of antibiotic-associated hemorrhagic colitis (cytotoxin positive): *NEJM 355:2418, 2006.*
Moderate diarrhea (≥4 unformed stools/day &/or systemic symptoms)		Antimotility agents *(see Comments)* + fluids		
Severe diarrhea (≥6 unformed stools/day, &/or temp ≥101°F, tenesmus, blood, or fecal leukocytes) **NOTE: Severe afebrile bloody diarrhea should ↑ suspicion of Shiga-toxin E. coli 0157:H7 & others** *(MMWR 58 (RR-12):1, 2009).*	Shigella, salmonella, C. jejuni, Shiga toxin + E. coli, toxin-positive C. difficile, Klebsiella oxytoca, E. histolytica. *For typhoid fever, see page 57*	**FQ** (**CIP** 500 mg po q12h or **Levo** 500 mg q24h) times 3–5 days *If recent antibiotic therapy* (C. difficile toxin colitis possible) **add:** **Metro** 500 mg po tid times 10–14 days	**TMP-SMX-DS** po bid times 3–5 days. Campylobacter resistance to TMP-SMX common in tropics. **Vanco** 125 mg po qid times 10–14 days	

[8] **Vanco** 1 gm IV q12h, (**parenteral β-lactam/β-lactamase inhibitors**; **AM-SB** 3 gm IV q6h, **PIP-TZ** 3.375 gm IV q6h or 4.5 gm IV q8h or 4 hr infusion of 3.375 gm q8h;TC-CL 3.1 gm IV q6h); **carbapenems: Doripenem** 500 mg (1-hr infusion) q8h, **ERTA** 1 gm IV q24h, **IMP** 0.5 gm IV q6h, **MER** 1 gm IV q8h, **daptomycin** 6 mg per kg IV q24h, **linezoid** 600 mg IV q12h, **aztreonam** 2 gm IV q8h. **CIP** 400 mg IV q12h, **Levo** 750 mg IV q24h, **Moxi** 400 mg IV q24h, **metro** 1 gm IV loading dose & then 0.5 gm IV q6h or 1 gm IV q12h.

Abbreviations on page 2. *NOTE: All dosage recommendations are for adults (unless otherwise indicated) and assume normal renal function.*

TABLE 1A (13)

ANATOMIC SITE/DIAGNOSIS/ MODIFYING CIRCUMSTANCES	ETIOLOGIES (usual)	SUGGESTED REGIMENS* PRIMARY	SUGGESTED REGIMENS* ALTERNATIVE[§]	ADJUNCT DIAGNOSTIC OR THERAPEUTIC MEASURES AND COMMENTS
GASTROINTESTINAL *(continued)*				
Gastroenteritis—Specific Therapy (results of culture, microscopy, toxin assay AVAILABLE) (Ref.: *NEJM 361:1560, 2009*)				
If culture negative, probably **Norovirus (Norwalk)** or rarely (in adults) **Rotavirus**—*see Norovirus, page 155* **NOTE: In 60 hospital pts with unexplained WBCs ≥15,000, 35% had C. difficile toxin present** *(AJM 115:543, 2003; CID 34:1585, 2002)*	**Aeromonas/Plesiomonas**	**CIP** 750 mg po bid x3 days.	**Azithro** 500 mg po once daily x3 days	Although no absolute proof, increasing evidence for Plesiomonas as cause of diarrheal illness *(NEJM 361:1560, 2009)*.
	Amebiasis (Entamoeba histolytica, Cyclospora, Cryptosporidia and **Giardia), see *Table 13A***			
	Campylobacter jejuni History of fever in 53-83%. Self-limited diarrhea in normal host.	**Azithro** 500 mg po q24h x 3 days.	**Erythro stearate** 500 mg po qid x 5 days or **CIP** 500 mg po bid (CIP resistance increasing).	**Post-Campylobacter Guillain-Barré;** assoc. 15% of cases *(Ln 366:1653, 2005)*. Assoc. with small bowel lymphoproliferative disease; may respond to antimicrobials *(NEJM 350:239, 2004)*. **Reactive arthritis** another potential sequelae. *See Traveler's diarrhea, page 18.*
	Campylobacter fetus Diarrhea uncommon. More systemic disease in debilitated hosts	**Gentamicin** *(see Table 10D)*	**AMP** 100 mg/kg IV div q6h or **IMP** 500 mg IV q6h	Draw blood cultures. Do not use erythro for C. fetus. In bacteremic pts, 32% resistant to FQs and 8% resistant to erythromycin *(CID 47:790, 2008)*. Meropenem inhibits C. fetus at low concentrations in vitro.
Differential diagnosis of toxin-producing diarrhea: • C. difficile • Klebsiella oxytoca • S. aureus • Shiga toxin producing E. coli (STEC) • Enterotoxigenic B. fragilis *(CID 47:797, 2008)* More on C. difficile: *Treatment review: CID 51:1306, 2010. SHEA/IDSA treatment guidelines: ICHE 31:431, 2010; ESCMID guidelines: Clin Microbiol Infect 15:1067, 2009.* *(Continued on next page)*	**C. difficile** toxin positive antibiotic-associated colitis. **Probiotics'** (lactobacillus or saccharomyces) inconsistent in prevention of C. difficile *(NEJM 359:1932, 2008)*.			
	po meds okay; WBC <15,000; no increase in serum creatinine.	**Metro** 500 mg po tid or 250 mg qid x 10-14 days	**Vanco** 125 mg po qid x 10-14 days **Teicoplanin**[NUS] 400 mg po bid x 10 days	**D/C antibiotic if possible; avoid antimotility agents, hydration, enteric isolation.** Recent review suggests antimotility agents can be used cautiously in certain pts with mild disease who are receiving rx *(CID 48: 598, 2009)*, but others believe there is insufficient data re safety of this approach *(CID 48: 606, 2009)*. Relapse in 10-20%. **Nitazoxanide** 500 mg po bid for 7–10 days equivalent to **Metro** po in phase 3 study[NAI] *(CID 43:421, 2006)*
	po meds okay; Sicker; WBC >15,000; ≥ 50% increase in baseline creatinine	**Vanco** 125 mg po qid x 10-14 days. To use IV **vanco po**, *see* Table 10C, *page 95*	**Metro** 500 mg po tid x 10 days	Vanco superior to metro in sicker pts. Relapse in 10-20% (not due to resistance: *JAC 56:988, 2005)*
	Post-treatment relapse	**1st relapse** **Metro** 500 mg po tid x 10 days	**2nd relapse** **Vanco** 125 mg po qid x 10-14 days, then immediately start taper (See Comments)	**Vanco** taper (all doses 125 mg po): week 1– bid, week 2 – q24h; week 3 – qod; then every 3rd day for 5 doses *(NEJM 359, 1932, 2008)*. Other options: 1) After initial vanco, **rifaximin**[NAI] 400-800 mg po daily divided bid or tid x 2 wks *(CID 44:846, 2007*, rifaximin-resistant C. diff. reported); 2) **nitazoxanide**[NAI] 500 mg bid x 10d *(JAC 59:705, 2007)*. **Last resort: stool transplant** *(CID 36:580, 2003)*.
	Post-op ileus; severe disease with toxic megacolon *(NEJM 359:1932, 2008)*.	**Metro** 500 mg IV q6h + **vanco** 500 mg q6h via nasogastric tube (or naso-small bowel tube) ± retrograde catheter in cecum. *See comment* for dosage.		For vanco instillation into bowel, add 500 mg vanco to 1 liter of saline and perfuse at 1-3 mL/min to maximum of 2 gm in 24 hrs *(CID 690, 2002)*. **Note: IV vanco not effective. IVIG:** Reports of benefit of 400 mg/kg x 1-3 doses *(JAC 53:882, 2004)* and lack of benefit *(Am J Inf Cont 35:131, 2007)*. Indications for colectomy, *see ICHE 31:431, 2010.* Reported successful use of tigecycline[NAI] IV to treat severe C. diff refractory to standard rx *(CID 48:1732, 2009)*.
	E. coli 0157:H7 History of bloody stools 63% shiga toxin producing E. Coli (STEC)	**NO TREATMENT** with antimicrobials or anti-motility drugs, may enhance toxin release and ↑ risk of hemolytic uremic syndrome (HUS) *(NEJM 342:1930 & 1990, 2000)*. Hydration important *(Ln 365:1073, 2005)*.		5–10% of pts develop HUS (approx. 10% with HUS die or have permanent renal failure; 50% HUS pts have some degree of renal impairment) *(CID 38:1298, 2004)*. Non O157:H7 STEC emerging: for lab diagnosis, *see MMWR 58 (RR-12), 2009.*
	Klebsiella oxytoca—antibiotic-associated diarrhea	Responds to stopping antibiotic		Suggested that stopping NSAIDs helps. Ref.: *NEJM 355:2418, 2006.*

Abbreviations on page 2. *NOTE: All dosage recommendations are for adults (unless otherwise indicated) and assume normal renal function.*

TABLE 1A (14)

ANATOMIC SITE/DIAGNOSIS/ MODIFYING CIRCUMSTANCES	ETIOLOGIES (usual)	SUGGESTED REGIMENS*		ADJUNCT DIAGNOSTIC OR THERAPEUTIC MEASURES AND COMMENTS
		PRIMARY	ALTERNATIVE[§]	
GASTROINTESTINAL/Gastroenteritis—Specific Therapy *(continued)*				
(Continued from previous page)	**Listeria monocytogenes**	Usually self-limited. Value of oral antibiotics (e.g., ampicillin or TMP-SMX) unknown, but their use might be reasonable in populations at risk for serious listeria infections *(CID 40:1327, 2005; Wien Klin Wochenschr 121:149, 2009)*. Those with bacteremia/meningitis require parenteral therapy: *see pages 8 & 57*.		Recognized as a cause of food-associated febrile gastroenteritis. Not detected in standard stool cultures *(NEJM 336:100 & 130, 1997)*. Percentage with complicating bacteremia/meningitis unknown. Among 292 children hospitalized during an outbreak, none developed sepsis *(NEJM 342:1236, 2000)*. Populations at ↑ risk of severe systemic disease: pregnant women, neonates, the elderly, and immunocompromised hosts *(MMWR 57:1097, 2008)*.
	Salmonella, non-typhi— For typhoid (enteric) fever, *see page 57* Fever in 71–91%, history of bloody stools in 34%	If pt asymptomatic or illness mild, antimicrobial therapy not indicated. **Treat if** <1 yr old or >50 yr old, if immunocompromised, if vascular grafts or prosthetic joints, bacteremic, hemoglobinopathy, or hospitalized with fever and severe diarrhea *(see typhoid fever, page 57)*.		
		(**CIP** 500 mg bid) or (**Levo** 500 mg q24h) x 7-10 days (14 days if immunocompromised)	**Azithro** 500 mg po once daily x 7 days (14 days if immunocompromised).	↑ resistance to TMP-SMX and chloro. Ceftriaxone, cefotaxime usually active *(see footnote, page 23, for dosage)*; ceftriaxone & FQ resistance in Asia *(AAC 53:2696, 2009)*. **Primary treatment of enteritis is fluid and electrolyte replacement.**
	Shigella Fever in 58%, history of bloody stools 51%	**CIP** 750 mg po bid x 3 days *See Comment for peds rx per dose*	**Azithro** 500 mg po once daily x 3 days	**Peds doses: Azithro** 10 mg/kg/day once daily x 3 days. For severe disease, ceftriaxone 50–75 mg/kg per day x 2–5 days. CIP suspension 10 mg/kg bid x 5 days. CIP superior to ceftriaxone in children *(LnID 3:537, 2003)*. **Immunocompromised children & adults: Treat for 7–10 days.** Azithro superior to cefixime in trial in children *(PIDJ 22:374, 2003)*.
	Staphylococcus aureus *See Comment*	**Vanco** 1 gm IV q12h + 125 mg po qid reasonable		Case reports of toxin-mediated pseudomembranous enteritis/colitis (pseudomembranes in small bowel) *(CID 39:747, 2004; Gastroent Hepatol 6:115, 2010)*. **Clinda** to stop toxin production reasonable if organism susceptible, but S. aureus and C. diff may occur simultaneously.
	Spirochetosis (Brachyspira pilosicoli)	Benefit of treatment unclear. Susceptible to **metro**, **ceftriaxone**, and **Moxi** *(AAC 47:2354, 2003)*.		Anaerobic intestinal spirochete that colonizes colon of domestic & wild animals plus humans. Case reports of diarrhea with large numbers of the organism present *(JCM 39:347, 2001; Am J Clin Path 120:828, 2003)*. Rarely, *B. pilosicoli* has been isolated from blood culture *(Ann Clin Micro Antimicrob 7:19, 2008)*.
	Vibrio cholerae Treatment decreases duration of disease, volume losses, & duration of excretion *(CID 37:272, 2003; Ln 363:223, 2004)*	**Primary therapy is rehydration.** Select antibiotics based on susceptibility of locally prevailing isolates. Options include: **Doxycycline** 300 mg po single dose **OR Azithromycin** 1 gm po single dose **OR Tetracycline** 500 mg po qid x 3 days **OR Erythromycin** 500 mg po qid x 3 days (these options are based on CDC recommendations for 2010 Haiti epidemic)	**For pregnant women: Azithromycin** 1 gm po single dose **OR Erythromycin** 500 mg po qid x 3 days **For children: Azithromycin** 20 mg/kg po as single dose; for other age-specific alternatives, *see CDC website http://www.cdc.gov/haiticholera/hcp_goingtohaiti.htm*	Antimicrobial therapy shortens duration of illness, but rehydration is paramount. When IV hydration is needed, use Ringer's lactate. Switch to PO repletion with Oral Rehydration Salts (ORS) as soon as able to take oral fluids. ORS are commercially available for reconstitution in potable water. If not available, WHO suggests a substitute can be made by dissolving ½ teaspoon salt and 6 level teaspoons of sugar per liter of potable water *(http://www.who.int/cholera/technical/en/)*. For additional practical considerations, *see Lancet 363:223, 2004*. CDC recommendations for other aspects of management developed for Haiti outbreak can be found at *http://www.cdc.gov/haiticholera/hcp_goingtohaiti.htm* Isolates from this outbreak demonstrate reduced susceptibility to ciprofloxacin and resistance to sulfisoxazole, nalidixic acid and furazolidone.
	Vibrio parahaemolyticus	Antimicrobial rx does not shorten course. Hydration.		Shellfish exposure common. Treat severe disease: **FQ, doxy, P Ceph 3**
	Vibrio vulnificus	Usual presentation is skin lesions & bacteremia; life-threatening; treat early: **ceftaz** + **doxy**—*see page 52; levo (AAC 46:3580, 2002)*.		
	Yersinia enterocolitica Fever in 68%, bloody stools in 26%	No treatment unless severe. If severe, combine **doxy** 100 mg IV bid + (**tobra** or **gent** 5 mg/kg per day once q24h). **TMP-SMX** or **FQs** are alternatives.		Mesenteric adenitis pain can mimic acute appendicitis. Lab diagnosis difficult: requires "cold enrichment" and/or yersinia selective agar. Desferrioxamine therapy increases severity, discontinue if pt on it. Iron overload states predispose to yersinia *(CID 27:1362 & 1367, 1998)*.

TABLE 1A (15)

ANATOMIC SITE/DIAGNOSIS/ MODIFYING CIRCUMSTANCES	ETIOLOGIES (usual)	SUGGESTED REGIMENS*		ADJUNCT DIAGNOSTIC OR THERAPEUTIC MEASURES AND COMMENTS
		PRIMARY	ALTERNATIVE[§]	
GASTROINTESTINAL *(continued)*				
Gastroenteritis—Specific Risk Groups–Empiric Therapy				
Anoreceptive intercourse				
Proctitis (distal 15 cm only)	Herpes viruses, gonococci, chlamydia, syphilis *See Genital Tract, page 20*			
Colitis	Shigella, salmonella, campylobacter, E. histolytica *(see Table 13A)*			*See specifc GI pathogens, Gastroenteritis, above.*
HIV-1 infected (AIDS): >10 days diarrhea	G. lamblia			*See Table 13A*
Acid-fast organisms:	Cryptosporidium parvum, Cyclospora cayetanensis			*See Table 13A*
Other:	Isospora belli, microsporidia (Enterocytozoon bieneusi, Septata intestinalis)			*See Table 13A*
Neutropenic enterocolitis or "typhlitis" *(CID 27:695 & 700, 1998)*	Mucosal invasion by **Clostridium septicum**. Occasionally caused by C. sordellii or P. aeruginosa	As for perirectal abscess. diverticulitis, pg 20. Ensure empiric regimen includes drug active vs. Clostridia species. Empiric regimen should have predictive activity vs. P. aeruginosa also.		Tender right lower quadrant may be clue, but tenderness may be diffuse or absent in immunocompromised host. Need surgical consult. Surgical resection controversial but may be necessary. **NOTE:** Resistance of clostridia to clindamycin reported. Broad-spectrum agents such as PIP-TZ, IMP, MER, DORI should cover most pathogens.
Traveler's diarrhea, self-medication. Patient usually afebrile *(CID 44:338 & 347, 2007)*	**Acute**: 60% due to diarrheagenic E. coli; shigella, salmonella, or campylobacter. C. difficile, amebiasis *(see Table 13)*. **If chronic**: cyclospora, cryptosporidia, giardia, isospora	**CIP** 750 mg po bid x 1-3 days or **other FQ** *(see footnote[9])* or **rifaximin** 200 mg po tid x 3 days		**Peds & pregnancy:** Avoid FQs. Azithro peds dose: 10 mg/kg/day single dose or ceftriaxone 50 mg/kg/day IV once daily x 3 days. Rifaximin approved for age 12 or older. Adverse effects similar to placebo.
		Add **Imodium**: 4 mg po x 1, then 2 mg after each loose stool to max.16 mg/day.		No loperamide if fever or blood in stool. **CIP and rifaximin** equivalent efficacy vs. non-invasive pathogens *(AJTMH 74:1060, 2006)*
Prevention of Traveler's diarrhea	Not routinely indicated. Current recommendation is to take **FQ** + **Imodium** with 1st loose stool.		Alternative during 1st 3 wk & only if activities are essential: **Rifaximin** 200 mg po bid *(AnIM 142:805 & 861, 2005)*.	

[9] **Other FQ** dosage po for self-rx traveler's diarrhea—mild disease: **Oflox** 300 mg po bid x 3 days. Once q24h x 3 days: **Levo** 500 mg once daily x 1-3 days; **Moxi**, 400 mg probably would work but not FDA-approved indication.

Abbreviations on page 2. *NOTE: All dosage recommendations are for adults (unless otherwise indicated) and assume normal renal function.*

TABLE 1A (16)

ANATOMIC SITE/DIAGNOSIS/ MODIFYING CIRCUMSTANCES	ETIOLOGIES (usual)	SUGGESTED REGIMENS* PRIMARY	SUGGESTED REGIMENS* ALTERNATIVE[§]	ADJUNCT DIAGNOSTIC OR THERAPEUTIC MEASURES AND COMMENTS
GASTROINTESTINAL *(continued)*				
Gastrointestinal Infections by Anatomic Site: Esophagus to Rectum				
Esophagitis	Candida albicans, HSV, CMV	*See* SANFORD GUIDE TO HIV/AIDS THERAPY *and Table 11A.*		
Duodenal/Gastric ulcer; gastric cancer, MALT lymphomas (not 2° NSAIDs) *(AnIM 148:923 & 962, 2008; Nature Clin Practice G-I; Hepatology 5:321, 2008; JAMA 300:1346, 2008).*	**Helicobacter pylori** *See Comment* Prevalence of pre-treatment resistance increasing	**Sequential therapy:** (**Rabeprazole** 20 mg – **amox** 1 gm) bid x 5 days, then (**rabeprazole** 20 mg + **clarithro** 500 mg + **tinidazole** 500 mg) bid for another 5 days. *See footnote*[10].	**Rx po for 14 days: Bismuth** *(see footnote*[11]*)*, bismuth subsalicylate 2 tabs qid + **tetracycline** 500 mg qid + **metro** 500 mg tid + **omeprazole** 20 mg bid.	**Treatment**: Due to 10-15% rate of clarithro resistance, failure of previously suggested triple therapy (PPI + clarithro + amox) is unacceptable 20%. Cure rate with sequential therapy is 90%. **Dx: Stool antigen**—Monoclonal EIA >90% sens. & 92% specific. *(Amer.J.Gastro. 101:921, 2006)* Other tests: if endoscoped, rapid urease &/or histology &/or culture; urea breath test, but some office-based tests underperform *(CID 48:1335, 2009)*. **Test of cure:** Repeat stool antigen and/or urea breath test >8 wks post-treatment. **Treatment:** Failure rate of triple therapy 20% due to clarithro resistance. Cure rate with sequential therapy 90%.
Small intestine: Whipple's disease *(NEJM 356:55, 2007; LnID 8:179, 2008)* *See Infective endocarditis, culture-negative, page 28*	Tropheryma whipplei	**Initial 10–14 days:** (**Pen G** 2 million units IV q4h + **streptomycin** 1 gm IM/IV q24h) OR **ceftriaxone** 2 gm IV q24h **Then, for approx. 1 year:** **TMP-SMX-DS** 1 tab po bid	**TMP-SMX-DS** 1 tab po bid if allergic to penicillin & cephalosporins. If sulfa-allergic: **Doxy** 100 mg po bid + hydroxychloroquine 200 mg po tid.	Therapy based on empiricism and retrospective analyses. Randomized trial reported that initial therapy with Meropenem 1 gm q8h was comparable to Ceftriaxone 2 gm q24h, each administered for 14 days and then followed by TMP-SMX for 12 months, in maintaining remission of Whipple's disease for at least 3 years *(Gastroenterology 138:478, 2010; editorial ibid 138:422, 2010)*. TMP-SMX: CNS relapses during therapy have been reported. Late relapses with resistance to TMP-SMX have been described *(J Antimicrobial Chemother 65:2005, 2010)*. Cultivated from CSF of patients with intestinal disease and no neurological findings *(J Infect Dis 188:797, 2003 & J Infect Dis 188:801, 2003)*. For review of Whipple's pathogenesis, *see Lancet Infect Dis 8:179, 2008.*
Inflammatory bowel disease (IBD)		• For mild-to-moderate disease, **sulfasalazine** is often used. For severe disease, anti-TNF agents are frequently used, which increase risk of reactivating latent infections. • In a randomized trial of mild-to-moderate Crohn's, **CIP** – **Metro** did not impart a statistically significant benefit when added to budesonide *(Gastro 123:33, 2002)*. • Exclude gastrointestinal infections that mimic (or complicate) IBD, such as E. histolytica, C. difficile, tuberculosis, CMV *(Heart Lung 34:291, 2005)*, Yersinia sp. *(Pediatrics 104:e36, 1999)*, Strongyloides *(Human Pathol 40:572, 2009)*. • When using anti-TNF agents screen for latent TB before use *(MMWR 53:683, 2004)*. If possible, delay anti-TNF drugs until TB prophylaxis is complete. For other risks, *see Lancet Infect Dis 8:601, 2008 and Aliment Pharmacol Ther 31:20, 2010.* Hepatitis B, CMV, histoplasmosis, and leishmaniasis are among other infections reported to have reactivated during anti-TNF therapy. • References: *Clin Infect Dis 44:256, 2007; Lancet 359:331, 2002; Aliment Pharmacol Ther 26:987, 2007*		

[10] Can substitute other proton pump inhibitors for omeprazole or rabeprazole--all bid: **esomeprazole** 20 mg (FDA-approved), **lansoprazole** 30 mg (FDA-approved), **pantoprazole** 40 mg (not FDA-approved for this indication).

[11] **3 bismuth preparations:** (1) In U.S., **bismuth subsalicylate (Pepto-Bismol)** 262 mg tabs; adult dose for helicobacter is 2 tabs (524 mg) qid. (2) Outside U.S., colloidal bismuth subcitrate (De-Nol) 120 mg chewable tablets; dose is 1 tablet qid. (3) Another treatment option: Ranitidine bismuth citrate 400 mg; give with metro 500 mg and clarithro 500 mg—all bid times 7 days. Worked despite metro/clarithro resistance *(Gastro 114:A323, 1998)*.

Abbreviations on page 2. *NOTE: All dosage recommendations are for adults (unless otherwise indicated) and assume normal renal function.*

TABLE 1A (17)

ANATOMIC SITE/DIAGNOSIS/ MODIFYING CIRCUMSTANCES	ETIOLOGIES (usual)	SUGGESTED REGIMENS* PRIMARY	ALTERNATIVE[§]	ADJUNCT DIAGNOSTIC OR THERAPEUTIC MEASURES AND COMMENTS
GASTROINTESTINAL/Gastrointestinal Infections by Anatomic Site: Esophagus to Rectum *(continued)*				
Diverticulitis, perirectal abscess, peritonitis *Also see Peritonitis, page 44* *CID 37:997, 2003*	Enterobacteriaceae, occasionally P. aeruginosa, Bacteroides sp., enterococci	**Outpatient rx—mild diverticulitis, drained perirectal abscess:** [(**TMP-SMX-DS** bid) or (**CIP** 750 mg bid or **Levo** 750 mg q24h)] + **metro** 500 mg q6h. All po x 7–10 days.	**AM-CL-ER** 1000/62.5 mg 2 tabs po bid x 7–10 days **OR** **Moxi** 400 mg po q24h x 7-10 days	Must "cover" both Gm-neg. aerobic & Gm-neg. anaerobic bacteria. **Drugs active only vs. anaerobic Gm-neg. bacilli:** clinda, metro. **Drugs active only vs. aerobic Gm-neg. bacilli:** APAG[12], P Ceph 2/3/4 *(see Table 10C, page 92)*, aztreonam, AP Pen, CIP, Levo. **Drugs active vs. both aerobic/anaerobic Gm-neg. bacteria:** cefoxitin, cefotetan, TC-CL, PIP-TZ, AM-SB, ERTA, Dori, IMP, MER, Moxi, & tigecycline. **Increasing resistance of Bacteroides species** *(AAC 51:1649, 2007)*: **Cefoxitin** / **Cefotetan** / **Clindamycin** — % Resistant: 5-30 / 17-87 / 19-35
		Mild-moderate disease—Inpatient—Parenteral Rx: (e.g., focal peri-appendiceal peritonitis, peri-diverticular abscess, endomyometritis) **PIP-TZ** 3.375 gm IV q6h **or** 4.5 gm IV q8h **or** **AM-SB** 3 gm IV q6h, **or TC-CL** 3.1 gm IV q6h **or ERTA** 1 gm IV q24h **or** **MOXI** 400 mg IV q24h	[(**CIP** 400 mg IV q12h) or (**Levo** 750 mg IV q24h)] + (**metro** 500 mg IV q6h or 1 gm IV q12h) **OR tigecycline** 100 mg IV 1st dose & then 50 mg IV q12h **OR Moxi** 400 mg IV q24h	Resistance to metro, PIP-TZ rare. Few case reports of metro resistance *(CID 40:e67, 2005; J Clin Micro 42:4127, 2004)*. If prior FQ exposure, increasing moxi resistance in Bacteriodes sp. on rectal swabs *(Abst 2008 ICAAC)*. **Ertapenem** poorly active vs. P. aeruginosa/Acinetobacter sp. **Concomitant surgical management important**, esp. with moderate-severe disease. **Role of enterococci remains debatable**. Probably pathogenic in infections of biliary tract. Probably need drugs active vs. enterococci in pts with valvular heart disease.
		Severe life-threatening disease, ICU patient: **IMP** 500 mg IV q6h **or MER** 1 gm IV q8h **or Dori** 500 mg q8h (1-hr infusion).	**AMP** + **metro** + (**CIP** 400 mg IV q12h or **Levo** 750 mg IV q24h) **OR** [**AMP** 2 gm IV q6h + **metro** 500 mg IV q6h + **aminoglycoside**[12] *(see Table 10D, page 101)*]	**Severe penicillin/cephalosporin allergy:** (**aztreonam** 2 gm IV q6h to q8h) + [**metro** (500 mg IV q6h) or (1 gm IV q12h)] **OR** [(**CIP** 400 mg IV q12h) or (**Levo** 750 mg IV q24h) + **metro**].
GENITAL TRACT: Mixture of empiric & specific treatment. Divided by sex of the patient. For sexual assault (rape), see ***Table 15A, page 176 & MMWR 59 (RR-12), 2010.*** **See Guidelines for Dx of Sexually Transmitted Diseases,** ***MMWR 59 (RR-12), 2010.***				
Both Women & Men: **Chancroid**	H. ducreyi	**Ceftriaxone** 250 mg IM single dose OR **azithro** 1 gm po single dose	**CIP** 500 mg bid po x 3 days OR **erythro base** 500 mg qid po x 7 days.	In HIV+ pts, failures reported with single dose azithro *(CID 21:409, 1995)*. Evaluate after 7 days, ulcer should objectively improve. Symptoms improve in 7 days. All patients treated for chancroid should be tested for HIV and syphilis.
Chlamydia, et al. non-gonococcal or post-gonococcal urethritis, cervicitis **NOTE: Assume concomitant N. gonorrhoeae** Chlamydia conjunctivitis, *see page 11*	Chlamydia 50%, Mycoplasma hominis. Other known etiologies (10–15%): trichomonas, herpes simplex virus, Mycoplasma genitalium. Ref: *JID 193:333, 336, 2006.*	(**Doxy** 100 mg bid po x 7 days) or (**azithro** 1 gm po as single dose). Evaluate & treat sex partner **In pregnancy: erythro base** 500 mg po qid x 7 days OR **amox** 500 mg po tid x 7 days.	(**Erythro base** 500 mg qid po x 7 days) or (**Oflox** 300 mg q12h po x 7 days) or (**Levo** 500 mg q24h x 7 days) **In pregnancy: azithro** 1 gm po x 1. **Doxy & FQs contraindicated**	**Diagnosis:** Nucleic acid amplification tests for C. trachomatis & N. gonorrhoeae on urine samples equivalent to cervix or urethra specimens *(AnIM 142:914, 2005)*. Test all urethritis/cervicitis pts for HIV & syphilis. For additional erythromycin regimens, *see MMWR (RR-11), 2006.* **Evaluate & treat sex partners.** Re-test for cure in pregnancy. Azithromycin 1 gm was superior to doxycycline for M. genitalium male urethritis *(CID 48:1649, 2009)*, but may select resistance leading to ↑ failure of multi-dose azithromycin retreatment regimens *(CID 48:1655, 2009)*.
Recurrent/persistent urethritis	**Occult trichomonas**, tetra-resistant U. urealyticum	**Metro** 2 gm po x 1	**Tinidazole** 2 gm po X 1 + **Azithromycin** 1 gm po X 1 (if not used for initial episode)	In men with NGU, 20% infected with trichomonas *(JID 188:465, 2003)*. *See above re M. genitalium.*

[12] **Aminoglycoside = antipseudomonal aminoglycosidic aminoglycoside, e.g., amikacin, gentamicin, tobramycin**

Abbreviations on page 2. *NOTE: All dosage recommendations are for adults (unless otherwise indicated) and assume normal renal function.*

TABLE 1A (18)

ANATOMIC SITE/DIAGNOSIS/ MODIFYING CIRCUMSTANCES	ETIOLOGIES (usual)	SUGGESTED REGIMENS*		ADJUNCT DIAGNOSTIC OR THERAPEUTIC MEASURES AND COMMENTS
		PRIMARY	ALTERNATIVE[§]	
GENITAL TRACT/Both Women & Men *(continued)*				
Gonorrhea *(MMWR 59 (RR-12): 49, 2010)*. **FQs no longer recommended for treatment of gonococcal infections *(MMWR 59 (RR-12):49, 2010)*.**				
Conjunctivitis (adult)	N. gonorrhoeae	**Ceftriaxone** 1 gm IM or IV single dose		Consider one-time saline lavage of eye.
Disseminated gonococcal infection (DGI, dermatitis-arthritis syndrome)	N. gonorrhoeae	(**Ceftriaxone** 1 gm IV q24h) or (**cefotaxime** 1 gm q8h IV) or (**ceftizoxime** 1 gm q8h IV)—*see Comment*	**Spectinomycin**[NUS] 2 gm IM q12h—*see Comment*.. FQs may be effective if susceptible organism.	Continue IM or IV regimen for 24hr after symptoms ↓; reliable pts may be discharged 24hr after sx resolve to complete 7 days rx with **cefixime[13] 400 mg po bid**. R/O meningitis/ endocarditis. **Treat presumptively for concomitant C. trachomatis**.
Endocarditis	N. gonorrhoeae	**Ceftriaxone** 1–2 gm IV q24h x 4 wk		Ref: *JID 157:1281, 1988*.
Pharyngitis	N. gonorrhoeae	**Ceftriaxone** 125 mg IM x 1	Due to resistance concerns, **do not use FQs**.	If chlamydia not ruled out: **Azithro** 1 gm po x 1 or **doxy** 100 mg po bid x 7 days. Some suggest test of cure culture after 1 wk. **Spectinomycin, cefixime, cefpodoxime & cefuroxime not effective**
Urethritis, cervicitis, proctitis (uncomplicated) For prostatitis, *see page 25*. **Diagnosis**: Nucleic acid amplification test (NAAT) on urine or urethral swab—*see AnIM 142:914, 2005*. ***NO FQs: MMWR 59 (RR-12):49, 2010.***	N. gonorrhoeae (50% of pts with urethritis, cervicitis have concomitant C. trachomatis —**treat for both unless NAAT indicates single pathogen**).	[(**Ceftriaxone** 125 mg IM x 1) or (**cefixime**[13] 400 mg po x 1) or (**cefpodoxime** 400 mg po x 1) **PLUS – if chlamydia infection not ruled out**: [(**Azithro** 2 gm po x 1) or (**doxy** 100 mg po q12h x 7 days] Severe pen/ceph allergy? Maybe **azithro**—see azithro comment. Understanding risk of FQ-resistance, could try FQ therapy with close follow-up.		Screen for syphilis. Other alternatives for **GC:** Spectinomycin[NUS] 2 gm IM x 1 Other single-dose cephalosporins: ceftizoxime 500 mg IM, cefotaxime 500 mg IM, cefoxitin 2 gm IM + probenecid 1 gm po. **Azithro** 1 gm po x 1 effective for chlamydia but need 2 gm po for GC; not recommended for GC due to GI side-effects, expense & rapid emergence of resistance.
Granuloma inguinale (Donovanosis)	Klebsiella (formerly Calymmatobacterium) granulomatis	**Doxy** 100 mg po bid x 3–4 wks	**TMP/SMX** one DS tablet bid x 3 wks **OR Erythro** 500 mg po qid x 3 wks OR **CIP** 750 mg po bid x 3 wks OR **azithro** 1 gm po q wk x 3 wks	Clinical response usually seen in 1 wk. **Rx until all lesions healed,** may take 4 wk. Treatment failures & recurrence seen with doxy & TMP-SMX. Report of efficacy with FQ and chloro. Ref.: *CID 25:24, 1997*. Relapse can occur 6-18 months after apparently effective Rx. If improvement not evidence in first few days, some experts add gentamicin 1 mg/kg IV q8h.
Herpes simplex virus	*See Table 14A, page 150*			
Human papilloma virus (HPV)	*See Table 14A, page 155*			
Lymphogranuloma venereum	Chlamydia trachomatis, serovars. L1, L2, L3	**Doxy** 100 mg po bid x 21 days	**Erythro** 0.5 gm po qid x 21 days or **Azithro** 1 gm po qwk X 3 weeks (clinical data lacking)	Dx based on serology; biopsy contraindicated because sinus tracts develop. Nucleic acid ampli tests for *C. trachomatis* will be positive. In MSM, presents as fever, rectal ulcer, anal discharge *(CID 39:996, 2004; Dis Colon Rectum 52:507, 2009)*.
Phthirus pubis **(pubic lice, "crabs")** & scabies	Phthirus pubis & Sarcoptes scabiei		*See Table 13, page 140*	

[13] Cefixime oral preparations now available as oral suspension, 200 mg/5 mL, and 400 mg tablets (Lupine Pharmaceuticals, (+1) 866-587-4617). *(MMWR 57:435, 2008)*.

TABLE 1A (19)

ANATOMIC SITE/DIAGNOSIS/ MODIFYING CIRCUMSTANCES	ETIOLOGIES (usual)	SUGGESTED REGIMENS*		ADJUNCT DIAGNOSTIC OR THERAPEUTIC MEASURES AND COMMENTS
		PRIMARY	ALTERNATIVE[§]	
GENITAL TRACT/Both Women & Men *(continued)*				
Syphilis *(JAMA 290:1510, 2003)*; **Syphilis & HIV:** *MMWR 59 (RR-12):26, 2010*				
Early: primary, secondary, or latent <1 yr	T. pallidum NOTE: Test all pts with syphilis for HIV; test all HIV patients for latent syphilis.	**Benzathine pen G (Bicillin L-A)** 2.4 million units IM x 1 or **Azithro** 2 gm po x 1 dose *(See Comment)*	(**Doxy** 100 mg po bid x 14 days) or (**tetracycline** 500 mg po qid x 14 days) or (**ceftriaxone** 1 gm IM/IV q24h x 8–10 days). Follow-up mandatory.	If early or congenital syphilis, **quantitative VDRL at 0**, 3, 6, 12 & 24 mo after rx. If 1° or 2° syphilis, VDRL should ↓ 2 tubes at 6 mo, 3 tubes 12 mo, & 4 tubes 24 mo. Update on congenital syphilis *(MMWR 59:413, 2010)*. Early latent: 2 tubes ↓ at 12 mo. With 1°, 50% will be RPR seronegative at 12 mo, 24% neg. FTA/ABS at 2–3 yrs *(AnIM 114:1005, 1991)*. If titers fail to fall, examine CSF; if CSF (+), treat as neurosyphilis; if CSF is negative, retreat with benzathine Pen G 2.4 m.u. IM weekly x 3 wks. **Azithro** 2 gm po x 1 dose (equivalent to **benzathine Pen** 2.4 M x 1 dose in early syphilis *(J Infect Dis 201:1729, 2010)*. **Azithro-resistant syphilis** documented in California, Ireland, & elsewhere *(CID 44:S130, 2007; AAC 54:583, 2010)*. NOTE: Use of **benzathine procaine penicillin** is inappropriate!!
More than 1 yr's duration (latent of indeterminate duration, cardiovascular, late benign gumma)	For penicillin desensitization method, *see Table 7, page 77* and *MMWR 59 (RR-12): 26, 2010.*	**Benzathine pen G (Bicillin L-A)** 2.4 million units IM q week x 3 = 7.2 million units total	**Doxy** 100 mg po bid x 28 days or **tetracycline** 500 mg po qid x 28 days; **Ceftriazone** 1 gm IV or IM daily for 10-14 days MAY be an alternative (No clinical data; consult an ID specialist)	No published data on efficacy of alternatives. **Indications for LP (CDC): neurologic symptoms, treatment failure, any eye or ear involvement, other evidence of active syphilis (aortitis, gumma, iritis).**
Neurosyphilis—Very difficult to treat. Includes ocular (retrobulbar neuritis) syphilis **All need CSF exam.**		**Pen G** 18-24 million units per day either as continuous infusion or as 3–4 million units IV q4h x 10–14 days.	(**Procaine pen G** 2.4 million units IM q24h + **probenecid** 0.5 gm po qid) both x 10–14 days—*See Comment*	**Ceftriaxone** 2 gm (IV or IM) q24h x 14 days. 23% failure rate reported *(AJM 93:481, 1992)*. For penicillin allergy: either desensitize to penicillin or obtain infectious diseases consultation. **Serologic criteria for response to rx: 4-fold or greater ↓ in VDRL titer over 6–12 mo.** *[CID 28 (Suppl. 1):S21, 1999]*.
HIV infection (AIDS) *CID 44:S130, 2007.*		Treatment same as HIV uninfected with closer follow-up. Treat early neurosyphilis for 10-14 days regardless of CD4 count: *MMWR 56:625, 2007.*		*See Syphilis discussion in MMWR 59 (RR-12), 2010.*
Pregnancy and syphilis		Same as for non-pregnant, some recommend 2nd dose (2.4 million units) **benzathine pen G** 1 wk after initial dose esp. in 3rd trimester or with 2° syphilis	Skin test for penicillin allergy. Desensitize if necessary, as parenteral pen G is only therapy with documented efficacy!	Monthly quantitative VDRL or equivalent. If 4-fold ↑, re-treat. Doxy, tetracycline contraindicated. Erythro not recommended because of high risk of failure to cure fetus.
Congenital syphilis *(Update on Congenital Syphilis: MMWR 59 (RR-12): 36, 2010)*	T. pallidum	**Aqueous crystalline pen G** 50,000 units/kg per dose IV q12h x 7 days, then q8h for 10 day total.	**Procaine pen G** 50,000 units/kg IM q24h for 10 days	Another alternative: Ceftriaxone ≤30 days old, 75 mg/kg IV/IM q24h (use with caution in infants with jaundice) or >30 days old 100 mg/kg IV/IM q24h. Treat 10–14 days. If symptomatic, ophthalmologic exam indicated. If more than 1 day of rx missed, restart entire course. **Need serologic follow-up!**
Warts, anogenital	*See Table 14, page 155*			

 NOTE: All dosage recommendations are for adults (unless otherwise indicated) and assume normal renal function.

TABLE 1A (20)

ANATOMIC SITE/DIAGNOSIS/ MODIFYING CIRCUMSTANCES	ETIOLOGIES (usual)	SUGGESTED REGIMENS*		ADJUNCT DIAGNOSTIC OR THERAPEUTIC MEASURES AND COMMENTS
		PRIMARY	ALTERNATIVE[§]	
GENITAL TRACT *(continued)*				
Women:				
Amnionitis, septic abortion	Bacteroides, esp. Prevotella bivius; Group B, A strepto-cocci; Enterobacteriaceae; C. trachomatis	[(**Cefoxitin** or **TC-CL** or **Dori**[NAI] or **IMP** or **MER** or **AM-SB** or **ERTA** or **PIP-TZ**) + **doxy**] **OR** [**Clinda** + (**aminoglycoside** or **ceftriaxone**)] *Dosage: see footnote[14]*		D&C of uterus. **In septic abortion**, Clostridium perfringens may cause fulminant intravascular hemolysis. **In postpartum patients** with enigmatic fever and/or pulmonary emboli, **consider septic pelvic vein thrombophlebitis** *(see Vascular, septic pelvic vein thrombophlebitis, page 62)*. After discharge: doxy or continue clinda. **NOTE:** IV clinda effective for C. trachomatis; no data on po clinda.
Cervicitis, mucopurulent Treatment based on results of nucleic acid amplification test	N. gonorrhoeae	Treat for Gonorrhea, *page 21*		Criteria for diagnosis: 1) (muco)purulent endocervical exudate and/or 2) sustained endocervical bleeding after passage of cotton swab. >10 WBC/hpf of vaginal fluid is suggestive. Intracellular gram-neg diplococci is specific but insensitive. If in doubt, send swab or urine for culture, EIA or nucleic acid amplification test and treat for both.
	Chlamydia trachomatis	Treat for non-gonococcal urethritis, *page 20*		
Endomyometritis/septic pelvic phlebitis				
Early postpartum (1st 48 hrs) (usually after C-section)	Bacteroides, esp. Prevotella bivius; Group B, A strepto-cocci; Enterobacteriaceae; C. trachomatis	[(**Cefoxitin** or **TC-CL** or **ERTA** or **IMP** or **MER** or **AM-SB** or **PIP-TZ**) + **doxy**] OR [**Clinda** + (**aminoglycoside** or **ceftriaxone**)] *Dosage: see footnote[14]*		*See Comments under Amnionitis, septic abortion, above*
Late postpartum (48 hrs to 6 wks) (usually after vaginal delivery)	Chlamydia trachomatis, M. hominis	**Doxy** 100 mg IV or po q12h times 14 days		Tetracyclines not recommended in nursing mothers; discontinue nursing. M. hominis sensitive to tetra, clinda, not erythro.
Fitzhugh-Curtis syndrome	C. trachomatis, N. gonorrhoeae	Treat as for pelvic inflammatory disease immediately below.		Perihepatitis (violin-string adhesions)
Pelvic actinomycosis; usually tubo-ovarian abscess	A. Israelii most common	**AMP** 50 mg/kg/day IV div 3-4 doses x 4-6 wks, then **Pen VK** 2-4 gm/day po x 3-6 mos.	**Doxy** or **ceftriaxone** or **clinda** or **erythro**	Complication of intrauterine device (IUD). Remove IUD. Can use **Pen G** 10-20 million units/day IV instead of **AMP** x 4-6 wks.
Pelvic Inflammatory Disease (PID), salpingitis, tubo-ovarian abscess				
Outpatient rx: limit to pts with temp <38°C, WBC <11,000 per mm³, minimal evidence of peritonitis, active bowel sounds & able to tolerate oral nourishment *CID 44:953 & 961, 2007; MMWR 59 (RR-12):63, 2010 & www.cdc.gov/std/treatment*	N. gonorrhoeae, chlamydia, bacteroides, Enterobacteria-ceae, streptococci, especially S. agalactiae Less commonly: G. vaginalis, Haemophilus influenzae, cytomegalovirus (CMV), M. hominis, U. urealyticum, and M. genitalium	**Outpatient rx:** [(**ceftriaxone** 250 mg IM or IV x 1) (± **metro** 500 mg po bid x 14 days) + (**doxy** 100 mg po bid x 14 days)]. **OR** (**cefoxitin** 2 gm IM with **probenecid** 1 gm po both as single dose) plus (**doxy** 100 mg po bid with **metro** 500 mg bid—both times 14 days)	**Inpatient regimens:** [(**Cefotetan** 2 gm IV q12h or **cefoxitin** 2 gm IV q6h) + (**doxy** 100 mg IV/po q12h)] (**Clinda** 900 mg IV q8h) + (**gentamicin** 2 mg/kg loading dose, then 1.5 mg/kg q8h or 4.5 mg/kg once per day), then **doxy** 100 mg po bid x 14 days	Another alternative parenteral regimen: **AM-SB** 3 gm IV q6h + **doxy** 100 mg IV/po q12h Remember: Evaluate and treat sex partner. FQs not recommended due to increasing resistance *(MMWR 59 (RR-12), 2010 & www.cdc.gov/std/treatment)*. Suggest initial inpatient evaluation/therapy for pts with tubo-ovarian abscess. For inpatient regimens, continue treatment until satisfactory response for ≥ 24-hr before switching to outpatient regimen.

[14] **P Ceph 2** (**cefoxitin** 2 gm IV q6–8h, **cefotetan** 2 gm IV q12h, **cefuroxime** 750 mg IV q8h); **TC-CL** 3.1 gm IV q4–6h; **AM-SB** 3 gm IV q6h; **PIP-TZ** 3.375 gm q6h or for nosocomial pneumonia: 4.5 gm IV q6h or 4-hr infusion of 3.375 gm q8h; **doxy** 100 mg IV/po q12h; **clinda** 450–900 mg IV q8h; **aminoglycoside** (**gentamicin**, *see Table 10D, page 101*); **P Ceph 3** (**cefotaxime** 2 gm IV q8h, **ceftriaxone** 2 gm IV q24h); **doripenem** 500 mg IV q8h (1-hr infusion); **ertapenem** 1 gm IV q24h; **IMP** 0.5 gm IV q6h; **MER** 1 gm IV q8h; **azithro** 500 mg IV q24h; **linezolid** 600 mg IV/po q12h; **vanco** 1 gm IV q12h

TABLE 1A (21)

ANATOMIC SITE/DIAGNOSIS/ MODIFYING CIRCUMSTANCES	ETIOLOGIES (usual)	SUGGESTED REGIMENS*		ADJUNCT DIAGNOSTIC OR THERAPEUTIC MEASURES AND COMMENTS
		PRIMARY	ALTERNATIVE[§]	
GENITAL TRACT/Women *(continued)*				
Vaginitis—*MMWR 59 (RR-12):63, 2010 or CID 35 (Suppl.2):S135, 2002*				
Candidiasis Pruritus, thick cheesy discharge, pH <4.5 *See Table 11A, page 106*	Candida albicans 80–90%. C. glabrata, C. tropicalis may be increasing—they are less susceptible to azoles	**Oral azoles: Fluconazole** 150 mg po x 1; **itraconazole** 200 mg po bid x 1 day	**Intravaginal azoles:** variety of strengths—from 1 dose to 7–14 days. Drugs available (all end in -azole): butocon, clotrim, micon, tiocon, tercon *(doses: Table 11A)*	Nystatin vag. tabs times 14 days less effective. Other rx for azole-resistant strains: gentian violet, boric acid. If recurrent candidiasis (4 or more episodes per yr): 6 mos. suppression with: fluconazole 150 mg po q week or itraconazole 100 mg po q24h or clotrimazole vag. suppositories 500 mg q week.
Trichomoniasis Copious foamy discharge, pH >4.5 Treat sexual partners—*see Comment*	Trichomonas vaginalis	**Metro** 2 gm as single dose or 500 mg po bid x 7 days OR **Tinidazole** 2 gm po single dose **Pregnancy**: *See Comment*	**For rx failure:** Re-treat with metro 500 mg po bid x 7 days; if 2nd failure: metro 2 gm po q24h x 3–5 days. If still failure, suggest ID consultation and/or contact CDC: 770-488-4115 or www.cdc.gov/std.	**Treat male sexual partners (2 gm metronidazole as single dose).** Nearly 20% men with NGU are infected with trichomonas *(JID 188:465, 2003)*. For alternative option in refractory cases, *see CID 33:1341, 2001.* **Pregnancy:** No data indicating metro teratogenic or mutagenic *[MMWR 51(RR-6), 2002]*. For discussion of treating trichomonas, including issues in pregnancy, *see MMWR 59 (RR-12), 2010; CID 44:S123, 2007*
Bacterial vaginosis Malodorous vaginal discharge, pH >4.5 Data on recurrence & review: *JID 193:1475,2006*	Etiology unclear: associated with Gardnerella vaginalis, mobiluncus, , Mycoplasma hominis, Prevotella sp., & Atopobium vaginae et al.	**Metro** 0.5 gm po bid x 7 days or **metro vaginal gel**[15] (1 applicator intra-vaginally) 1x/day x 5 days OR **Tinidazole** (2 gm po once daily x 2 days or 1 gm po once daily x 5 days)	**Clinda** 0.3 gm bid po x 7 days or 2% **clinda vaginal cream** 5 gm intravaginally at bedtime x 7 days or **clinda ovules** 100 mg intravag-inally at bedtime x 3 days.	Reported 50% ↑ in cure rate if abstain from sex or use condoms: *CID 44:213 & 220, 2007.* Treatment of male sex partner **not** indicated unless balanitis present. Metro extended release tabs 750 mg po q24h x 7 days available; no published data. **Pregnancy:** Oral **metro** or oral **clinda** 7-day regimens *(see Canadian OBGYN practice guidelines in JObstetGynCan 30:702, 2008)* Atopobium resistant to metro in vitro; susceptible to clinda *(BMC Inf Dis 6:51, 2006);* importance unclear.
Men:				
Balanitis	Candida 40%, Group B strep, gardnerella	**Metro** 2 gm po as a single dose OR **Fluc** 150 mg po x1 OR **itra** 200 mg po bid x 1 day.		Occurs in 1/4 of male sex partners of women infected with candida. Exclude circinate balanitis (Reiter's syndrome). Plasma cell balanitis (non-infectious) responds to hydrocortisone cream.
Epididymo-orchitis *Reviews in Brit J Urol Int 87:747, 2001; Andrologia 40:76, 2008.*				
Age <35 years	N. gonorrhoeae, Chlamydia trachomatis	**Ceftriaxone** 250 mg IM x 1 + **doxy** 100 mg po bid x 10 days		Also: bed rest, scrotal elevation, and analgesics. Enterobacteriaceae occasionally encountered. All patients treated for epididymo-orchitis < 35 yrs of age should be tested for HIV and syphilis.
Age >35 years or homosexual men (insertive partners in anal intercourse)	Enterobacteriaceae (coli-forms)	[**Levo** 500-750 mg IV/po once daily] OR [(**cipro** 500 mg po bid) or (400 mg IV twice daily)] for 10-14 days.	**AM-SB**, **P Ceph 3**, **TC-CL**, **PIP-TZ** *(Dosage: see footnote page 23)*	Midstream pyuria and scrotal pain and edema. Also: bed rest, scrotal elevation, and analgesics. NOTE: Do urine NAAT (nucleic acid amplification test) to ensure absence of N. gonorrhoeae with concomitant risk of FQ-resistant gonorrhoeae or of chlamydia if using agents without reliable activity. Other causes include: mumps, brucella, TB, intravesicular BCG, B. pseudomallei, coccidioides, Behcet's *(see Brit J Urol Int 87:747, 2001)*.
Non-gonococcal urethritis	*See Chlamydia et al, Non-gonococcal urethritis, Table 1A(17), page 20*			

[15] 1 applicator contains 5 gm of gel with 37.5 mg metronidazole

Abbreviations on page 2. *NOTE: All dosage recommendations are for adults (unless otherwise indicated) and assume normal renal function.*

TABLE 1A (22)

ANATOMIC SITE/DIAGNOSIS/ MODIFYING CIRCUMSTANCES	ETIOLOGIES (usual)	SUGGESTED REGIMENS*		ADJUNCT DIAGNOSTIC OR THERAPEUTIC MEASURES AND COMMENTS
		PRIMARY	ALTERNATIVE[§]	
GENITAL TRACT/Men *(continued)*				
Prostatitis—Review: *CID 50:1641, 2010.*				
Acute Uncomplicated (with risk of STD; age < 35 yrs)	N. gonorrhoeae, C. trachomatis	(**ceftriaxone** 250 mg IM x 1 OR **cefixime** 400 mg po X 1) then **doxy** 100 mg bid x 10 days.		FQs no longer recommended for gonococcal infections. Test for HIV. In AIDS pts, prostate may be focus of Cryptococcus neoformans.
Uncomplicated with low risk of STD	Enterobacteriaceae (coliforms)	**FQ** *(dosage: see Epididymo-orchitis, >35 yrs, above)* or **TMP-SMX** 1 DS tablet (160 mg TMP) po bid x 10–14 days (minimum). Some authorities recommend 4 weeks of therapy.		Treat as acute urinary infection, 14 days (not single dose regimen). Some authorities recommend 3–4 wk therapy. If uncertain, do urine test for C. trachomatis and of N. gonorrhoeae. If resistant enterobacteriaceae, use ERTA 1 gm IV qd. If resistant pseudomonas, use IMP or MER (500 mg IV q6 or q8 respectively)
Chronic bacterial	Enterobacteriaceae 80%, enterococci 15%, P. aeruginosa	**FQ** (**CIP** 500 mg po bid x 4-6 wks **Levo** 750 mg po q24h x 4 wk—*see Comment*)	**TMP-SMX-DS** 1 tab po bid x 1-3 mo	With treatment failures consider infected prostatic calculi. FDA approved dose of levo is 500 mg; editors prefer higher dose.
Chronic prostatitis/chronic pain syndrome (New NIH classification, *JAMA 282:236, 1999*)	The most common prostatitis syndrome. Etiology is unknown, molecular probe data suggest infectious etiology *(Clin Micro Rev 11: 604, 1998)*.	**α-adrenergic blocking agents are controversial** *(AnIM 133:367, 2000)*.		Pt has sx of prostatitis but negative cultures and no cells in prostatic secretions Rev.: *JAC 46:157, 2000.* In randomized double-blind study, CIP and an alpha-blocker of no benefit *(AnIM 141:581 & 639, 2004)*.
HAND *(Bites: See Skin)*				
Paronychia				
Nail biting, manicuring	Staph. aureus (maybe MRSA)	Incision & drainage; do culture	**TMP-SMX-DS** 1-2 tabs po bid while waiting for culture result.	*See Table 6 for alternatives.* Occasionally--candida, gram-negative rods.
Contact with oral mucosa—dentists, anesthesiologists, wrestlers	Herpes simplex (Whitlow)	**Acyclovir** 400 mg tid po x 10 days	**Famciclovir** or **valacyclovir** should work, *see Comment*	Gram stain and routine culture negative. Famciclovir/valacyclovir doses used for primary genital herpes should work; *see Table 14, page 150*
Dishwasher (prolonged water immersion)	Candida sp.	**Clotrimazole** (topical)		Avoid immersion of hands in water as much as possible.
HEART				
Infective endocarditis—Native valve—empirical rx awaiting cultures—No IV illicit drugs	**NOTE: Diagnostic criteria** include evidence of continuous bacteremia (multiple positive blood cultures), new murmur (worsening of old murmur) of valvular insufficiency, definite emboli, and echocardiographic (transthoracic or transesophageal) evidence of valvular vegetations. Refs.: *Circulation 111:3167, 2005; Ln 363:139, 2004.* For antimicrobial prophylaxis, *see Table 15C, page 181.*			
Valvular or congenital heart disease but no modifying circumstances *See Table 15C, page 181 for prophylaxis*	Viridans strep 30–40%, "other" strep 15–25%, enterococci 5–18%, staphylococci 20-35% (including coag-neg staphylococci--*CID 46:232, 2008*).	[(**Pen G** 20 million units IV q24h, continuous or div. q4h) or (**AMP** 12 gm IV q24h, continuous or div. q4h) + (**nafcillin** or **oxacillin** 2 gm IV q4h) + **gentamicin** 1 mg/kg IM or IV q8h *(see Comment)*]	(**Vanco** 15 mg/kg[16] IV q12h (not to exceed 2 gm q24h unless serum levels monitored) + **gentamicin** 1 mg/kg[16] IM or IV q8h) **OR dapto** 6 mg/kg IV q24h	If patient not acutely ill and not in heart failure, we prefer to wait for blood culture results. If initial 3 blood cultures neg. after 24–48 hrs, obtain 2–3 more blood cultures before empiric therapy started. **Nafcillin/oxacillin + gentamicin** may not cover enterococci, hence addition of penicillin G pending cultures. When blood cultures +, modify regimen to specific therapy for organism. **Gentamicin** used for synergy; peak levels need not exceed 4 mcg per mL. **Surgery indications:** heart failure, paravalvular infection, resistant organism *(JACC 48:e1, 2006)*; in selected pts, emboli, esp if after one week of therapy *(AHJ 154:1086, 2007)* and large mobile vegetation.

[16] Assumes estimated creatinine clearance ≥80 mL per min., *see Table 17.*

TABLE 1A (23)

ANATOMIC SITE/DIAGNOSIS/ MODIFYING CIRCUMSTANCES	ETIOLOGIES (usual)	SUGGESTED REGIMENS*		ADJUNCT DIAGNOSTIC OR THERAPEUTIC MEASURES AND COMMENTS
		PRIMARY	ALTERNATIVE[§]	
HEART *(continued)*				
Infective endocarditis—Native valve—IV illicit drug use ± evidence rt-sided endocarditis —empiric therapy	S. aureus*(MSSA & MRSA)*. All others rare	**Vanco** 30-60 mg/kg per day in 2-3 divided doses to achieve target trough concentrations of 15-20 mcg/mL recommended for serious infections.	**Dapto** 6 mg/kg IV q24h Approved for right-sided endocarditis.	**Quinupristin-dalfopristin** cidal vs. S. aureus if both constituents active. In controlled clinical trial, **dapto** equivalent to vanco plus 4 days of gentamicin for right-sided endocarditis *(NEJM 355:653, 2006)*.
Infective endocarditis—Native valve—culture positive *(NEJM 345:1318, 2001; CID 36:615, 2003; JAC 54:971, 2004*[17]*)*				
Viridans strep, S. bovis *(S. gallolyticus)* with **penicillin G MIC ≤0.1 mcg/mL** **NOTE:** New name for *S. bovis, biotype 1* is *S. gallolyticus subsp. gallolyticus (JCM 46:2966, 2008)*.	**Viridans strep, S. bovis**	[(**Pen G** 12–18 million units/day IV, divided q4h **x 2 wk**) PLUS (**gentamicin** IV 1 mg/kg q8h IV **x 2 wks**)] **OR** (**Pen G** 12–18 million units/day IV, divided - q4h **x 4 wk**) **OR** (**ceftriaxone** 2 gm IV q24h **x 4 wk**)	(**Ceftriaxone** 2 gm IV q24h + **gentamicin** 1 mg per kg IV q8h both **x 2 wks**). If allergy pen G or ceftriax, use **vanco** 15 mg/kg IV q12h to 2 gm/day max unless serum levels measured **x 4 wks**	Target **gent levels:** peak 3 mcg/mL, trough <1 mcg/mL. If very obese pt, recommend consultation for dosage adjustment. Infuse vanco over ≥1 hr to avoid "red man" syndrome. **S. bovis suggests occult bowel pathology (new name: S. gallolyticus).** Since relapse rate may be greater in pts ill for >3 mos. prior to start of rx, the penicillin-gentamicin synergism theoretically may be advantageous in this group. **NOTE: Dropped option of continuous infusion of Pen G due to instability of penicillin in acidic IV fluids, rapid renal clearance and rising MICs *(JAC 53:675, 2004)*.**
Viridans strep, S. bovis (S. gallolyticus) with **penicillin G MIC >0.1 to <0.5 mcg/mL**	**Viridans strep, S. bovis, nutritionally variant streptococci, (e.g. S. abiotrophia) tolerant strep**[18]	**Pen G** 18 million units/day IV (divided q4h) **x 4 wks PLUS gentamicin** 1 mg/kg IV q8h **x 2 wks** **NOTE: Low dose of gentamicin**	**Vanco** 15 mg/kg IV q12h to max. 2 gm/day unless serum levels documented **x 4 wks**	Can use cefazolin for pen G in pt with allergy that is not IgE-mediated (e.g., anaphylaxis). Alternatively, can use vanco. *(See Comment above on gent and vanco)* **NOTE: If necessary to remove infected valve & valve culture neg., 2 weeks antibiotic treatment post-op sufficient *(CID 41:187, 2005)*.**
For viridans strep or S. bovis with **pen G MIC ≥0.5** and enterococci susceptible to AMP/pen G, vanco, gentamicin **NOTE:** Inf. Dis. consultation suggested	**"Susceptible" enterococci, viridans strep, S. bovis, nutritionally variant streptococci** (new names are: Abiotrophia sp. & Granulicatella sp.)	[(**Pen G** 18–30 million units per 24h IV, divided q4h **x 4–6 wks**) **PLUS** (**gentamicin** 1–1.5 mg/kg q8h IV **x 4–6 wks**)] **OR** (**AMP** 12 gm/day IV, divided q4h + **gent** as above **x 4–6 wks**)	**Vanco** 15 mg/kg IV q12h to max of 2 gm/day unless serum levels measured **PLUS gentamicin** 1–1.5 mg/kg q8h IV **x 4–6 wks** **NOTE: Low dose of gent**	**4 wks of rx if symptoms <3 mos.; 6 wks of rx if symptoms >3 mos.** Vanco for pen-allergic pts; do not use cephalosporins. Do **not** give gent once-q24h for enterococcal endocarditis. Target gent levels: peak 3 mcg/mL, trough <1 mcg/mL. Vanco target serum levels: peak 20–50 mcg/mL, trough 5–12 mcg/mL. **NOTE:** Because of ↑ frequency of resistance *(see below)*, all enterococci causing endocarditis should be tested in vitro for susceptibility to penicillin, gentamicin and vancomycin plus β lactamase production.
Enterococci: MIC streptomycin >2000 mcg/mL; MIC gentamicin >500-2000 mcg/mL; no resistance to penicillin	**Enterococci, high-level aminoglycoside resistance**	**Pen G** or **AMP** IV as above **x 8–12 wks** (approx. 50% cure)	If prolonged pen G or AMP fails, consider surgical removal of infected valve. *See Comment*	10–25% E. faecalis and 45–50% E. faecium resistant to high gent levels. May be sensitive to streptomycin, check MIC. Case report of success with combination of AMP, IMP, and vanco *(Scand J Inf Dis 29:628, 1997)*. **Cure rate of 67% with IV AMP 2 gm q4h plus ceftriaxone 2 gm q12h x 6 wks *(AnIM 146:574, 2007)*.** Theory is sequential blocking of PBPs 4&5 (Amp) and 2&3 (ceftriaxone).
Enterococci: pen G MIC >16 mcg/mL; no gentamicin resistance	**Enterococci, intrinsic pen G/AMP resistance**	**Vanco** 15 mg/kg IV q12h (check levels if >2 gm) **PLUS gent** 1–1.5 mg/kg q8h **x 4–6 wks** *(see Comment)*		Desired vanco serum levels: trough 5–12 mcg/mL. **Gentamicin** used for synergy; peak levels need not exceed 4 mcg/mL.

[17] Ref. for Guidelines of British Soc. for Antimicrob. Chemother. Includes drugs not available in U.S.: flucloxacillin IV, teicoplanin IV: *JAC 54:971, 2004*.
[18] Tolerant streptococci = MBC 32-fold greater than MIC

TABLE 1A (24)

ANATOMIC SITE/DIAGNOSIS/ MODIFYING CIRCUMSTANCES	ETIOLOGIES (usual)	SUGGESTED REGIMENS*		ADJUNCT DIAGNOSTIC OR THERAPEUTIC MEASURES AND COMMENTS
		PRIMARY	ALTERNATIVE[§]	
HEART/Infective endocarditis—Native valve—culture positive *(continued)*				
Enterococci: Pen/AMP resistant + high-level gent/strep resistant + vanco resistant; usually VRE **Consultation suggested**	**Enterococci, vanco-resistant, usually E. faecium**	No reliable effective rx. Can try **quinupristin-dalfopristin** (Synercid) or **linezolid**—*see Comment and Table 5*	**Teicoplanin** active against a subset of vanco-resistant enterococci. Teicoplanin is not available in U.S. **Dapto** is an option.	**Synercid** activity limited to E. faecium and is usually bacteriostatic, therefore expect high relapse rate. Dose: 7.5 mg per kg IV (via central line) q8h. **Linezolid** active most enterococci, but bacteriostatic. Dose: 600 mg IV or po q12h. Linezolid failed in pt with E. faecalis endocarditis *(CID 37:e29, 2003)*. **Dapto** is bactericidal in vitro; clinical experience in *CID 41:1134, 2005.*
Staphylococcal endocarditis Aortic &/or mitral valve infection—MSSA Surgery indications: *see Comment page 25.*	**Staph. aureus, methicillin-sensitive** **Note: Low dose of gentamicin for only 3-5 days**	**Nafcillin (oxacillin)** 2 gm IV q4h **x 4–6 wks PLUS gentamicin** 1 mg/kg IV q8h **x 3–5 days**	[(**Cefazolin** 2 gm IV q8h **x 4–6 wk**) **PLUS (gentamicin** 1 mg/kg IV q8h **x 3–5 days**). **Low dose of gent] OR Vanco** 15 mg/kg IV q12h (check levels if >2 gm per day) **x 4–6 wks**	If IgE-mediated penicillin allergy, 10% cross-reactivity to cephalosporins *(AnIM 141:16, 2004)*. **Cefazolin** failures reported *(CID 37:1194, 2003)*. American Heart Association guidelines list addition of low dose **gentamicin** as optional *(http://circ.ahajournals.org/cgi/content/full/111/23/e394)*. The benefit of low dose gentamicin in improving outcome is unproven and even low-dose gentamicin for only a few days is nephrotoxic *(CID 48:713, 2009)*; if used at all it should be administered **for no more than 3-5 days**.
Aortic and/or mitral valve—MRSA	**Staph. aureus, methicillin-resistant**	**Vanco** 30-60 mg/kg per day in 2-3 divided doses to achieve target trough concentrations of 15-20 mcg/mL recommended for serious infections.	**Dapto** not FDA-approved for left-sided endocarditis	In clinical trial *(NEJM 355:653, 2006)*, high failure rate with both vanco and dapto in small numbers of pts. For other alternatives, *see Table 6, pg 75.*
Tricuspid valve infection (usually IVDUs): MSSA	**Staph. aureus, methicillin-sensitive**	**Nafcillin (oxacillin)** 2 gm IV q4h **PLUS gentamicin** 1 mg/kg IV q8h **x 2 wks. NOTE: low dose of gent**	**If penicillin allergy: Vanco** 15 mg/kg IV q12h + low-dose **gent** 1 mg/kg IV q8h x 2 wks **OR Dapto** 6 mg/kg IV q24h (avoid if concomitant left-sided endocarditis). 8-12 mg/kg IV q24h used in some cases, but not FDA approved.	**2-week regimen not long enough if metastatic infection (e.g., osteo) or left-sided endocarditis.** **Daptomycin**: Approved for bacteremia and in **right-sided** endocarditis based on randomized study *(NEJM 355:653 & 727, 2006)*.
Tricuspid valve--MRSA	**Staph. aureus, methicillin-resistant**	**Vanco** 30-60 mg/kg per day in 2-3 divided doses to achieve target trough concentrations of 15-20 mcg/mL recommended for serious infections **x 4-6 wks**	**Dapto** 6 mg/kg IV q24h x 4-6 wk equiv to **vanco** for rt-sided endocarditis; both vanco & dapto did poorly if lt-sided endocarditis *(NEJM 355: 653, 2006). (See Comments & table 6, page 75)*	**Quinupristin-dalfopristin** another option. **Linezolid:** Limited experience *(see JAC 58:273, 2006)* in patients with few treatment options; 64% cure rate; clear failure in 21%; thrombocytopenia in 31%. **Dapto** dose of 8-12 mg/kg may help in selected cases, but not FDA-approved
Slow-growing fastidious Gm-neg. bacilli--any valve	**HACEK group** *(see Comments)*. Change to HACEK if add Bartonella.	**Ceftriaxone** 2 gm IV q24h **x 4 wks** (Bartonella resistant – *see below*).	**AMP** 12 gm q24h (continuous or div. q4h) **x 4 wks** + **gentamicin** 1 mg/kg IV/IM q8h **x 4 wks.**	**HACEK (acronym for Haemophilus parainfluenzae, H. (aphrophilus) aggregatibacter, Actinobacillus, Cardiobacterium, Eikenella, Kingella)**. H. aphrophilus resistant to vanco, clinda and methicillin. Penicillinase-positive HACEK organisms should be susceptible to AM-SB + gentamicin.
Bartonella species--any valve	B. henselae, B. quintana	[**Ceftriaxone** 2 gm IV q24h x 6 wks + **gentamicin** 1 mg/kg q8h x 14 days] + **doxy** 100 mg IV/po bid x 6 wks.		**Dx:** Immunofluorescent antibody titer ≥1:800; blood cultures only occ. positive, or PCR of tissue from surgery. **Surgery:** Over ½ pts require valve surgery; relation to cure unclear. B. quintana transmitted by body lice among homeless.

 NOTE: All dosage recommendations are for adults (unless otherwise indicated) and assume normal renal function.

TABLE 1A (25)

ANATOMIC SITE/DIAGNOSIS/ MODIFYING CIRCUMSTANCES	ETIOLOGIES (usual)	SUGGESTED REGIMENS*		ADJUNCT DIAGNOSTIC OR THERAPEUTIC MEASURES AND COMMENTS
		PRIMARY	ALTERNATIVE[§]	
HEART *(continued)*				
Infective endocarditis— "culture negative" Fever, valvular disease, and ECHO vegetations ± emboli and neg. cultures. Rev.: *Medicine 84:162, 2005*		Etiology in 348 cases studied by serology, culture, histopath, & molecular detection: C. burnetii 48%, Bartonella sp. 28%, and rarely (Abiotrophia elegans (nutritionally variant strep), Mycoplasma hominis, Legionella pneumophila, Tropheryma whipplei—together 1%), & rest without etiology identified (most on antibiotic). Ref.: *NEJM 356:715, 2007.*		
Infective endocarditis—Prosthetic valve—empiric therapy (cultures pending) S. aureus now most common etiology *(JAMA 297:1354, 2007).*				
Early (<2 mo post-op)	S. epidermidis, S. aureus. Rarely, Enterobacteriaceae, diphtheroids, fungi	**Vanco** 15 mg/kg IV q12h + **gentamicin** 1 mg/kg IV q8h + **RIF** 600 mg po q24h		Early surgical consultation advised especially if etiology is S. aureus, evidence of heart failure, presence of diabetes and/or renal failure, or concern for valve ring abscess *(JAMA 297:1354, 2007; CID 44:364, 2007).*
Late (>2 mo post-op)	S. epidermidis, viridans strep, enterococci, S. aureus			
Infective endocarditis— Prosthetic valve—positive blood cultures **Surgical consultation advised:** Indications for surgery: severe heart failure, S. aureus infection, prosthetic dehiscence, resistant organism, emboli due to large vegetation *(JACC 48:e1, 2006).*	Staph. epidermidis	(**Vanco** 15 mg /kg IV q12h + **RIF** 300 mg po q8h) **x 6 wks** + **gentamicin** 1 mg/kg IV q8h **x 14 days**.		If S. epidermidis is susceptible to nafcillin/oxacillin in vitro (not common), then substitute nafcillin (or oxacillin) for vanco.
	Staph. aureus	Methicillin sensitive: (**Nafcillin** 2 gm IV q4h + **RIF** 300 mg po q8h) **times 6 wks** + **gentamicin** 1 mg per kg IV q8h **times 14 days.** Methicillin resistant: (**Vanco** 1 gm IV q12h + **RIF** 300 mg po q8h) **times 6 wks** + **gentamicin** 1 mg per kg IV q8h **times 14 days.**		
	Viridans strep, enterococci	*See infective endocarditis, native valve, culture positive, page 26*		
	Enterobacteriaceae or P. aeruginosa	**Aminoglycoside** (**tobra** if P. aeruginosa) + (**AP Pen** or **P Ceph 3 AP** or **P Ceph 4**)		In theory, could substitute CIP for APAG, but no clinical data.
	Candida, aspergillus	*Table 11, page 104*		High mortality. Valve replacement plus antifungal therapy standard therapy but some success with antifungal therapy alone.
Infective endocarditis—Q fever *LnID 10:527, 2010; NEJM 356:715, 2007.*	Coxiella burnetii	**Doxy** 100 mg po bid + **hydroxychloroquine** 600 mg/day for at least 18 mo *(Mayo Clin Proc 83:574, 2008).* *Pregnancy: Need long term* **TMP-SMX** *(see CID 45:548, 2007).*		**Dx:** Phase I IgG titer >800 plus clinical evidence of endocarditis. Treatment duration: 18 mos for native valve, 24 mos for prosthetic valve. Monitor serologically for 5 yrs.
Pacemaker/defibrillator infections	S. aureus (40%), S. epidermidis (40%), Gram-negative bacilli (5%), fungi (5%).	**Device removal** + **vanco** 1 gm IV q12h + **RIF** 300 mg po bid	**Device removal** + **dapto** 6 mg per kg IV q24h[NAI] ± **RIF** *(no data)* 300 mg po bid	**Duration of rx after device removal:** For "pocket" or subcutaneous infection, 10–14 days; if lead-assoc. endocarditis, 4–6 wks depending on organism. Ref: *Mayo Clin Proc 83:46, 2008.*
Pericarditis, purulent— empiric therapy *Ref: Medicine 88: 52, 2009.*	Staph. aureus, Strep. pneumoniae, Group A strep, Enterobacteriaceae	**Vanco + CIP** *(Dosage, see footnote[19])*	**Vanco + CFP** *(see footnote[19])*	Drainage required if signs of tamponade. Forced to use empiric vanco due to high prevalence of MRSA.
Rheumatic fever with carditis Ref.: *Ln 366:155, 2005*	Post-infectious sequelae of Group A strep infection (usually pharyngitis)	ASA, and usually prednisone 2 mg/kg po q24h for symptomatic treatment of fever, arthritis, arthralgia. May not influence carditis.		Clinical features: Carditis, polyarthritis, chorea, subcutaneous nodules, erythema marginatum. *Prophylaxis: see page 57*
Ventricular assist device-related infection Ref: *LnID 6:426, 2006*	S. aureus, S. epidermidis, aerobic gm-neg bacilli, Candida sp	After culture of blood, wounds, drive line, device pocket and maybe pump: **Vanco** 1 gm IV q12h + (**Cip** 400 mg IV q12h or **levo** 750 mg IV q24h) + **fluconazole** 800 mg IV q24h.		Can substitute **daptomycin** 6 mg/kg/d for **vanco, cefepime** 2 gm IV q12h for FQ, and (**vori, caspo, micafungin or anidulafungin**) for **fluconazole**.

[19] **Aminoglycosides** *(see Table 10D, page 101),* **IMP** 0.5 gm IV q6h, **MER** 1 gm IV q8h, **nafcillin** or **oxacillin** 2 gm IV q4h, **TC-CL** 3.1 gm IV q6h, **PIP-TZ** 3.375 gm IV q6h or 4.5 gm q8h, **AM-SB** 3 gm IV q6h, **P Ceph** 1 (cephalothin 2 gm IV q4h or cefazolin 2 gm IV q8h), **CIP** 750 mg po bid or 400 mg IV bid, **vanco** 1 gm IV q12h, **RIF** 600 mg po q24h, **aztreonam** 2 gm IV q8h, **CFP** 2 gm IV q12h

 NOTE: All dosage recommendations are for adults (unless otherwise indicated) and assume normal renal function.

TABLE 1A (26)

ANATOMIC SITE/DIAGNOSIS/ MODIFYING CIRCUMSTANCES	ETIOLOGIES (usual)	SUGGESTED REGIMENS*		ADJUNCT DIAGNOSTIC OR THERAPEUTIC MEASURES AND COMMENTS
		PRIMARY	ALTERNATIVE[§]	
JOINT—*Also see Lyme Disease, page 55*				
Reactive arthritis				
Reiter's syndrome *(See Comment for definition)*	Occurs wks after infection with C. trachomatis, Campylobacter jejuni, Yersinia enterocolitica, Shigella/Salmonella sp.	Only treatment is non-steroidal anti-inflammatory drugs		Definition: Urethritis, conjunctivitis, arthritis, and sometimes uveitis and rash. Arthritis: asymmetrical oligoarthritis of ankles, knees, feet, sacroiliitis. Rash: palms and soles—keratoderma blennorrhagia; circinate balanitis of glans penis. HLA-B27 positive predisposes to Reiter's.
Poststreptococcal reactive arthritis *(See Rheumatic fever, above)*	Immunologic reaction after strep pharyngitis: (1) arthritis onset in <10 days, (2) lasts months, (3) unresponsive to ASA	Treat strep pharyngitis and then NSAIDs (prednisone needed in some pts)		A reactive arthritis after a β-hemolytic strep infection in absence of sufficient Jones criteria for acute rheumatic fever. Ref.: *Mayo Clin Proc 75:144, 2000.*
Septic arthritis: Treatment requires both adequate drainage of purulent joint fluid and appropriate antimicrobial therapy. **There is no need to inject antimicrobials into joints**. Empiric therapy after collection of blood and joint fluid for culture; review Gram stain of joint fluid.				
Infants <3 mo (neonate)	Staph. aureus, Enterobacteriaceae, Group B strep, N. gonorrhoeae	**If MRSA not a concern:** (**Nafcillin** or **oxacillin**) + **P Ceph 3**	**If MRSA a concern: Vanco + P Ceph 3**	Blood cultures frequently positive. Adjacent bone involved in 2/3 pts. Group B strep and gonococci most common community-acquired etiologies.
		(Dosage, see Table 16, page 137)		
Children (3 mo–14 yr)	Staph. aureus 27%, S. pyogenes & S. pneumo 14%, H. influenzae 3%, Gm-neg. bacilli 6%, other (GC, N. meningitidis) 14%, unknown 36%	**Vanco** + **P Ceph 3** until culture results available *See Table 16 for dosage* Steroids—*see Comment*		Marked ↓ in H. influenzae since use of conjugate vaccine. **NOTE:** Septic arthritis due to salmonella has no association with sickle cell disease, unlike salmonella osteomyelitis. 10 days of therapy as effective as a 30-day treatment course if there is a good clinical response and CRP levels normalize quickly *(CID 48:1201, 2009)*.
Adults *(review Gram stain): See page 55 for Lyme Disease Lyme Disease and page 55 for gonococcal arthritis*				
Acute monoarticular				
At risk for sexually-transmitted disease	**N. gonorrhoeae** *(see page 21)*, S. aureus, streptococci, rarely aerobic Gm-neg. bacilli	**Gram stain negative: Ceftriaxone** 1 gm IV q24h or **cefotaxime** 1 gm IV q8h or **ceftizoxime** 1 gm IV q8h	If Gram stain shows Gm+ cocci in clusters: **vanco** 1 gm IV q12h; if >100 kg, 1.5 gm IV q12h	For treatment comments, *see Disseminated GC, page 21*
Not at risk for sexually-transmitted disease	S. aureus, streptococci, Gm-neg. bacilli	**All empiric choices guided by Gram stain** **Vanco + P Ceph 3**	**Vanco + (CIP or Levo)**	Differential includes gout and chondrocalcinosis (pseudogout). **Look for crystals in joint fluid.** **NOTE:** *See Table 6 for MRSA treatment.*
		For treatment duration, see Table 3, page 66 *For dosage, see footnote page 31*		
Chronic monoarticular	Brucella, nocardia, mycobacteria, fungi	*See Table 2 & Table 12*		
Polyarticular, usually acute	**Gonococci**, B. burgdorferi, acute rheumatic fever; viruses, e.g., hepatitis B, rubella vaccine, parvo B19	Gram stain usually negative for GC. If sexually active, culture urethra, cervix, anal canal, throat, blood, joint fluid, and then: **ceftriaxone** 1 gm IV q24h		If GC, usually associated petechiae and/or pustular skin lesions and tenosynovitis. Consider Lyme disease if exposure areas known to harbor infected ticks. *See page 55.* Expanded differential includes gout, pseudogout, reactive arthritis (HLA-B27 pos.).
Septic arthritis, post intra-articular injection	MSSE/MRSE 40%, MSSA/MRSA 20%, P. aeruginosa, Propionibacteria, mycobacteria	**NO empiric therapy.** Arthroscopy for culture/sensitivity, crystals, washout		Treat based on culture results x 14 days (assumes no foreign body present).

Abbreviations on page 2. *NOTE: All dosage recommendations are for adults (unless otherwise indicated) and assume normal renal function.*

TABLE 1A (27)

ANATOMIC SITE/DIAGNOSIS/ MODIFYING CIRCUMSTANCES	ETIOLOGIES (usual)	SUGGESTED REGIMENS* PRIMARY	ALTERNATIVE[§]	ADJUNCT DIAGNOSTIC OR THERAPEUTIC MEASURES AND COMMENTS
JOINT *(continued)*				
Infected prosthetic joint *See surgical options in Comments* ***Drug dosages in footnote***[20] ***For dental prophylaxis, see Table 15B*** Ref: *NEJM 361:787, 2009*	Cultures pending	**No empiric therapy.** Need culture & sens. results. Can ↑ yield of culture by sonication *(NEJM 357:654, 2007)*. Surgical options in Comment.		**Surg. options: 1. 2-stage:** Remove infected prosthesis & leave spacer, antimicrobics, then new prosthesis. Highest cure rate *(CID 42:216, 2006)*. **2. 1-stage:** Removal of infected prosthesis, debridement, new prosthesis, then antibiotics. Long-term success in ~80% of selected cases; extending therapy beyond 6 months may not improve outcome as duration of therapy not predictive of recurrence *(JAC 63:1264, 2009)*. **3. Extensive debridement & leave prosthesis in place** plus antibiotic therapy; 53% failure rate, esp. if ≥8 days of symptoms *(CID 42:471, 2006)* **4. Remove prosthesis & treat ± bone fusion of joint. Last option:** debridement and chronic antimicrobic suppression.
	S. pyogenes: Gps A, B, or G; viridans strep	Debridement & prosthesis retention; (**Pen G** or **ceftriax**) IV x 4 wks. Cured 17/19 pts *(CID 36:847, 2003)*.		
	Gram-negative bacilli: *CID 49:1036, 2009*	35 of 47 patients in remission with debridement & prolonged IV to po therapy *(AAC 53:4772, 2009)*.		
	MSSE/MSSA--see surgical options	(**Nafcillin/oxacillin** IV + **RIF** po) x 6 wks	(**Vanco** IV + **RIF** po) **OR** (**Dapto** IV + **RIF** po) x 6 wk	**RIF** bactericidal vs. surface-adhering, slow-growing, & biofilm-producing bacteria. Never use **RIF** alone due to rapid development of resistance. **RIF + Fusidic acid**[NUS] (dosage in footnote) another option *(Cl.Micro.&Inf. 12(53):93, 2006)*.
	MRSE/MRSA--see surgical options	(**Vanco** IV + **RIF** po) x 6 wks	[(**CIP** or **Levo**—if susceptible—po) + (**RIF** po)] **OR** (**linezolid** po) **OR (Dapto + RIF) x 6 wk**	Limited linezolid experience is favorable *(JAC 55:387, 2005)*. Watch for toxicity if over 2 wks of therapy, *Table 10C, page 96*. **Dapto** experience: *IDCP 14:144, 2006*
	Propioni bacterium acnes	No clear consensus: **Vanco** or **ceftriaxone**	**Dapto** or **penicillin**	Also susceptible in vitro to carbapenems, linezolid *(AAC 50:2728, 2006)*. 15% resistant to clindamycin *(Clin Micro & Infection 11:204, 2005)*.
	P. aeruginosa	**Ceftaz** IV + (**CIP** or **Levo** po)		
Rheumatoid arthritis	**TNF inhibitors** (adalimumab, certolizumab, etanercept, golimumab, infliximab) ↑ risk of TBc, fungal infection and malignancy. *(LnID 8:601, 2008; Med Lett 51:55, 2009)*. Treat latent TBc first. Tocilizumab (IL-6 receptor inhibitor) may also increase infection risk.			
Septic bursitis: Olecranon bursitis; prepatellar bursitis	Staph. aureus >80%, M. tuberculosis (rare), M. marinum (rare)	(**Nafcillin** or **oxacillin** 2 gm IV q4h or **dicloxacillin** 500 mg po qid) if **MSSA** *Other doses, see footnote page 31*	(**Vanco** 1 gm IV q12h or **linezolid** 600 mg po bid) if **MRSA**	Immunosuppression, not duration of therapy, is a risk factor for recurrence; 7 days of therapy may be sufficient for immunocompetent patients undergoing one-stage bursectomy *(JAC 65:1008, 2010)*.
KIDNEY, BLADDER AND PROSTATE				
Acute uncomplicated urinary tract infection (cystitis-urethritis) in females [NOTE: Routine urine culture not necessary; self-rx works *(AnIM 135:9, 2001)*].				
NOTE: Resistance of E. coli to TMP-SMX approx. 15–20% & correlates with microbiological/ clinical failure. **Recent reports of E. coli resistant to FQs as well.** 5-day **nitrofurantoin** ref: *ArcIM 167:2207, 2007*	Enterobacteriaceae (E. coli), Staph. saprophyticus, enterococci	**<20% of Local E. coli resistant to TMP-SMX & no allergy**: **TMP-SMX-DS** bid x 3 days; if sulfa allergy, **nitrofurantoin** 100 mg po bid x 5 days or **fosfomycin** 3 gm po x one dose. All plus **Pyridium**	**>20% Local E. coli resistant to TMP-SMX or sulfa allergy**: then 3 days of **CIP** 250 mg bid, **CIP-ER** 500 mg q24h, **Levo** 250 mg q24h OR **Moxi** 400 mg q24h **OR Nitrofurantoin** 100 mg bid OR single 3 gm dose of **fosfomycin.** All plus **Pyridium**	7-day rx recommended **in pregnancy** [discontinue or do not use sulfonamides (TMP-SMX) near term (2 weeks before EDC) because of potential ↑ in kernicterus]. If failure on 3-day course, culture and rx 2 weeks. **Fosfomycin** 3 gm po times 1 less effective vs. E. coli than multi-dose TMP-SMX or FQ. Fosfo active vs. E. faecalis; poor activity vs. other coliforms. **Moxifloxacin**: Not approved for UTIs. Moxi equivalent to comparator drugs in unpublished clinical trials (on file with Bayer). Therapy of **ESBL producing E. coli and Klebsiella spp.** problematic because of multiple drug resistances: ESBL producers susceptible to fosfomycin, ertapenem, and combo of amox-clav + cefdinir in vitro *(AAC 53:1278, 2009)*. **Phenazopyridine (Pyridium)**—non-prescription—may relieve dysuria: 200 mg po tid times 2 days. Hemolysis if G6PD deficient.

[20] **Aqueous Pen G** 2 million units IV q4h; **cefazolin** 1 gm IV q8h; **ceftriaxone** 2 gm IV q24h; **nafcillin** or **oxacillin** 2 gm IV q4h; **vancomycin** 1 gm IV q12h; **Daptomycin** 6 mg/kg IV q24h; **RIF** 300 mg IV/po bid; **CIP** 750 mg IV/po bid; **Levo** 750 mg IV/po q24h; **ceftazidime** 2 gm IV q8h; **Fusidic Acid**[NUS] 500 mg po/IV tid; **clindamycin** 900 mg IV q8h.

 NOTE: All dosage recommendations are for adults (unless otherwise indicated) and assume normal renal function.

TABLE 1A (28)

ANATOMIC SITE/DIAGNOSIS/ MODIFYING CIRCUMSTANCES	ETIOLOGIES (usual)	SUGGESTED REGIMENS*		ADJUNCT DIAGNOSTIC OR THERAPEUTIC MEASURES AND COMMENTS
		PRIMARY	ALTERNATIVE[§]	
KIDNEY, BLADDER AND PROSTATE/Acute uncomplicated urinary tract infection (cystitis-urethritis) in females *(continued)*				
Risk factors for STD, Dipstick: positive leukocyte esterase or hemoglobin, neg. Gram stain	C. trachomatis	**Azithro** 1 gm po single dose	**Doxy** 100 mg po bid 7 days	Pelvic exam for vaginitis & herpes simplex, urine LCR/PCR for GC and C. trachomatis.
Recurrent (3 or more episodes/ year) in young women	Any of the above bacteria	Eradicate infection, then **TMP-SMX** 1 single-strength tab po q24h long term		A cost-effective alternative to continuous prophylaxis is self-administered single dose rx (TMP-SMX DS, 2 tabs, 320/1600 mg) at symptom onset. Another alternative: 1 DS tablet TMP-SMX post-coitus.
Child: ≤5 yrs old & grade 3–4 reflux	Coliforms	[**TMP-SMX** (2 mg TMP/10 mg SMX) per kg po q24h] or (**nitrofurantoin** 2 mg per kg po q24h). **CIP** approved as alternative drug ages 1–17 yrs.		
Recurrent UTI in postmenopausal women	E. coli & other Enterobacteriaceae, enterococci, S. saprophyticus	Treat as for uncomplicated UTI. Evaluate for potentially correctable urologic factors—see *Comment*. **Nitrofurantoin** more effective than vaginal cream in decreasing frequency, but Editors worry about pulmonary fibrosis with long-term NF rx.		Definition: ≥3 culture + symptomatic UTIs in 1 year or 2 UTIs in 6 months. Urologic factors: (1) cystocele, (2) incontinence, (3) ↑ residual urine volume (≥50 mL).
Acute uncomplicated pyelonephritis (usually women 18–40 yrs, temperature >102°F, definite costovertebral tenderness. [NOTE: Culture of urine and blood indicated prior to therapy]. **If male, look for obstructive uropathy or other complicating pathology.**				
Moderately ill (outpatient) **NOTE:** May need one IV dose due to nausea. Resistance of E. coli to TMP/SMX 13-45% in collaborative ER study *(CID 47:1150, 2008)*.	Enterobacteriaceae (most likely E. coli), enterococci (Gm stain of **uncentrifuged** urine may allow identification of Gm-neg. bacilli vs. Gm+ cocci)	**FQ** po times 5-7 days: **CIP** 500 mg bid or **CIP-ER** 1000 mg q24h, **Levo** 750 mg q24h, **Oflox** 400 mg bid, **Moxi**[NAI] 400 mg q24h possibly ok—see comment.	**AM-CL**, **O Ceph**, or **TMP-SMX-DS po.** Treat for 14 days. Dosage in footnote[21] Beta-lactams not as effective as FQs: *JAMA 293:949, 2005*	In randomized double-blind trial, bacteriologic and **clinical success higher for 7 days of CIP than for 14 days of TMP-SMX**; failures correlated with TMP-SMX in vitro resistance. Since **CIP** worked with 7-day rx, suspect other FQs effective with 7 days of therapy; **Levo** 750 mg FDA-approved for 5 days.
Acute pyelonephritis-- Hospitalized	E. coli most common, enterococci 2nd in frequency	**FQ** (IV) or (**AMP** + **gentamicin**) or **ceftriaxone** or **PIP-TZ**. Treat for 14 days.	**TC-CL** or **AM-SB** or **PIP-TZ** or **ERTA** or **DORI**; 500 mg q8h. Treat for 14 days.	Treat IV until pt afebrile 24–48 hrs, then complete 2-wk course with oral drugs (as *Moderately ill, above*). **DORI** approved for 10 day treatment.
		Dosages in footnote[21]. Do not use cephalosporins for suspect or proven enterococcal infection		**If pt hypotensive, prompt imaging (Echo or CT) is recommended to ensure absence of obstructive uropathy.** **NOTE: Cephalosporins & ertapenem not active vs. enterococci.**
Complicated UTI/catheters Obstruction, reflux, azotemia, transplant, **Foley catheter-related, R/O obstruction ; multi-drug resistant gram-neg bacilli.** *For IDSA Guidelines: CID 50:625, 2010.*	Enterobacteriaceae, P. aeruginosa, enterococci rarely S. aureus *(CID 42:46 2006)*	(**AMP** + **gent**) or **PIP-TZ** or **TC-CL** or **DORI** or **IMP** or **MER** for up to 2–3 wks	(IV **FQ**: **CIP**, **Gati**, **Levo**) or **Ceftaz** or **CFP** for up to 2–3 wks	Not all listed drugs predictably active vs. enterococci or *P. aeruginosa*. **CIP** approved in children (1-17 yrs) as alternative. Not 1st choice secondary to increased incidence joint adverse effects. Peds dose: 6-10 mg/kg (400 mg max) **IV** q8h or 10-20 mg/kg (750 mg max) **po** q12h.
		Switch to po **FQ** or **TMP-SMX** when possible *For dosages, see footnote[21].*		Increasing number of multi-drug resistant gram-negative bacilli. For treatment options, *see JAC 65 (Suppl 3): 25, 2010.*

[21] **AM-CL** 875/125 mg po q12h or 500/125 mg po tid or 2000 /125 mg po bid *Antipseudomonal penicillins*: **AM-SB** 3 gm IV q6h **PIP** 3 gm IV q4-6h; **PIP-TZ** 3.375 gm IV q4-6h (4.5 gm IV q6h for pseudomonas pneumonia); **TC-CL** 3.1 gm IV q6h; *Antipseudomonal cephalosporins*: **ceftaz** 2 gm IV q8h; **CFP** 2 gm IV q12h; **aztreonam** 2 gm IV q8h; *Carbapenems*: **DORI** 500 mg IV q8h (1 hr infusion); **ERTA** 1 gm IV q24h; **IMP** 0.5 gm IV q12h (max 4 gm/day); **MER** 1 gm IV q8h; *Parenteral cephalosporins*: **cefotaxime** 1 gm IV q12h (2 gm IV q4h for severe infection); **cefoxitin** 2 gm IV q8h; **ceftriaxone** 1-2 gm IV q24h; *Oral cephalosporins-- see Table 10C, page 95*; **dicloxacillin** 500 mg po q6h; *FQs*: **CIP** 400 mg IV q12h; **Gati**[NUS] 400 mg IV q24h; **levo** 750 mg IV q24h; **gentamicin**-- *see Table 10D, page 101*; **linezolid** 600 mg IV/po q12h; **metro** 500 mg po q6h or 15 mg/kg IV q12h (max 4 gm/day); **nafcillin/oxacillin** 2 gm IV q4h; **TMP-SMX** 2 mg/kg (TMP component) IV q6h; **vanco** 1 gm IV q12h (if over 100 kg, 1.5 gm IV q12h).

Abbreviations on page 2. *NOTE: All dosage recommendations are for adults (unless otherwise indicated) and assume normal renal function.*

TABLE 1A (29)

ANATOMIC SITE/DIAGNOSIS/ MODIFYING CIRCUMSTANCES	ETIOLOGIES (usual)	SUGGESTED REGIMENS*		ADJUNCT DIAGNOSTIC OR THERAPEUTIC MEASURES AND COMMENTS
		PRIMARY	ALTERNATIVE[§]	
KIDNEY, BLADDER AND PROSTATE *(continued)*				
Asymptomatic bacteriuria. IDSA Guidelines: *CID 40:643, 2005; U.S. Preventive Services Task Force AnIM 149:43, 2008.*				
Preschool children		Base regimen on C&S, not empirical		Diagnosis requires ≥10^5 CFU per mL urine of same bacterial species in 2 specimens obtained 3–7 days apart.
Pregnancy	Aerobic Gm-neg. bacilli & Staph. hemolyticus	Screen 1st trimester. If positive, rx 3–7 days with **amox**, **nitrofurantoin**, **O Ceph**, **TMP-SMX**, or **TMP** alone		Screen monthly for recurrence. Some authorities treat continuously until delivery (stop TMP-SMX 2 wks before EDC). ↑ resistance of E. coli to TMP-SMX.
Before and after invasive urologic intervention, e.g., Foley catheter	Aerobic Gm-neg. bacilli	Obtain urine culture and then rx 3 days with **TMP-SMX DS**, bid. For prevention of UTI: Consider removal after 72 hrs *(CID 46:243 & 251, 2008).*		Clinical benefit of antimicrobial-coated Foley catheters is uncertain *(AnIM 144:116, 2006).*
Neurogenic bladder – see "spinal cord injury" below		No therapy in asymptomatic patient; intermittent catheterization if possible		Ref.: *AJM 113(1A):67S, 2002*—Bacteriuria in spinal cord injured patient.
Asymptomatic, advanced age, male or female Ref: *CID 40:643, 2005*		No therapy indicated unless in conjunction with surgery to correct obstructive uropathy; measure residual urine vol. in females; prostate exam/PSA in males. No screening recommended in men and non-pregnant women *(AnIM 149:43, 2008).*		
Malacoplakia	E. coli	**Bethanechol chloride** + (**CIP** or **TMP-SMX**)		Chronic pyelo with abnormal inflammatory response. *See CID 29:444, 1999.*
Perinephric abscess				
Associated with staphylococcal bacteremia	Staph. aureus	If **MSSA, Nafcillin/ oxacillin** or **cefazolin** *(Dosage, see footnote page 30)*	If **MRSA: Vanco** 1 gm IV q12h **OR dapto** 6 mg/kg IV q24h	Drainage, surgical or image-guided aspiration
Associated with pyelonephritis	Enterobacteriaceae	*See pyelonephritis, complicated UTI, above*		Drainage, surgical or image-guided aspiration
Post Renal Transplant Obstructive Uropathy *(CID 46:825, 2008)*	Corynebacterium urealyticum	**Vanco** or **Teicoplanin**[NUS]		Organism can synthesize struvite stones. Requires 48-72 hr incubation to detect in culture
Prostatitis		*See prostatitis, page 25*		
Spinal cord injury pts with UTI	E. coli, Klebsiella sp., enterococci	**CIP** 250 mg po bid x 14 days		If fever, suspect assoc. pyelonephritis. Microbiologic cure greater after 14 vs. 3 days of CIP *(CID 39:658 & 665, 2004)*; for asymptomatic bacteriuria *see AJM 113(1A):675, 2002.*
LIVER *(for spontaneous bacterial peritonitis, see page 44)*				
Cholangitis		*See Gallbladder, page 15*		
Cirrhosis & variceal bleeding	Esophageal flora	(**Norfloxacin** 400 mg po bid or **CIP** 400 mg IV q12h) x max. of 7 days	**Ceftriaxone** 1 gm IV once daily for max. of 7 days	Short term prophylactic antibiotics in cirrhotics with G-I hemorr, with or without ascites, decreases rate of bacterial infection & ↑ survival *(Hepatology 46:922, 2007).*
Hepatic abscess Klebsiella liver abscess ref.: *CID 47:642, 2008*	Enterobacteriaceae (esp. Klebsiella sp.), bacteroides, enterococci, Entamoeba histolytica, Yersinia enterocolitica (rare), Fusobacterium necrophorum *(Lemierre's). For echinococcus, see Table 13, page 139. For cat-scratch disease (CSD), see pages 43 & 54*	**Metro** + (**ceftriaxone** or **cefoxitin** or **TC-CL** or **PIP-TZ** or **AM-SB** or **CIP** or **levo**. *(Dosage, see footnote[21] on page 31)* **AMP** + **aminoglycoside** + **metro** traditional & effective but AMP-resistant Gm-neg. bacilli ↑ and aminoglycoside toxicity an issue.	**Metro** (for amoeba) + either **IMP**, **MER** or **Dori** *(Dosage, see footnote[21] on page 31)*	**Serological tests for amebiasis should be done on all patients;** if neg., surgical drainage or percutaneous aspiration. In pyogenic abscess, ½ have identifiable GI source or underlying biliary tract disease. If amoeba serology positive, treat with **metro** alone without surgery. Empiric **metro** included for both E. histolytica & bacteroides. **Hemochromatosis** associated with Yersinia enterocolitica liver abscess; regimens listed are effective for yersinia. Klebsiella pneumonia genotype K1 associated ocular & CNS Klebsiella infections *(CID 45:284, 2007).*
Hepatic encephalopathy	Urease-producing gut bacteria	**Rifaxamin** 550 mg po bid (take with lactulose)		Refs: *NEJM 362:1071, 2010; Med Lett 52:87, 2010.*

Abbreviations on page 2. *NOTE: All dosage recommendations are for adults (unless otherwise indicated) and assume normal renal function.*

TABLE 1A (30)

ANATOMIC SITE/DIAGNOSIS/ MODIFYING CIRCUMSTANCES	ETIOLOGIES (usual)	SUGGESTED REGIMENS*		ADJUNCT DIAGNOSTIC OR THERAPEUTIC MEASURES AND COMMENTS
		PRIMARY	ALTERNATIVE[§]	
LIVER *(continued)*				
Leptospirosis	Leptospirosis, *see page 57*			
Peliosis hepatis in AIDS pts	Bartonella henselae and B. quintana	*See page 54*		
Post-transplant infected "biloma"	Enterococci (incl. VRE), candida, Gm-neg. bacilli (P. aeruginosa 8%), anaerobes 5%	**Linezolid** 600 mg IV bid + **CIP** 400 mg IV q12h + **fluconazole** 400 mg IV q24h	**Dapto** 6 mg/kg per day + **Levo** 750 mg IV q24h + **fluconazole** 400 mg IV q24h	Suspect if fever & abdominal pain post-transplant. Exclude hepatic artery thrombosis. Presence of candida and/or VRE bad prognosticators.
Viral hepatitis	Hepatitis A, B, C, D, E, G	*See Table 14, page 146*		
LUNG/Bronchi				
Bronchiolitis/wheezy bronchitis (expiratory wheezing)				
Infants/children (≤ age 5) See *RSV, Table 14B page 157* Ref: *Ln 368:312, 2006*	**Respiratory syncytial virus** (RSV) 50%, parainfluenza 25%, human metapneumovirus	Antibiotics not useful, mainstay of therapy is oxygen. Ribavirin for severe disease: 6 gm vial (20 mg/mL) in sterile H_2O by SPAG-2 generator over 18-20 hrs daily times 3-5 days.		RSV most important. Rapid diagnosis with antigen detection methods. For prevention a humanized mouse monoclonal antibody, **palivizumab**. *See Table 14, page 157*. RSV immune globulin is no longer available. Review: *Red Book of Peds 2006, 27th Ed.*
Bronchitis				
Infants/children (≤ age 5)	< Age 2: Adenovirus; age 2–5: Respiratory syncytial virus, parainfluenza 3 virus, human metapneumovirus		Antibiotics indicated only with associated sinusitis or heavy growth on throat culture for S. pneumo., Group A strep, H. influenzae or no improvement in 1 week. Otherwise rx is symptomatic.	
Adolescents and adults with acute tracheobronchitis (Acute bronchitis) Ref.: *NEJM 355:2125, 2006*	Usually viral. M. pneumoniae 5%; C. pneumoniae 5%. *See Persistent cough, below*	**Antibiotics not indicated.** Antitussive ± inhaled bronchodilators		Purulent sputum alone not an indication for antibiotic therapy. Expect cough to last 2 weeks. If fever/rigors, get chest x-ray.
Persistent cough (>14 days), afebrile during community outbreak: Pertussis (whooping cough) 10–20% adults with cough >14 days have pertussis *(MMWR 54 (RR-14), 2005)*. Review: *Chest 130:547, 2006*	Bordetella pertussis & occ. Bordetella parapertussis. Also consider asthma, gastroesophageal reflux, post-nasal drip	**Peds doses: Azithro/ clarithro** OR **erythro estolate**[22] OR **erythro base**[22] OR **TMP/SMX** *(doses in footnote[22])*	**Adult doses: Azithro** po 500 mg day 1, 250 mg q24h days 2–5 OR **erythro estolate** 500 mg po qid times 14 days OR **TMP-SMX-DS** 1 tab po bid times 14 days OR (**clarithro** 500 mg po bid or 1 gm **ER** q24h times 7 days)	**3 stages of illness:** catarrhal (1–2 wks), paroxysmal coughing (2–4 wks), and convalescence (1–2 wks). Treatment may abort or eliminate pertussis in catarrhal stage, but does not shorten paroxysmal stage. **Diagnosis:** PCR on nasopharyngeal secretions or ↑ pertussis-toxin antibody. **Rx aimed at eradication of NP carriage.** In non-outbreak setting, likelihood of pertussis increased if post-tussive emeris or inspiratory whoop present *(JAMA 304:890, 2010)*.
Pertussis: Prophylaxis of household contacts	Drugs and doses as per treatment immediately above			Recommended by Am. Acad. Ped. Red Book 2006 for all household or close contacts; community-wide prophylaxis not recommended.

[22] **ADULT DOSAGE: AM-CL** 875/125 mg po bid or 500/125 mg po q8h or 2000/125 mg po bid; **azithro** 500 mg po x 1 dose, then 250 mg q24h x 4 days or 500 mg po q24h x 3 days; *Oral cephalosporins*: **cefaclor** 500 mg po q8h or 500 mg extended release q12h; **cefdinir** 300 mg po q12h or 600 mg po q24h; **cefditoren** 200 mg tabs—2 tabs bid; **cefixime** 400 mg po q24h; **cefpodoxime proxetil** 200 mg po q12h; **cefprozil** 500 mg po q12h; **ceftibuten** 400 mg po q24h; **cefuroxime axetil** 250 or 500 mg q12h; **loracarbef** 400 mg po q12h; **clarithro** extended release 1000 mg po q24h; **doxy** 100 mg po bid; **erythro base** 40 mg/kg/day po div q6h; **erythro estolate** 40 mg/kg/day po div qid; *FQs*: **CIP** 750 mg po q12h; **gemi** 320 mg po q24h; **levo** 500 mg po q24h; **moxi** 400 mg po q24h; **TMP-SMX** 1 DS tab po bid.
PEDS DOSAGE: azithro 10 mg/kg/day po on day 1, then 5 mg/kg po q24h x 4 days; **clarithro** 7.5 mg/kg po q12h; **erythro base** 40 mg/kg/day div q6h; **erythro estolate** 40 mg/kg/day div q8-12h; **TMP-SMX** (>6 mos. of age) 8 mg/kg/day (TMP component) div bid.

Abbreviations on page 2. *NOTE: All dosage recommendations are for adults (unless otherwise indicated) and assume normal renal function.*

TABLE 1A (31)

ANATOMIC SITE/DIAGNOSIS/ MODIFYING CIRCUMSTANCES	ETIOLOGIES (usual)	SUGGESTED REGIMENS*		ADJUNCT DIAGNOSTIC OR THERAPEUTIC MEASURES AND COMMENTS
		PRIMARY	ALTERNATIVE[§]	
LUNG/Bronchi/Bronchitis *(continued)*				
Acute bacterial exacerbation of chronic bronchitis (ABECB), adults (almost always smokers with COPD) Ref: *NEJM 359:2355, 2008.*	Viruses 20–50%, C. pneumoniae 5%, M. pneumoniae <1%; role of S. pneumo, H. influenzae & M. catarrhalis controversial. Tobacco use, air pollution contribute. Non-pathogenic H. haemolyticus may be mistaken for H. influenza *(JID 195:81, 2007).*	**Severe ABECB** = ↑ dyspnea, ↑ sputum viscosity/purulence, ↑ sputum volume. For severe ABECB: (1) consider chest x-ray, esp. if febrile &/or low O_2 sat.; (2) inhaled anticholinergic bronchodilator; (3) oral corticosteroid; taper over 2 wks *(Cochrane Library 3, 2006)*; (4) D/C tobacco use; (5) non-invasive positive pressure ventilation. **Role of antimicrobial therapy debated even for severe disease**. **For mild or moderate disease, no antimicrobial treatment** or maybe amox, doxy, TMP-SMX, or O Ceph. **For severe disease,** AM-CL, azithro/clarithro, or O Ceph or FQs with enhanced activity vs. drug-resistant S. pneumo (Gemi, Levo, or Moxi). ***Drugs & doses in footnote.*** **Duration** varies with drug: range 3–10 days. Limit Gemi to 5 days to decrease risk of rash.		
Fever, cough, myalgia during influenza season *(See NEJM 360:2605, 2009 regarding novel H1N1 influenza A)*	Influenza A & B	*See Influenza, Table 14A, page 154.*		**Complications: Influenza pneumonia, secondary bacterial pneumonia** Community MRSA and MSSA, *S. pneumoniae, H. influenzae.*
Bronchiectasis. Ref: *Chest 134:815, 2008* Acute exacerbation	H. influ., P. aeruginosa, and rarely S. pneumo.	**Gemi**, **levo**, or **moxi** x 7-10 days. *Dosage in footnote*[22].		Many potential etiologies: obstruction, ↓ immune globulins, cystic fibrosis, dyskinetic cilia, tobacco, prior severe or recurrent necrotizing bronchitis: e.g. pertussis.
Prevention of exacerbation	Not applicable	One option: **Erythro** 500 mg po bid or **azithro** 250 mg q24h x 8 wks.		
Specific organisms	Aspergillus *(see Table 11)* MAI *(Table 12)* and P. aeruginosa *(Table 5)*.			
Pneumonia: CONSIDER TUBERCULOSIS IN ALL PATIENTS; ISOLATE ALL SUSPECT PATIENTS				
Neonatal: Birth to 1 month	**Viruses:** CMV, rubella, H. simplex **Bacteria:** Group B strep, listeria, coliforms, S. aureus, P. aeruginosa **Other:** Chlamydia trachomatis, syphilis	**AMP** + **gentamicin** ± **cefotaxime**. Add **vanco** if MRSA a concern. For chlamydia therapy, **erythro** 12.5 mg per kg po or IV qid times 14 days.		Blood cultures indicated. Consider C. trachomatis if afebrile pneumonia, staccato cough, IgM >1:8; therapy with erythro or sulfisoxazole. If MRSA documented, **vanco**, **TMP-SMX**, & **linezolid** alternatives. **Linezolid** dosage from birth to age 11 yrs is **10 mg per kg q8h**.
Age 1–3 months Pneumonitis syndrome. Usually afebrile	C. trachomatis, RSV, parainfluenza virus 3, human metapneumovirus, Bordetella, S. pneumoniae, S. aureus (rare)	**Outpatient: po erythro** 12.5 mg/kg q6h x 14 days or po **azithro** 10 mg/kg x dose, then 5 mg/kg x 4 days.	**Inpatient: If afebrile erythro** 10 mg/kg IV q6h or **azithro** 2.5 mg/kg IV q12h *(see Comment)*. **If febrile**, add **cefotaxime** 200 mg/kg per day div q8h	Pneumonitis syndrome: cough, tachypnea, dyspnea, diffuse infiltrates, afebrile. Usually requires hospital care. Reports of hypertrophic pyloric stenosis after erythro under age 6 wks; not sure about azithro; bid azithro dosing theoretically might ↓ risk of hypertrophic pyloric stenosis. If lobar pneumonia, give AMP 200–300 mg per kg per day for S. pneumoniae. No empiric coverage for S. aureus, as it is rare etiology.
		For **RSV**, *see Bronchiolitis, page 33*		

(Continued on next page)

 NOTE: All dosage recommendations are for adults (unless otherwise indicated) and assume normal renal function.

TABLE 1A (32)

ANATOMIC SITE/DIAGNOSIS/ MODIFYING CIRCUMSTANCES	ETIOLOGIES (usual)	SUGGESTED REGIMENS*		ADJUNCT DIAGNOSTIC OR THERAPEUTIC MEASURES AND COMMENTS
		PRIMARY	ALTERNATIVE§	
LUNG/Bronchi/Pneumonia *(continued)*				
Age 4 months–5 years For RSV, *see bronchiolitis, page 33, & Table 14*	RSV, human metapneumovirus, other resp. viruses, S. pneumo, H. flu, mycoplasma, S. aureus (rare), M. tbc	**Outpatient: Amox** 100 mg/kg/day div q8h. **Inpatient (not ICU):** No antibiotic if viral or IV **AMP** 200 mg/kg per day div q6h	**Inpatient (ICU): Cefotaxime** 200 mg per kg per day IV div q8h plus **azithro** 5 mg/kg (max 500 mg/day) IV q24h plus **vanco** (for CA-MRSA) 40 mg/kg/day div q6h.	Common "other" viruses: rhinovirus, influenza, parainfluenza, adenovirus. Often of mild to moderate severity. S. pneumo, non-type B H. flu in 4–20%. Treat for 10–14 days. Ref: *http://www.cincinnatichildrens.org/svc/alpha/h/health-policy/ev-based pneumonia.htm*
Age 5 years–15 years, Non-hospitalized, immuno-competent	Mycoplasma, Chlamydophila pneumoniae, S. pneumoniae, Mycobacterium tuberculosis. Respiratory viruses: mixed, e.g., influenza. Bacterial/viral infection in 23% Legionella: especially in pts with malignancy Ln Inf Dis 6:529, 2006	[(**Amox** 100 mg/kg per day) + (**Clarithro** 500 mg po bid or 1 gm ER q24h; Peds dose: 7.5 mg/kg q12h)] **OR** (**azithro** 0.5 gm po x 1, then 0.25 gm/day; Peds dose: 10 mg/kg per day, max. of 500 mg po, then 5 mg/kg per day, max. 250 mg)	(**Amox** 100 mg/kg per day) + [**Doxy** 100 mg po bid (if pt >8 yrs old) or **erythro** 500 mg po qid. (Peds dose: 10 mg/kg po q6h)]	If otherwise healthy and if not concomitant with (or post-) influenza, S. pneumoniae & S. aureus uncommon in this subset; suspect S. pneumo if sudden onset and large amount of purulent sputum. **Macrolide-resistant S. pneumo** an issue. Higher prevalence of macrolide-resistant S. pneumo in pts <5 yrs old. Also reports of macrolide-resistant M. pneumoniae. Mycoplasma PCR/viral culture usually not done for outpatients. **Mycoplasma requires 2–3 wks of therapy,** C. pneumoniae up to 6 wks. Macrolide-resistant *M. pneumo* reported. **Linezolid** approved for peds use for pen-susceptible & multi-drug resistant S. pneumo (including bacteremia) & methicillin-resistant S. aureus.
		Recent review of several studies recommended amoxicillin 50 mg/kg per day in two divided doses for 3 to 5 days as first-line therapy and TMP-SMX, 8 mg/kg of TMP, in 2 divided doses, as second-line, for non-severe pneumonia *(Lancet Infect Dis. 9:185, 2009)*.		
Children, hospitalized, immunocompetent— 2–18 yrs	S. pneumoniae, viruses, mycoplasma; consider S. aureus if abscesses or necrotizing, esp. during influenza season	**Ceftriaxone** 50 mg per kg per day IV (to max. 2 gm per day) + **azithro** 10 mg per kg per day up to 500 mg IV div q12h. Add anti-staph drug if evidence of lung necrosis: **vanco** 40 mg/kg/day divided q8h.		**Alternatives are a problem in children:** If proven S. pneumo resistant to azithro & ceftriaxone (or severe ceftriaxone allergy): IV vanco, linezolid, or off-label respiratory FQ. No doxy under age 8. Linezolid reported efficacious in children.

(Continued on next page)

Abbreviations on page 2. *NOTE: All dosage recommendations are for adults (unless otherwise indicated) and assume normal renal function.*

TABLE 1A (33)

ANATOMIC SITE/DIAGNOSIS/ MODIFYING CIRCUMSTANCES	ETIOLOGIES (usual)	SUGGESTED REGIMENS*		ADJUNCT DIAGNOSTIC OR THERAPEUTIC MEASURES AND COMMENTS
		PRIMARY	ALTERNATIVE[§]	
LUNG/Bronchi/Pneumonia *(continued)*				
Adults (over age 18)— IDSA/ATS Guideline for CAP in adults: ***CID 44 (Suppl 2): S27-S72, 2007.***				
Community-acquired, not hospitalized **Prognosis prediction: CURB-65** *(AnIM 118:384, 2005)*: C: confusion = 1 pt U. BUN >19 mg/dl = 1 pt R. RR >30 min = 1 pt B. BP <90/60 = 1 pt Age ≥65 = 1 pt **If score = 1, ok for outpatient therapy; if >1, hospitalize.** The higher the score, the higher the mortality. Lab diagnosis of invasive pneumococcal disease: *CID 46:926, 2008.*	Varies with clinical setting. **No co-morbidity:** Atypicals—M. pneumoniae, et al.[23], S. pneumo, viral **Co-morbidity:** Alcoholism: S. pneumo, anaerobes, coliforms Bronchiectasis: *see Cystic fibrosis, page 40* COPD: H. influenzae, M. catarrhalis, S. pneumo IVDU: Hematogenous S. aureus Post-CVA aspiration: Oral flora, incl. S. pneumo Post-obstruction of bronchi: S. pneumo, anaerobes Post- influenza: S. pneumo. and S. aureus	**No co-morbidity:** **Azithro** 0.5 gm po times 1, then 0.25 gm per day **OR azithro-ER** 2 gm times 1 **OR clarithro** 500 mg po bid or **clarithro-ER** 1 gm po q24h **OR doxy** 100 mg po bid **OR if prior antibiotic within 3 months: (azithro** or **clarithro)** + **(amox** 1 gm po tid or high dose **AM-CL OR Respiratory FQ**	**Co-morbidity present: Respiratory FQ** *(see footnote[24])* OR [(**azithro** or **clarithro**) + (high dose **amox**, high dose **AM-CL**, **cefdinir**, **cefpodoximе**, **cefprozil**)] *Doses in footnote[25]*	**Azithro/clarithro:** <u>Pro</u>: appropriate spectrum of activity; more in vitro resistance than clinical failure; q24h dosing; better tolerated than erythro. <u>Con</u>: Overall S. pneumo resistance in vitro 20–30% and may be increasing. If pen G resist. S. pneumo, up to 50%+ resistance to azithro/clarithro. Increased risk of macrolide resistance with prior use. **Amoxicillin:** <u>Pro</u>: Active 90–95% S. pneumo at 3–4 gm per day. <u>Con</u>: No activity atypicals or β-lactamase positive organisms. **AM-CL:** <u>Pro</u>: Spectrum of activity includes β-lactamase positive organisms. <u>Con</u>: No activity atypicals. **Cephalosporins—po:** Cefditoren, cefpodoxime, cefprozil, cefuroxime & others—*see footnote[25]*. <u>Pro</u>: Active 75–85% S. pneumo & H. influenzae. Cefuroxime least active & higher mortality rate when S. pneumo resistant. <u>Con</u>: Inactive vs. atypical pathogens . **Doxycycline:** <u>Pro</u>: Active vs. S. pneumo but resistance may be increasing. Active vs. H. influenzae, atypicals, & bioterrorism agents (anthrax, plague, tularemia). <u>Con</u>: Resistance of S. pneumo 18–20%. Sparse clinical data. **FQs—Respiratory FQs:** Moxi, levo & gemi <u>Pro</u>: In vitro & clinically effective vs. pen-sensitive & pen-resistant S. pneumo. **NOTE: dose of Levo is 750 mg q24h.** Q24H dosing. Gemi only available po. <u>Con</u>: Geographic pockets of resistance with clinical failure. Important Drug-drug interactions *(see Table 22A, page 200)*. Reversible rash in young females given Gemi for >7 days. **Ceftriaxone/cefotaxime:** <u>Pro</u>: Drugs of choice for pen-sens. S. pneumo, active H. influenzae, M. catarrhalis, & MSSA <u>Con</u>: Not active atypicals or pneumonia due to bioterrorism pathogens. <u>Add</u> macrolide for atypicals and perhaps their anti-inflammatory activity. **Ceftaroline:** (FDA approved at a dose of 600 mg q12h IV for 5-7 days for hospitalized patients with CAP): <u>Pro</u>: Higher cure rates than ceftriaxone (85.5% vs 68.6%) in registration trials for CAP patients with S. pneumo, multidrug resistant strains in particular *(CID 51:1401, 2010)* and 6% (1.4-10.7% 95%CI) higher cure rate overall in an integrated analysis of the two trials. <u>Con</u>: More expensive; no data for MRSA yet.
		Duration of rx: S. pneumo—Not bacteremic: until afebrile 3 days —Bacteremic: 10–14 days reasonable C. pneumoniae—Unclear. Some reports suggest 21 days. Some bronchitis pts required 5–6 wks of clarithro *(J Med Micro 52:265, 2003)* Legionella—10–21 days Necrotizing pneumonia 2° to coliforms, S. aureus, anaerobes: ≥2 weeks **Cautions:** **1. If local macrolide resistance to S. pneumoniae >25%, use alternative empiric therapy.** **2. Esp. during influenza season, look for S. aureus.**		
Community-acquired, hospitalized—NOT in the ICU Empiric therapy Treat for minimum of 5 days, afebrile for 48-72 hrs, with stable BP, adequate oral intake, and room air O_2 saturation of >90% *(COID 20:177, 2007)*.	Etiology by co-morbidity & risk factors *as above*. Culture sputum & blood. S. pneumo, urine antigen reported helpful *(CID 40: 1608, 2005)*. Legionella urine antigen indicated. In general, the sicker the pt, the more valuable culture data. Look for S. aureus.	**Ceftriaxone** 1 gm IV q24h + **azithro** 500 mg IV q24h OR **Ertapenem** 1 gm q24h plus **azithro** 500 mg IV q24h	**Levo** 750 mg IV q24h or **Moxi** 400 mg IV q24h **Gati** 400 mg IV q24h (gati no longer marketed in US due to hypo- and hyperglycemic reactions)	
		No rigid time window for first dose; if in ER, first dose in ER. If diagnosis of pneumonia vague, OK for admitting diagnosis of "uncertain." *(Chest 130:16, 2006)*.		

[23] Atypical pathogens: Chlamydophila pneumoniae, C. psittaci, Legionella sp., M. pneumoniae, C. burnetii (Q fever) (Ref.: *LnID 3:709, 2003)*

[24] Respiratory FQs with enhanced activity vs. S. pneumo with high-level resistance to penicillin: **Gati**[NUS] 400 mg IV/po q24h (no longer marketed in US due to hypo- and hyperglycemic reactions), **Gemi** 320 mg po q24h, **Levo** 750 mg IV/po q24h, **Moxi** 400 mg IV/po q24h. Ketolide: **telithro** 800 mg po q24h (physicians warned about rare instances of hepatotoxicity).

[25] **O Ceph** dosage: **Cefdinir** 300 mg po q12h, **cefditoren pivoxil** 200 mg, 2 tabs po bid, **cefpodoxime proxetil** 200 mg po q12h, **cefprozil** 500 mg po q12h, **high dose amox** 1 gm po tid; **high dose AM-CL**—use **AM-CL-ER** 1000/62.5 mg, 2 tabs po bid.

 NOTE: All dosage recommendations are for adults (unless otherwise indicated) and assume normal renal function.

TABLE 1A (34)

ANATOMIC SITE/DIAGNOSIS/ MODIFYING CIRCUMSTANCES	ETIOLOGIES (usual)	SUGGESTED REGIMENS*		ADJUNCT DIAGNOSTIC OR THERAPEUTIC MEASURES AND COMMENTS
		PRIMARY	ALTERNATIVE[§]	
LUNG/Bronchi/Pneumonia/Adults (over age 18) *(continued)*				
Community-acquired, hospitalized—IN ICU Empiric therapy **NOTE:** Not all ICU admissions meet IDSA/ATS CAP Guideline criteria for severe CAP. Do not believe that all ICU pneumonia patients need 2 drugs with activity vs. gram-negative bacilli. Hence, 4 example clinical settings are outlined: **severe COPD; post-influenza, suspect gm-neg bacilli; risk of pen-resistant S. pneumo**	**Severe COPD** pt with pneumonia: S. pneumoniae, H. influenzae, Moraxella sp., Legionella sp. Rarely S. aureus. Culture sputum, blood and maybe pleural fluid. Look for respiratory viruses. Urine antigen for both Legionella and S. pneumoniae. Sputum PCR for Legionella.	**Levo** 750 mg IV q24h or **Moxi** 400 mg IV q24h **Gati** not available in US due to hypo- and hyperglycemic reactions Addition of a macrolide to beta-lactam empiric regimens lowers mortality for patients with bacteremic pneumococcal pneumonia *(CID 36:389, 2003)*. Benefit NOT found with use of FQ or tetracycline for "atypicals" *(Chest 131:466, 2007)*. Combination therapy benefited patients with concomitant "shock." *(CCM 35:1493 & 1617, 2007)*.	[**Ceftriaxone** 1 gm IV q24h + **azithro** 500 mg IV q24h] or **ERTA** 1 gm q24h IV + **azithro** 500 mg IV q24h *(see Comment)*	**Various studies** indicate improved outcome when azithro added to a β-lactam *(CID 36:389 & 1239, 2003; ArIM 164:1837, 2001 & 159:2562, 1999)*. Similar results in prospective study of critically ill pts with pneumococcal bacteremia *(AJRCCM 170:440, 2004)*. **Ertapenem** could substitute for ceftriaxone; need azithro for atypical pathogens. Do not use if suspect P. aeruginosa. **Legionella:** Not all Legionella species detected by urine antigen; if suspicious culture or PCR on airway secretions. Value of specific diagnosis: *CID 46:1356 & 1365, 2008*. In patients with normal sinus rhythm and not receiving beta-blockers, relative bradycardia suggests Legionella, psittacosis, Q-fever, or typhoid fever *(Clin Micro Infect 6:633, 2000)*.
Community-acquired, hospitalized—IN ICU Empiric therapy	**If concomitant with or post-influenza**, S. aureus and S. pneumoniae possible.	**Vanco** 1 gm IV q12h + (**Levo** 750 mg IV q24h or **moxi** 400 mg IV q24h)	**Linezolid** 600 mg IV bid + (**levo** or **moxi**)	Sputum gram stain may help. *S. aureus* post-influenza ref: *EID 12:894, 2006* Empiric therapy vs. MRSA decreases risk of mortality *(CCM 34:2069, 2006)*
Community-acquired, hospitalized—IN ICU Empiric therapy	**Suspect aerobic gm-neg bacilli:** eg, P. aeruginosa and/or life-threatening infection *(see comment)*. Hypoxic and/or hypotensive "Cover" S. pneumo & Legionella	Anti-pseudomonal beta-lactam[26] + (respiratory **FQ or aminoglycoside**). Add **azithro** if no FQ *Drugs and doses in footnote[26].*	If severe IgE-mediated beta-lactam allergy **aztreonam** + **FQ** or (**aztreonam + aminoglycoside + azithro**).	At risk for gm-neg rod pneumonia due to: alcoholism with necrotizing pneumonia, underlying chronic bronchiectasis (e.g. cystic fibrosis), chronic tracheostomy and/or mechanical ventilation, febrile neutropenia and pulmonary infiltrates, septic shock, underlying malignancy, or organ failure.
	Risk of Pen G-resistant S. pneumoniae 2° antibiotic use in last 3 months.	High dose IV **amp (or Pen G)** + **azithro** + **respiratory FQ**	Beta-lactam allergy: **vanco** + **respiratory FQ**	**If Pen G MIC>4 mg/mL, vanco. Very rare event.**
Health care-associated pneumonia (HCAP) Ref: *CID 46 (Suppl 4): S296, 2008.*	HCAP used to designate large diverse population of pts with many co-morbidities who reside in nursing homes, other long-term care facilities, require home IV therapy or are dialysis pts. Pneumonia in these pts frequently resembles hospital-acquired pneumonia *(see next section)*.			

[26] Antipseudomonal beta-lactams: **Aztreonam** 2 gm IV q6h; **piperacillin** 3 gm IV q4h; **piperacillin/tazobactam** 3.375 gm IV q4h or 4.5 gm IV q6h or 4-hr infusion of 3.375 gm q8h(high dose for Pseudomonas); **cefepime** 2 gm IV q12h; **ceftazidime** 2 gm IV q8h; **doripenem** 500 mg IV q8h as 1 or 4 hr infusion; **imipenem/cilastatin** 500 mg IV q6h; **meropenem** 1 gm IV q8h; **gentamicin or tobramycin** *(see Table 10D, pg 101)*. FQ for P. aeruginosa: **CIP** 400 mg IV q8h or **levo** 750 mg IV once daily. **Respitatory FQs: levofloxacin** 750 mg IV q24h or **moxifloxacin** 400 mg IV q24h; **high-dose ampicillin** 2 gm IV q6h; **azithromycin** 500 mg IV q24h; **vanco** 1 gm IV q12h.

TABLE 1A (35)

ANATOMIC SITE/DIAGNOSIS/ MODIFYING CIRCUMSTANCES	ETIOLOGIES (usual)	SUGGESTED REGIMENS*		ADJUNCT DIAGNOSTIC OR THERAPEUTIC MEASURES AND COMMENTS
		PRIMARY	ALTERNATIVE§	
LUNG/Bronchi/Pneumonia/Adults (over age 18) *(continued)*				
Hospital-acquired—usually with mechanical ventilation (VAP) (empiric therapy) Refs: *U.S. Guidelines: AJRCCM 171:388, 2005; U.S. Review: JAMA 297:1583, 2007; Canadian Guidelines: Can J Inf Dis Med Micro 19:19, 2008; British Guidelines: JAC 62:5, 2008*	Highly variable depending on clinical setting: S. pneumo, S. aureus, Legionella, coliforms, P. aeruginosa, stenotrophomonas, acinetobacter[27], anaerobes all possible	(**IMP** 0.5 gm IV q6h or **DORI**[NAI] 500 mg IV q8H (1 or 4-hr infusion) or **MER** 1 gm IV q8h)[27] plus, if suspect legionella or bioterrorism, **respiratory FQ (Levo or Moxi)** **NOTE**: *Regimen not active vs.* ***MRSA***—see specific rx below *See Comment regarding diagnosis* ***Dosages:*** *See footnote*[26]. Duration of therapy, *see footnote*[29]	If suspect P. aeruginosa, empirically start 2 anti-P. are drugs to increase likelihood that at least one will be active, e.g.: (**IMP** or **CFP** or **PIP-TZ**[28]) + (**CIP** or **tobra**). Ref: *CCM 35:1888, 2007*	**Dx of ventilator-associated pneumonia:** Fever & lung infiltrates often **not** pneumonia. Quantitative cultures helpful: bronchoalveolar lavage (>10^4 per mL pos.) or protect. spec. brush (>10^3 per mL pos.) Ref.: *AJRCCM 165:867, 2002; AnIM 132:621, 2000.* **Microbial etiology:** No empiric regimen covers all possibilities. Regimens listed active majority of **S. pneumo**, **legionella**, & **most coliforms**. Regimens **not active vs. MRSA, Stenotrophomonas & others;** *see below: Specific therapy when culture results known.* **Ventilator-associated pneumonia—Prevention:** Keep head of bed elevated 30° or more. Remove N-G, endotracheal tubes as soon as possible. If available, continuous subglottic suctioning. Chlorhexidine oral care. Refs.: *Chest 130:251, 2006; AJRCCM 173:1297, 1348, 2006.* **Misc. clarithro** accelerated resolution of VAP *(CID 46:1157, 2008)*. Silver-coated endotracheal tubes reported to reduce incidence of VAP *(JAMA 300:805 & 842, 2008)*.
Hospital- or community-acquired, neutropenic pt (<500 neutrophils per mm³)	Any of organisms listed under community- & hospital-acquired + fungi (aspergillus). *See Table 11*	*See Hospital-acquired, immediately above*. Vanco not included in initial therapy unless high suspicion of infected IV access or drug-resistant S. pneumo. Ampho not used unless still febrile after 3 days or high clinical likelihood. *See Comment*		See consensus document on management of febrile neutropenic pt: *CID 34:730, 2002*.
Adults—Selected specific therapy after culture results (sputum, blood, pleural fluid, etc.) available. *Also see Table 2, page 63*				
Acinetobacter *baumannii* *(See also Table 5);* Ref: *NEJM 358:1271, 2008*	Patients with VAP	Use **IMP** if susceptible	If **IMP** resistant: **colistin** (polymyxin E). In U.S.: 2.5-5 mg/kg/day div into 2-4 doses	Sulbactam portion of AM-SB often active; dose: 3 gm IV q6h. Reported more efficacious than colistin. *(JAC 61:1369, 2008 & J Inf 56:432, 2008)*. Colistin summary: *LnID 8:403, 2008*
Burkholderia (Pseudomonas) pseudomallei (etiology of melioidosis) Can cause primary or secondary skin infection *(CID 47:603, 2008)*.	Gram-negative	**Initial parenteral rx:** **Ceftazidime** 30–50 mg per kg IV q8h or **IMP** 20 mg per kg IV q8h. Rx minimum 10 days & improving, then po therapy → *see Alternative column*	**Post-parenteral po rx:** **Adults** *(see Comment for children)*: **Chloro** 10 mg per kg q6h times 8 wks; **Doxy** 2 mg per kg bid times 20 wks; **TMP-SMX** 5 mg per kg (TMP component) bid times 20 wks	**Children ≤8 yrs old & pregnancy:** For oral regimen, use **AM-CL-ER** 1000/62.5, 2 tabs po bid times 20 wks. Even with compliance, relapse rate is 10%. Max. daily ceftazidime dose: 6 gm. Tigecycline: No clinical data but active in vitro *(AAC 50:1555, 2006)*
Haemophilus influenzae	β-lactamase negative	**AMP** IV, **amox** po, **TMP-SMX**, **azithro/clarithro**, **doxy**		25–35% strains β-lactamase positive. ↑ resistance to both TMP-SMX and doxy. *See Table 10C, page 92 for dosages*. High % of commensal H. hemolyticus misidentified as H. influenza *(JID 195:81, 2007)*.
	β-lactamase positive	**AM-CL**, **O Ceph 2/3**, **P Ceph 3**, **FQ** Dosage: *Table 10C*		
Klebsiella sp.—ESBL pos. & other coliforms[30]	β-lactamase positive	**Dori, IMP** or **MER**; if resistant, **polymyxin E (colistin) or B** Usually several weeks of therapy.		ESBL[30] inactivates all cephalosporins, β-lactam/β-lactamase inhibitor drug activ. not predictable; co-resistance to all FQs & often aminoglycosides.

[27] If Acinetobacter sp., **susceptibility to IMP & MER** may be discordant *(CID 41:758, 2005)*.
[28] **PIP-TZ** for P. aeruginosa pneumonia : 3.375 gm IV over 4 hrs & repeat q8h *(CID 44:357, 2007)* plus **tobra.**
[29] Dogma on duration of therapy not possible with so many variables: ie, certainty of diagnosis, infecting organism, severity of infection and number/serverity of co-morbidities. Agree with efforts to de-escalate & shorten course. Treat at least 7-8 days. Need clinical evidence of response: fever resolution, improved oxygenation, falling WBC. Refs: *AJRCCM 171:388, 2005; CID 43:S75, 2006; COID 19:185, 2006.*
[30] **ESBL** = Extended spectrum beta-lactamase

 NOTE: All dosage recommendations are for adults (unless otherwise indicated) and assume normal renal function.

TABLE 1A (36)

ANATOMIC SITE/DIAGNOSIS/ MODIFYING CIRCUMSTANCES	ETIOLOGIES (usual)	SUGGESTED REGIMENS*		ADJUNCT DIAGNOSTIC OR THERAPEUTIC MEASURES AND COMMENTS
		PRIMARY	ALTERNATIVE§	
LUNG/Pneumonia/Adults— Selected specific therapy after culture results (sputum, blood, pleural fluid, etc.) available *(continued)*				
Legionella species Relative bradycardia common feature	**Hospitalized/ immunocompromised**	**Azithro** 500 mg **IV** or **Levo** 750 mg **IV** or **Moxi** 400 mg **IV**. *See Table 10C, pages 96 & 98 for dosages.* Treat for 7–14 days *(CID 39:1734, 2004)*		Legionella website: www.legionella.org. Two studies support superiority of **Levo** over macrolides *(CID 40:794 & 800, 2005), although not FDA-approved.*
Moraxella catarrhalis	93% β-lactamase positive	**AM-CL**, **O Ceph 2/3**, **P Ceph 2/3**, **macrolide**[31], **FQ**, **TMP-SMX**. **Doxy** another option. *See Table 10C, page 92 for dosages*		
Pseudomonas aeruginosa	Often ventilator-associated	**(PIP-TZ** 3.375 gm IV q4h or prefer 4-hr infusion of 3.375 gm q8h) + **tobra** 5 mg/kg IV once q24h *(see Table 10D, page 101)*. Could substitute anti-pseudomonal **cephalosporin** or **carbapenem** (**DORI**, **IMP**, **MER**) for **PIP-TZ** if pt. strain is susceptible.		**NOTE: PIP-TZ** for P. aeruginosa *(CID 44:357, 2007)*; other options: **CFP** 2 gm IV q 12h; **CIP** 400 mg IV q8h + **PIP-TZ**; **IMP** 500 mg IV q6h + **CIP** 400 mg IV q12h; if multi-drug resistant, **polymyxin**—parenteral & perhaps by inhalation, 80 mg bid *(CID 41:754, 2005)*.
Staphylococcus aureus Duration of treatment: 2-3 wks if just pneumonia; 4-6 wks if concomitant endocarditis and/or osteomyelitis. *IDSA Guidelines, CID 52 (Feb 1):1, 2011.*	Nafcillin/oxacillin susceptible	**Nafcillin/oxacillin** 2 gm IV q4h	**Vanco** 1 gm IV q12h or **linezolid** 600 mg IV q12h	Increase dose of vancomycin to achieve target concentrations of 15-20 mcg/ml. Some authorities recommend a 25-30 mg/kg loading dose (actual body weight in severely ill patients *(CID 49:325, 2009)*. Linezolid non-inferior to vancomycin in 2 randomized trials with subset analysis suggesting improved survival in MRSA pneumonia. Ongoing trial compares linezolid to vanco for MRSA pneumonia.
	MRSA	**Vanco** 1 g q12h IV or **Linezolid** 600 mg q12h	**Dapto** probably not an option; pneumonia developed during dapto rx *(CID 49:1286, 2009)*.	
Stenotrophomonas maltophilia		**TMP-SMX**	**TC-CL** ± **aztreonam**	Potential synergy: **TMP-SMX** + **TC-CL**.
Streptococcus pneumoniae	Penicillin-susceptible	**AMP** 2 gm IV q6h, **amox** 1 gm po tid, **macrolide**[31], **pen G** IV[32], **doxy**, **O Ceph 2**, **P Ceph 2/3**. *See Table 10C, page 92 for other dosages.* Treat until afebrile, 3-5 days (min. of 5 days).		
	Penicillin-resistant, high level	**FQs** with enhanced activity: **Gemi**, **Levo**, **Moxi**; **P Ceph 3** (resistance rare); high-dose IV **AMP**; **vanco** IV—*see Table 5, page 74 for more data*. If all options not possible (e.g., allergy), linezolid active: 600 mg IV or po q12h. *Dosages Table 10C.* Treat until afebrile, 3-5 days (min. of 5 days). In CAP trial, Ceftaroline 600 mg IV q12h superior to Ceftriaxone *(CID 51:641, 2010)*.		
Yersinia pestis (Plague) *CID 49:736, 2009*	Aerosol Y. pestis	**Gentamicin** 5 mg/kg IV q24h	**Doxy** 200 mg IV times 1, then 100 mg IV bid	TMP-SMX used as prophylaxis for plague pneumonia *(CID 40:1166, 2005)*. Chloro effective but potentially toxic. Cephalosporins and FQs effective in animal models.
LUNG—Other Specific Infections				
Actinomycosis	A. Israelii and rarely others	**AMP** 50 mg/kg/day IV div in 3-4 doses x 4-6 wks, then **Pen VK** 2-4 gm/day po x 3-6 wks	**Doxy** or **ceftriaxone** or **clinda** or **erythro**	Can use **Pen G** instead of AMP: 10-20 million units/day IV x 4-6 wks.

[31] **Macrolide** = azithromycin, clarithromycin and erythromycin.
[32] **IV Pen G dosage:** no meningitis, 2 million units IV q4h. If concomitant meningitis, 4 million units IV q4h.

TABLE 1A (37)

ANATOMIC SITE/DIAGNOSIS/ MODIFYING CIRCUMSTANCES	ETIOLOGIES (usual)	SUGGESTED REGIMENS*		ADJUNCT DIAGNOSTIC OR THERAPEUTIC MEASURES AND COMMENTS
		PRIMARY	ALTERNATIVE[§]	
LUNG—Other Specific Infections *(continued)*				
Anthrax **Inhalation** (applies to oropharyngeal & gastrointestinal forms): **Treatment** (Cutaneous: *See page 49)* Ref: *www.bt.cdc.gov*	Bacillus anthracis **To report possible bioterrorism event: 770-488-7100** Plague, tularemia: *See page 42.* Chest x-ray: mediastinal widening & pleural effusion	**Adults (including pregnancy): (CIP** 400 mg IV q12h) or (**Levo** 500 mg IV q24h) or (**doxy** 100 mg IV q12h) **plus (clindamycin** 900 mg IV q8h &/or **RIF** 300 mg IV q12h). Switch to po when able & lower CIP to 500 mg po bid; clinda to 450 mg po q8h; & RIF 300 mg po bid. Treat times 60 days.	**Children:** (**CIP** 10 mg/kg IV q12h or 15 mg/kg po q12h) or (**Doxy**: >8 y/o & >45 kg: 100 mg IV q12h; >8 y/o & ≤45 kg: 2.2 mg/kg IV q12h; ≤8 y/o: 2.2 mg/kg IV q12h) **plus clindamycin** 7.5 mg/kg IV q6h **and/or RIF** 20 mg/kg (max. 600 mg) IV q24h. Treat times 60 days. *See Table 16, page 187 for oral dosage.*	1. Clinda may block toxin production 2. Rifampin penetrates CSF & intracellular sites. 3. If isolate shown penicillin-susceptible: a. **Adults: Pen G** 4 million units IV q4h b. **Children: Pen G** <12 y/o: 50,000 units per kg IV q6h; >12 y/o: 4 million units IV q4h c. Constitutive & inducible β-lactamases—do not use pen or amp alone. 4. Do not use cephalosporins or TMP-SMX. 5. Erythro, azithro activity borderline; clarithro active. 6. No person-to-person spread. 7. Antitoxins in development 8. Moxi should work, but no clinical data 9. Case report of survival with use of anthrax immunoglobulin *(CID 44:968, 2007).*
Anthrax, prophylaxis	Info: www.bt.cdc.gov	**Adults (including pregnancy) or children >50 kg: (CIP** 500 mg po bid or **Levo** 500 mg po q24h) x 60 days. **Children <50 kg: CIP** 20–30 mg/kg per day div q12h x 60 days or **levo** 8 mg/kg q12h x 60 days	**Adults (including pregnancy): Doxy** 100 mg po bid x 60 days. **Children** *(see Comment)*: **Doxy** >8 y/o & >45 kg: 100 mg po bid; >8 y/o & ≤45 kg: 2.2 mg/kg po bid; ≤8 y/o: 2.2 mg/kg po bid. All for 60 days.	1. Once organism shows suscept. to penicillin, switch to amoxicillin 80 mg per kg per day div. q8h (max. 500 mg q8h); pregnant pt to amoxicillin 500 mg po tid. 2. Do **not** use cephalosporins or TMP-SMX. 3. Other FQs (Gati, Moxi) & clarithro should work but no clinical experience.
Aspiration pneumonia ± lung abscess	Transthoracic culture in 90 pts—% of total isolates: anaerobes 34%, Gm-pos. cocci 26%, S. milleri 16%, Klebsiella pneumoniae 25%, nocardia 3%	**PIP-TZ** 3.375 gm IV q6h or 4-hr infusion of 3.375 gm q8h *(CID 44:357, 2007).*	**Ceftriaxone** 1 gm IV q24h plus **metro** 500 mg IV q6h or 1 gm IV q12h	Suggested regimens based on retrospective evaluation of 90 pts with cultures obtained by transthoracic aspiration *(CID 40:915 & 923, 2005).* Surprising frequency of Klebsiella pneumoniae. **Moxi** 400 mg IV/po q24h another option *(CID 41:764, 2005).* **Clindamycin** 300 mg po tid is also effective for infection due to oral anaerobes or streptococci
Chronic pneumonia with fever, night sweats and weight loss	M. tuberculosis, coccidioidomycosis, histoplasmosis	*See Table 11, Table 12.* For risk associated with TNF inhibitors, *see CID 41(Suppl.3):S187, 2005.*		HIV+, foreign-born, alcoholism, contact with TB, travel into developing countries
Cystic fibrosis **Acute exacerbation of pulmonary symptoms** Ref: *AJRCCM 180:802, 2009* *(Continued on next page)*	S. aureus or H. influenzae early in disease; P. aeruginosa later in disease	**For P. aeruginosa:** (Peds doses) **Tobra** 3.3 mg/kg q8h or 12 mg/kg IV q24h. Combine tobra with (**PIP** or **ticarcillin** 100 mg/kg q6h) **or ceftaz** 50 mg/kg IV q8h to max of 6 gm per day. If resistant to above, **CIP/Levo** used if P. aeruginosa susceptible. *See footnote[33] & Comment*	**For S. aureus: (1) MSSA—oxacillin/nafcillin** 2 gm IV q4h *(Peds dose, Table 16).* **(2) MRSA—vanco** 1 gm q12h & check serum levels. *See Comment*	Cystic Fibrosis Foundation Guidelines: 1. Combination therapy for P. aeruginosa infection. 2. Once-daily dosing for aminoglycosides. 3. Need more data on continuous infusion beta-lactam therapy. 4. Routine use of steroid not recommended. For chronic suppression of P. aeruginosa, **inhaled phenol-free tobra** 300 mg bid x 28 days, then no rx x 28 days, then repeat cycle *(AJRCCM 167:841, 2003).* Inhaled aztreonam lysine in Phase III trials.

[33] Other options: (Tobra + aztreonam 50 mg per kg IV q8h); (IMP 15–25 mg per kg IV q6h + tobra); **CIP commonly used in children**, e.g., CIP IV/po + ceftaz IV *(LnID 3:537, 2003).*

TABLE 1A (38)

ANATOMIC SITE/DIAGNOSIS/ MODIFYING CIRCUMSTANCES	ETIOLOGIES (usual)	SUGGESTED REGIMENS*		ADJUNCT DIAGNOSTIC OR THERAPEUTIC MEASURES AND COMMENTS
		PRIMARY	ALTERNATIVE[§]	
LUNG—Other Specific Infections *(continued)*				
(Continued from previous page)	Burkholderia (Pseudomonas) cepacia	**TMP-SMX** 5 mg per kg (TMP) IV q6h	**Chloro** 15–20 mg per kg IV/po q6h	B. cepacia has become a major pathogen. Patients develop progressive respiratory failure, 62% mortality at 1 yr. **Fail to respond to aminoglycosides**, piperacillin, & ceftazidime. Patients with B. cepacia should be isolated from other CF patients.
		For other alternatives, see Table 2		
Empyema. Refs.: Pleural effus on review: *CID 45:1480, 2007*				
Neonatal	Staph. aureus	*See Pneumonia, neonatal, page 34*		Drainage indicated.
Infants/children (1 month–5 yrs)	Staph. aureus, Strep. pneumoniae, H. influenzae	*See Pneumonia, age 1 month–5 years, page 34*		Drainage indicated.
Child >5 yrs to ADULT—Diagnostic thoracentesis; chest tube for empyemas				
Acute, usually parapneumonic *For dosage, see Table 10 or footnote page 23* Microbiologic diagnosis: *CID 42:1135, 2006.*	Strep. pneumoniae, Group A strep	**Cefotaxime** or **ceftriaxone** *(Dosage, see footnote[14] page 23)*	**Vanco**	In large multicenter double-blind trial, **intrapleural streptokinase** did not improve mortality, reduce the need for surgery or the length of hospitalization *(NEJM 352:865, 2005)*. Success using S. pneumoniae urine antigen test on pleural fluid *(Chest 131:1442, 2007)*.
	Staph. aureus: Check for MRSA	**Nafcillin** or **oxacillin** if MSSA	**Vanco** or **linezolid** if MRSA.	Usually complication of S. aureus pneumonia &/or bacteremia.
	H. influenzae	**Ceftriaxone**	**TMP-SMX** or **AM-SB**	Pleomorphic Gm-neg. bacilli. ↑ resistance to TMP-SMX.
Subacute/chronic	Anaerobic strep, Strep. milleri, Bacteroides sp., Enterobacteriaceae, M. tuberculosis	**Clinda** 450–900 mg IV q8h + **ceftriaxone**	**Cefoxitin** or **IMP** or **TC-CL** or **PIP-TZ** or **AM-SB** *(Dosage, see footnote[14] page 23)*	If organisms not seen, treat as subacute. Drainage. R/O tuberculosis or tumor. Pleural biopsy with culture for mycobacteria and histology if TBc suspected.
Human immunodeficiency virus infection (HIV+): See *Sanford Guide to HIV/AIDS Therapy*				
CD4 T-lymphocytes <200 per mm³ or clinical AIDS Dry cough, progressive dyspnea, & diffuse infiltrate **Prednisone first if suspect pneumocystis *(see Comment)***	Pneumocystis carini most likely; also M. tbc, fungi, Kaposi's sarcoma, & lymphoma NOTE: AIDS pts may develop pneumonia due to DRSP or other pathogens—*see next box below*	*Rx listed here is for* **severe** *pneumocystis; see Table 13, page 135 for po regimens for* **mild** *disease.* **Prednisone 1st *(see Comment)*, then:** **TMP-SMX** [IV: 15 mg per kg per day div q8h (TMP component) or po: 2 DS tabs q8h], total of 21 days	(**Clinda** 600 mg IV q8h + **primaquine** 30 mg po q24h) or (**pentamidine isethionate** 4 mg per kg per day IV) times 21 days. *See Comment*	**Diagnosis (induced sputum or bronchial wash) for:** histology or monoclonal antibody strains or PCR. Serum beta-glucon (Fungitell) levels under study *(CID 46:1928 & 1930, 2008)*. **Prednisone 40 mg bid po times 5 days then 40 mg q24h po times 5 days then 20 mg q24h po times 11 days is indicated with PCP (pO_2 <70 mmHg), should be given at initiation of anti-PCP rx; don't wait until pt's condition deteriorates.** If PCP studies negative, consider bacterial pneumonia, TBc, cocci, histo, crypto, Kaposi's sarcoma or lymphoma. **Pentamidine not active vs. bacterial pathogens. NOTE: Pneumocystis resistant to TMP-SMX, albeit rare, does exist.**
CD4 T-lymphocytes normal Acute onset, purulent sputum & pulmonary infiltrates ± pleuritic pain. **Isolate pt until TBc excluded: Adults**	Strep. pneumoniae, H. influenzae, aerobic Gm-neg. bacilli (including P. aeruginosa), Legionella rare, M. tbc	Ceftriaxone 1 gm IV q24h (over age 65 1 gm IV q24h) + **azithro**. Could use **Levo,** or **Moxi** IV as alternative *(see Comment)*		If Gram stain of sputum shows Gm-neg. bacilli, options include **P Ceph 3 AP**, **TC-CL**, **PIP-TZ**, **IMP**, or **MER**. **FQs**: **Levo** 750 mg po/IV q24h; **Moxi** 400 mg po/IV q24h. Gati not available in US due to hypo- & hyperglycemic reactions.
As above: Children	Same as adult with HIV + lymphoid interstitial pneumonia (LIP)	As for HIV+ adults with pneumonia. If diagnosis is LIP, rx with steroids.		In children with AIDS, LIP responsible for 1/3 of pulmonary complications, usually >1 yr of age vs. PCP, which is seen at <1 yr of age. Clinically: clubbing, hepatosplenomegaly, salivary glands enlarged (take up gallium), lymphocytosis.

 NOTE: All dosage recommendations are for adults (unless otherwise indicated) and assume normal renal function.

TABLE 1A (39)

ANATOMIC SITE/DIAGNOSIS/ MODIFYING CIRCUMSTANCES	ETIOLOGIES (usual)	SUGGESTED REGIMENS*		ADJUNCT DIAGNOSTIC OR THERAPEUTIC MEASURES AND COMMENTS
		PRIMARY	ALTERNATIVE[§]	
LUNG—Other Specific Infections *(continued)*				
Nocardia pneumonia Expert Help: Wallace Lab (+1) 903-877-7680; CDC (+1) 404-639-3158 Ref: *Medicine 88:250, 2009.*	N. asteroides, N. brasiliensis	**TMP-SMX** 15 mg/kg/day IV/po in 2-4 divided doses + **Imipenem** 500 mg IV q6h for first 3-4 weeks then **TMP-SMX** 10 mg/kg/day in 2-4 divided doses x 3-6 mo.	**IMP** 500 mg IV q6h + **amikacin** 7.5 mg/kg IV q12h x 3-4 wks & then po **TMP-SMX**	**Duration:** 3 mos. if immunocompetent; 6 mos. if immunocompromised. **Measure peak sulfonamide levels**: Target is 100-150 mcg/mL 2 hrs post po dose. **Linezolid** active in vitro *(An Pharmacother 41:1694, 2007)*. In vitro resistance to TMP-SMX may be increasing *(Clin Infect Dis 51:1445, 2010)*, but whether this is associated with worse outcomes is not known.
Tularemia **Inhalational tularemia** Ref.: *JAMA 285:2763, 2001& www.bt.cdc.gov*	Francisella tularemia **Treatment**	(**Streptomycin** 15 mg per kg IV bid) or (**gentamicin** 5 mg per kg IV qd) times 10 days	**Doxy** 100 mg IV or po bid times 14–21 days or **CIP** 400 mg IV (or 750 mg po) bid times 14–21 days	For pediatric doses, *see Table 16, page 187*. Pregnancy: *as for non-pregnant adults*. **Tobramycin** should work.
	Post-exposure prophylaxis	**Doxy** 100 mg po bid times 14 days	**CIP** 500 mg po bid times 14 days	For pediatric doses, *see Table 16, page 187*. Pregnancy: *As for non-pregnant adults*
Viral (interstitial) pneumonia suspected ***See Influenza, Table 14A, page 154.*** Ref: *Chest 133:1221, 2008.*	Consider: **Influenza**, adenovirus, coronavirus (SARS), hantavirus, metapneumovirus, parainfluenza virus, respiratory syncytial virus	**Oseltamivir** 75 mg po bid for 5 days or **zanamivir** two 5 mg inhalations twice a day for 5 days.		No known efficacious drugs for adenovirus, coronavirus (SARS), hantavirus, metapneumovirus, parainfluenza or RSV. Need travel (SARS) & exposure (Hanta) history. RSV and human metapneumovirus as serious as influenza in the elderly *(NEJM 352:1749 & 1810, 2005; CID 44:1152 & 1159, 2007)*.
LYMPH NODES (approaches below apply to lymphadenitis without an obvious primary source)				
Lymphadenitis, acute				
Generalized	Etiologies: EBV, early HIV infection, syphilis, toxoplasma, tularemia, Lyme disease, sarcoid, lymphoma, systemic lupus erythematosus, and **Kikuchi-Fujimoto** disease. Complete history and physical examination followed by appropriate serological tests. Treat specific agent(s).			
Regional				
Cervical—see cat-scratch disease (CSD), below	CSD (B. henselae), Grp A strep, Staph. aureus, anaerobes, M. TBc (scrofula), M. avium, M. scrofulaceum, M. malmoense, toxo, tularemia	History & physical exam directs evaluation. If nodes fluctuant, aspirate and base rx on Gram & acid-fast stains. **Kikuchi-Fujimoto** disease causes fever and benign self-limited adenopathy; the etiology is unknown *(CID 39:138, 2004)*.		
Inguinal				
Sexually transmitted	HSV, chancroid, syphilis, LGV			
Not sexually transmitted	GAS, SA, tularemia, CSD, Y. pestis (plague)	Consider bubonic plague & glandular tularemia.		
Axillary	GAS, SA, CSD, tularemia, Y. pestis, sporotrichosis	Consider bubonic plague & glandular tularemia.		
Extremity, with associated nodular lymphangitis	Sporotrichosis, leishmania, Nocardia brasiliensis, Mycobacterium marinum, Mycobacterium chelonae, tularemia	Treatment varies with specific etiology		A distinctive form of lymphangitis characterized by subcutaneous swellings along inflamed lymphatic channels. Primary site of skin invasion usually present; regional adenopathy variable.

 NOTE: All dosage recommendations are for adults (unless otherwise indicated) and assume normal renal function.

TABLE 1A (40)

ANATOMIC SITE/DIAGNOSIS/ MODIFYING CIRCUMSTANCES	ETIOLOGIES (usual)	SUGGESTED REGIMENS*		ADJUNCT DIAGNOSTIC OR THERAPEUTIC MEASURES AND COMMENTS
		PRIMARY	ALTERNATIVE[§]	
LYMPH NODES/Lymphadenitis, acute/Regional *(continued)*				
Nocardia lymphadenitis & skin abscesses	N. asteroides, N. brasiliensis	**TMP-SMX** 5-10 mg/kg/day based on TMP IV/po div in 2-4 doses	**Sulfisoxazole** 2 gm po qid or **minocycline** 100-200 mg po bid.	**Duration:** 3 mos. if immunocompetent; 6 mos. if immunocompromised. **Linezolid:** 600 mg po bid reported effective *(An Pharmacother 41:1694, 2007)*.
Cat-scratch disease—immunocompetent patient Axillary/epitrochlear nodes 46%, neck 26%, inguinal 17%	Bartonella henselae	**Azithro** dosage—**Adults** (>45.5 kg): 500 mg po x 1, then 250 mg/day x 4 days. **Children** (<45.5 kg): liquid azithro 10 mg/kg x 1, then 5 mg/kg per day x 4 days. Rx is controversial	No therapy; resolves in 2–6 mos. Needle aspiration relieves pain in suppurative nodes. Avoid I&D.	**Clinical:** Approx. 10% nodes suppurate. Atypical presentation in <5% pts, i.e., lung nodules, liver/spleen lesions, Parinaud's oculoglandular syndrome, CNS manifestations in 2% of pts (encephalitis, peripheral neuropathy, retinitis), FUO. **Dx:** Cat exposure. Positive IFA serology. Rarely need biopsy. **Rx:** Only 1 prospective randomized blinded study, used azithro with ↑ rapidity of resolution of enlarged lymph nodes *(PIDJ 17:447, 1998)*. **Note:** In elderly, endocarditis more frequent; lymphadenitis less frequent *(CID 41:969, 2005)*.
MOUTH				
Aphthous stomatitis, recurrent	Etiology unknown	Topical steroids (Kenalog in Orabase) may ↓ pain and swelling; if AIDS, *see* SANFORD GUIDE TO HIV/AIDS THERAPY.		
Buccal cellulitis Children <5 yrs	H. influenzae	**Cefuroxime** or **ceftriaxone** *Dosage: see Table 16, page 187*	**AM-CL** or **TMP-SMX**	With Hib immunization, invasive H. influenzae infections have ↓ by 95%. Now occurring in infants prior to immunization.
Candida Stomatitis ("Thrush")	C. albicans	**Fluconazole**	Echinocandin	*See Table 11, page 104*
Herpetic stomatitis	Herpes simplex virus 1 & 2	*See Table 14*		
Submandibular space infection, bilateral (Ludwig's angina)	Oral anaerobes, facultative streptococci	(**PIP-TZ** or **TC-CL**) or (**Pen G** IV + **Metro** IV)	**Clinda** 600 mg IV q6-8h (for Pen-allergic pt)	Ensure adequate airway
Ulcerative gingivitis (Vincent's angina or Trench mouth)	Oral anaerobes + vitamin deficiency	**Pen G** po/IV + **Metro** po/IV	**Clinda**	Replete vitamins (A-D). Can mimic scurvy. Severe form is NOMA (Cancrum oris)*(Ln 368:147, 2006)*
MUSCLE				
"Gas gangrene". Contaminated traumatic wound. Can be spontaneous without trauma.	Cl. perfringens, other histo-toxic Clostridium sp.	(**Clinda** 900 mg IV q8h) + (**pen G** 24 million units/day div. q4–6h IV)	**Ceftriaxone** 2 gm IV q12h or **erythro** 1 gm q6h IV (not by bolus)	Surgical debridement primary therapy. **Hyperbaric oxygen** adjunctive: efficacy debated, consider if debridement not complete or possible. Clinda decreases toxin production.
Pyomyositis	Staph. aureus, Group A strep, (rarely Gm-neg. bacilli), variety of anaerobic organisms	(**Nafcillin** or **oxacillin** 2 gm IV q4h) or [**P Ceph 1** (**cefazolin** 2 gm IV q8h)] if **MSSA**	**Vanco** 1 gm IV q12h if **MRSA**	Common in tropics; rare, but occurs, in temperate zones. Follows exercise or muscle injury, *see Necrotizing fasciitis*. Now seen in HIV/AIDS. Add **metro** if anaerobes suspected or proven.

 NOTE: All dosage recommendations are for adults (unless otherwise indicated) and assume normal renal function.

TABLE 1A (41)

ANATOMIC SITE/DIAGNOSIS/ MODIFYING CIRCUMSTANCES	ETIOLOGIES (usual)	SUGGESTED REGIMENS*		ADJUNCT DIAGNOSTIC OR THERAPEUTIC MEASURES AND COMMENTS
		PRIMARY	ALTERNATIVE[§]	
PANCREAS: Review: *NEJM 354:2142, 2006.*				
Acute alcoholic (without necrosis) (idiopathic) pancreatitis	Not bacterial	None No necrosis on CT	1–9% become infected but prospective studies show no advantage of prophylactic antimicrobials. Observe for pancreatic abscesses or necrosis which require therapy.	
Post-necrotizing pancreatitis; infected pseudocyst; pancreatic abscess	Enterobacteriaceae, enterococci, S. aureus, S. epidermidis, anaerobes, candida	Need culture of abscess/infected pseudocyst to direct therapy; **PIP-TZ** is reasonable empiric therapy		Can often get specimen by fine-needle aspiration.
Antimicrobic prophylaxis, necrotizing pancreatitis	As above	If > 30% pancreatic necrosis on CT scan (with contrast), initiate antibiotic therapy: **IMP** 0.5-1 gm IV q6h or **MER** 1 gm IV q8h. No need for empiric Fluconazole. If patient worsens CT guided aspiration for culture & sensitivity. Controversial: *Cochrane Database Sys Rev 2003: CD 002941; Gastroenterol 126:977, 2004; Ann Surg 245:674, 2007.*		
PAROTID GLAND				
"Hot" tender parotid swelling	S. aureus, S. pyogenes, oral flora, & aerobic Gm-neg. bacilli (rare), mumps, rarely enteroviruses/ influenza: **Nafcillin** or **oxacillin** 2 gm IV q4h if MSSA; **vanco** if MRSA			Predisposing factors: stone(s) in Stensen's duct, dehydration. Therapy depends on ID of specific etiologic organism.
"Cold" non-tender parotid swelling	Granulomatous disease (e.g., mycobacteria, fungi, sarcoidosis, Sjögren's syndrome), drugs (iodides, et al.), diabetes, cirrhosis, tumors			History/lab results may narrow differential; may need biopsy for diagnosis
PERITONEUM/PERITONITIS: *Reference—CID 50:133, 2010*				
Primary (spontaneous bacterial peritonitis, SBP) *Hepatology 49:2087, 2009.* Dx: Pos. culture & ≥ 250 neutrophils/mm³ of ascitic fluid	Enterobacteriaceae 63%, S. pneumo 9%, enterococci 6–10%, anaerobes <1%. Extended β-lactamase (ESBL) positive Klebsiella species.	[**Cefotaxime** 2 gm IV q8h (if life-threatening, q4h)] or [**TC-CL** or **PIP-TZ** or **AM-SB**] OR [**ceftriaxone** 2 gm IV q24h] or [**ERTA** 1 gm IV q24h] **If resistant E. coli/Klebsiella species (ESBL+), then:** (**DORI**, **ERTA**, **IMP** or **MER**) or (**FQ: CIP**, **Levo**, **Moxi**) *(Dosage in footnote[34])*. Check in vitro susceptibility.		One-year **risk of SBP** in pts with ascites and cirrhosis as high as 29% *(Gastro 104: 1133, 1993)*. Diagnosis of SBP: 30–40% of pts have neg. cultures of blood and ascitic fluid. % pos. cultures ↑ if 10 mL of pt's ascitic fluid added to blood culture bottles *(JAMA 299:1166, 2008)*. **Duration of rx unclear**. Suggest 2 wks if blood culture +. One report suggests repeat paracentesis after 48 hrs of cefotaxime. If PMNs <250/mm³ & ascitic fluid sterile, success with 5 days of treatment *(AJM 97:169, 1994)*. **IV albumin** (1.5 gm/kg at dx & 1 gm/kg on day 3) may ↓ frequency of renal impairment (p 0.002) & ↓ hospital mortality (p 0.01) *(NEJM 341:403, 1999)*.
Prevention of SBP *(Amer J Gastro 104:993, 2009)*: Cirrhosis & ascites *For prevention after UGI bleeding, see Liver, page 32*		**TMP-SMX-DS** 1 tab po 5 days/wk or **CIP** 750 mg po q wk	**TMP-SMX** ↓ peritonitis or spontaneous bacteremia from 27% to 3% *(AnIM 122:595, 1995)*. Ref. for CIP: *Hepatology 22:1171, 1995*	

[34] Parenteral **IV therapy** for peritonitis: **TC-CL** 3.1 gm q6h, **PIP-TZ** 3.375 gm q6h or 4.5 gm q8h or 4-hr infusion of 3.375 gm q8h *(See Table 10)*, **Dori** 500 mg IV q8h (1-hr infusion), **IMP** 0.5-1 gm q6h, **MER** 1 gm q8h, **FQ** [**CIP** 400 mg q12h, **Oflox** 400 mg q12h, **Levo** 750 mg q24h, **Moxi** 400 mg q24h], **AMP** 1 gm q6h, **aminoglycoside** *(see Table 10D, page 101)*, **cefotetan** 2 gm q12h, **cefoxitin** 2 gm q8h, **P Ceph 3** (**cefotaxime** 2 gm q4–8h, **ceftriaxone** 1–2 gm q24h, **ceftizoxime** 2 gm q4–8h), **P Ceph 4** (**CFP** 2 gm q12h, **cefpirome**[NUS] 2 gm q12h), **clinda** 600–900 mg q8h, **metro** 1 gm loading then 0.5 gm q6h or 1 gm q12h, **AP Pen** (**ticarcillin** 4 gm q6h, **PIP** 4 gm q6h, **aztreonam** 2 gm q8h)

    NOTE: All dosage recommendations are for adults (unless otherwise indicated) and assume normal renal function.

TABLE 1A (42)

ANATOMIC SITE/DIAGNOSIS/ MODIFYING CIRCUMSTANCES	ETIOLOGIES (usual)	SUGGESTED REGIMENS*		ADJUNCT DIAGNOSTIC OR THERAPEUTIC MEASURES AND COMMENTS
		PRIMARY	ALTERNATIVE[§]	
PERITONEUM/PERITONITIS *(continued)*				
Secondary (bowel perforation, ruptured appendix, ruptured diverticula) Ref: *CID 50:133, 2010*	Enterobacteriaceae, Bacteroides sp., enterococci, P. aeruginosa (3-15 %). If VRE documented, dapto may work *(Int J Antimicrob Agents 32:369, 2008)*.	**Mild-moderate disease—Inpatient—parenteral rx:** (e.g., focal periappendiceal peritonitis, peridiverticular abscess, endomyometritis). Usually need surgery for source control. **PIP-TZ** 3.375 gm IV q6h or 4.5 gm IV q8h or 4-hr infusion of 3.375 gm q8h **OR** **TC-CL** 3.1 gm IV q6h **OR** **ERTA** 1 gm IV q24h **OR** **MOXI** 400 mg IV q24h **Severe life-threatening disease—ICU patient:** Surgery for source control + **IMP** 500 mg IV q6h or **MER** 1 gm IV q8h or **DORI** 500 mg IV q8h (1-hr infusion). *See Comments.* **Concomitant surgical management important.**	[**(CIP** 400 mg IV q12h or **Levo** 750 mg IV q24h) **+ (metro** 1 gm IV q12h)] or (**CFP** 2 gm q12h + **metro**) or **tigecycline** 100 mg IV times 1 dose, then 50 mg q12h [**AMP + metro – (CIP** 400 mg IV q8h or **Levo** 750 mg IV q24h)] **OR** [**AMP** 2 gm IV q6h + **metro** 500 mg IV q6h + **aminoglycoside** *(see Table 10D, page 1C1)*]	Must "cover" both Gm-neg. aerobic & Gm-neg. anaerobic bacteria. Empiric coverage of MRSA, enterococci and candida not necessary unless culture indicates infection. Cover enterococci if valvular heart disease. **Drugs active only vs. anaerobic Gm-neg. bacilli:** metro. **Drugs active only vs. aerobic Gm-neg. bacilli:** aminoglycosides, P Ceph 2/3/4, aztreonam, AP Pen, CIP, Levo. **Drugs active vs. both aerobic/anaerobic Gm-neg. bacteria:** cefoxitin, TC-CL, PIP-TZ, AM-SB, Dori, IMP, MER, Moxi. Increasing resistance (R) of Bacteroides species *(AAC 51:1649, 2007)*: **Cefoxitin** / **Cefotetan** / **Clindamycin** **% R** 5-30 / 17-87 / 19-35 Essentially no resistance: **metro**, **PIP-TZ**. Case reports of metro resistance: *CID 40:e67, 2005; JCM 42:4127, 2004.* **Ertapenem** not active vs. P. aeruginosa/ Acinetobacter species. If absence of ongoing fecal contamination, **aerobic/anaerobic culture** of peritoneal exudate/abscess may be of help in guiding specific therapy. Less need for aminoglycosides. **With severe pen allergy**, can "cover" Gm-neg. aerobes with **CIP** or **aztreonam. Remember DORI/IMP/MER are β-lactams.** IMP dose increased to 1 gm q6h if suspect P. aeruginosa and pt. is critically ill. If VRE documented, daptomycin may work *(Int J Antimicrobial Agents 32:369, 2008)*.
Abdominal actinomycosis	A. Israelii and rarely others	**AMP** 50 mg/kg/day IV div in 3-4 doses x 4-6 wks, then **Pen VK** 2-4 gm/day po x 3-6 mos.	**Doxy** or **ceftriaxone** or **clinda** or **erythro**	Presents as mass +/- fistula tract after abdominal surgery, e.g., for ruptured appendix. Can use IV Pen G instead of AMP: 10-20 million units/day IV x 4-6 wks.
Associated with chronic ambulatory peritoneal dialysis (Abdominal pain, cloudy dialysate, dialysate WBC >100 cell/μL with >50% neutrophils)	Staph. aureus (most common), Staph. epidermidis, P. aeruginosa 7%, Gm-neg. bacilli 11%, sterile 20%, M. fortuitum (rare)	If of moderate severity can rx by adding drug to dialysis fluid—*see Table 17 for dosage*. Reasonable empiric combinations: (**vanco** + **ceftazidime**) or (**vanco** + **gent**). If severely ill, rx with same drugs IV (adjust dose for renal failure, *Table 17*) & via addition to dialysis fluid. *See Perit Dialysis Int 25:107, 2005 & 29:5, 2009.* **After Dx**, treat empirically by adding drug to dialysate. Vanco or Cefazolin (Gm-pos cocci), Ceftaz, Cefepime, CIP or Gent (Gm-neg bacilli). Dose continuously or intermittently: *See Table 19.*		For diagnosis: concentrate several hundred mL of removed dialysis fluid by centrifugation. Gram stain concentrate and then inject into aerobic/anaerobic blood culture bottles. A positive Gram stain will guide initial therapy. If culture shows Staph. epidermidis, good chance of "saving" dialysis catheter; **if multiple Gm-neg. bacilli cultured, consider catheter-induced bowel perforation and need for catheter removal.** *See Perit Dialysis Int 25:107, 2005 & 29:5, 2009.*

 NOTE: All dosage recommendations are for adults (unless otherwise indicated) and assume normal renal function.

TABLE 1A (43)

ANATOMIC SITE/DIAGNOSIS/ MODIFYING CIRCUMSTANCES	ETIOLOGIES (usual)	SUGGESTED REGIMENS*		ADJUNCT DIAGNOSTIC OR THERAPEUTIC MEASURES AND COMMENTS
		PRIMARY	ALTERNATIVE[§]	
PHARYNX				
Pharyngitis/Tonsillitis				
Exudative or Diffuse Erythema				
Without significant cough or congestion	Group A, C, G Strep.; Fusobacterium (in research studies); Infectious Mono; Primary HIV; *N. gonorrhea*; Respiratory viruses	(**Pen V** po x 10 days or **Benzathine Pen** 1.2 million units IM x 1 dose) OR (**Cefdinir** or **Cefpodoxime**) x 5 days. **Doses in footnote**[35] (adult and peds) (Durations are FDA-approved).	Pen allergic: **Clinda** 300-450 mg po q6-8h x 5 days. **Azithro**, **Clarithro** are alternatives, but resistant *S. pyogenes* reported *(CID 41:599, 2005; JAC 63:42, 2009)*. Sulfonamides and Tetracyclines not active.	Dx: Rapid Strep test. No need for post-treatment test of cure rapid strep test or culture. Complications of Strep pharyngitis: 1) Acute rheumatic fever 46 – follows Grp A *S. pyogenes* infection, rare after Grp C/G infection. *See footnote*[36]. For prevention, start treatment within 9 days of onset of symptoms. *See Ln 366:155, 2005.* 2) Children age < 7 yrs at risk for post-streptococcal glomerulophlebitis. 3) Pediatric autoimmune neuropsychiatric disorder associated with Grp A Strep (PANDAS) infection. 4) Peritonsillar abscess; Suppurative phlebitis.
	Gonococcal pharyngitis	**Ceftriaxone** 125 mg IM x 1 dose + (**Azithro** or **Doxy**)*(See Comment)*	FQs not recommended due to resistance *(MMWR 56:332, 2007)*	Risk of concomitant genital C. trachomatis: add either Azithro 1 gm po x 1 dose or Doxy 100 mg po bid x 7 days. Not effective in pharynx: spectinomycin, cefixime, cefpodoxime and cefuroxime.
	Proven *S. pyogenes* recurrence	**Cefdinir** or **Cefpodoxime**	**AM-CL** or **Clinda**	
	Grp A infections: 6 in 1 yr; 4 in 2 consecutive yrs	Tonsillectomy reasonable *(BMJ 334:939, 2007)*		
Peritonsillor abscess – Serious complication of exudative pharyngitis	**F. necrophorum** (44%) Grp A Strep (33%) Grp C/G Strep (9%) *(CID 49:1467, 2009)*	Surgical drainage plus **PIP-TZ** or **TC-CL**	Pen allergic: **Clinda** IV	**Avoid macrolides: Fusobacterium is resistant.** Reports of beta-lactamase production by oral anaerobes *(Anaerobe 9:105, 2003)*.
Other complications	*See parapharyngeal space infection and jugular vein suppurative phlebitis (below)*			
Membranous pharyngitis: think Diphtheria	*C. diphtheria*	[**Antitoxin** + **Erythro** 20–25 mg/kg IV q12h x 7–14 days *(JAC 35:717, 1995)*] or [**Benzyl pen G** 50,000 units/kg/day x 5 days, then po **Pen VK** 50 mg/kg per day x 5 days]		Diphtheria occurs in immunized individuals. Antibiotics may ↓ toxin production, ↓ spread of organisms. Penicillin superior to erythro in randomized trial *(CID 27:845, 1998)*.

[35] **Treatment of Group A, C & G strep: Treatment durations are from approved package inserts. Subsequent studies indicate efficacy of shorter treatment courses. All po unless otherwise indicated. PEDIATRIC DOSAGE; Benzathine penicillin** 25,000 units per kg IM to max. 1.2 million units; **Pen V** 25–50 mg per kg per day div. q6h times10 days; **amox ER** 775 mg po once daily x 10 days; **AM-CL** 45 mg per kg per day div. q12h times 10 days; **erythro estolate** 20 mg per kg div. bid or **succinate** 40 mg per kg per day div. bid times 10 days; **cefuroxime axetil** 20 mg per kg per day div. bid for 4–10 days *(PIDJ 14:295, 1995)*; **cefpodoxime proxetil** 10 mg per kg div. bid times10 days; **cefdinir** 7 mg per kg q12h times 5–10 days or 14 mg per kg q24h times 10 days; **cefprozil** 15 mg per kg per day div. bid times 10 days; **clarithro** 15 mg per kg per day div. bid times 10 days; **azithro** 12 mg per kg once daily times 5 days; **clinda** 20–30 mg per kg per day div. q8h times 10 days **ADULT DOSAGE; Benzathine penicillin** 1.2 million units IM times 1; **Pen V** 500 mg bid or 250 mg qid times 10 days; **erythro**, dosage varies—with erythro base 500 mg qid times 10 days; **cefditoren** 200 mg bid times 10 days; **cefuroxime axetil** 250 mg bid times 4 days; **cefpodoxime proxetil** 100 mg bid times 4 days; **cefdinir** 300 mg q12h times 5–10 days or 600 mg q24h times 10 days; **cefditoren** 200 mg bid; **cefprozil** 500 mg q24h times 10 days; **NOTE:** All **O Ceph 2** drugs approved for 10-day rx of strep. pharyngitis; increasing number of studies show efficacy of 4–6 days; **clarithro** 250 mg bid times 10 days; **azithro** 500 mg times 1 and then 250 mg q24h times 4 days or 500 mg q24h times 3 days.

[36] Primary rationale for therapy is eradication of Group A strep (GAS) and prevention of acute rheumatic fever (ARF). Benzathine penicillin G has been shown in clinical trials to ↓ rate of ARF from 2.8 to 0.2%. This was associated with clearance of GAS on pharyngeal cultures *(CID 19:1110, 1994)*. Subsequent studies have been based on cultures, not actual prevention of ARF. Treatment decreases duration of symptoms.

 NOTE: All dosage recommendations are for adults (unless otherwise indicated) and assume normal renal function.

TABLE 1A (44)

ANATOMIC SITE/DIAGNOSIS/ MODIFYING CIRCUMSTANCES	ETIOLOGIES (usual)	SUGGESTED REGIMENS*		ADJUNCT DIAGNOSTIC OR THERAPEUTIC MEASURES AND COMMENTS
		PRIMARY	ALTERNATIVE§	
PHARYNX/Pharyngitis/Tonsillitis *(continued)*				
Vesicular, ulcerative pharyngitis (viral)	Coxsackie A9, B1-5, ECHO (multiple types), Enterovirus 71, Herpes simplex 1,2	Antibacterial agents not indicated. For HSV-1,2: **acyclovir** 400 mg tid po x 10 days		
Epiglottitis				
Children	H. influenzae (rare), S. pyogenes, S. pneumoniae, S. aureus	**Peds dosage: Cefotaxime** 50 mg per kg IV q8h or **ceftriaxone** 50 mg per kg IV q24h	**Peds dosage: AM-SB** 100–200 mg/kg per day div q6h or **TMP-SMX** 8–12 mg TMP component /kg per day div q12h	Have tracheostomy set "at bedside." **Chloro** is effective, but potentially less toxic alternative agents available. Review (adults): *JAMA 272:1358, 1994.*
Adults	Group A strep, H. influenzae (rare)	**Adult dosage:** *See footnote*[37]		
Parapharyngeal space infection; peritonsillor abscess [Spaces include sublingual, submandibular (Ludwig's angina), lateral pharyngeal, retropharyngeal, pretracheal]				
Poor dental hygiene, dental extractions, foreign bodies (e.g., toothpicks, fish bones) Ref: *CID 49:1467, 2009*	Polymicrobic: Strep sp., anaerobes, Eikenella corrodens. Anaerobes outnumber aerobes 10:1.	[(**Clinda** 600–900 mg IV q8h) or (**pen G** 24 million units/day by cont. infusion or div q4–6h IV] + **metro** 1 gm load and then 0.5 gm IV q6h)	**Cefoxitin** 2 gm IV q8h or **clinda** 600-900 mg IV q8h or **TC-CL** or **PIP-TZ** or **AM-SB** *(Dosage, see footnote*[37]*)*	Close observation of airway, 1/3 require intubation. MRI or CT to identify abscess; **surgical drainage. Metro** may be given 1 gm IV q12h. Complications: infection of carotid (rupture possible) & jugular vein phlebitis.
Jugular vein suppurative phlebitis (Lemierre's syndrome) *Eur J Clin Micro Inf Dis 27:779, 2008.*	Fusobacterium necrophorum in vast majority	**Pen G** 24 million units q24h by cont. infusion or div. q4–6h	**Clinda** 600–900 mg IV q8h. **Avoid macrolides: fusobacterium resistance**	Emboli: pulmonary and systemic common. Erosion into carotid artery can occur. Lemierre described F. necrophorum in 1936; other anaerobes & Gm-positive cocci are less common etiologies of suppurative phlebitis.
Laryngitis (hoarseness)	Viral (90%)	Not indicated		
SINUSES, PARANASAL				
Sinusitis, acute; current terminology: acute rhinosinusitis				
Obstruction of sinus ostia, viral infection, allergens Refs.: *Otolaryn-Head & Neck Surgery 130:S1, 2004; JAMA 301:1798, 2009.* For rhinovirus infections (common cold), *see Table 14, page 157*	S. pneumoniae 33%, H. influenzae 32%, M. catarrhalis 9%, Group A strep 2%, anaerobes 6%, viruses 15%, Staph. aureus 10%: *CID 45:e121, 2007.* **By CT scans, sinus mucosa inflamed in 87% of viral URIs; only 2% develop bacterial rhinosinusitis**	Reserve antibiotic therapy for pts given decongestants/ analgesics for 10 days who have (1) maxillary/facial pain & (2) purulent nasal discharge; if severe illness (pain, fever), treat sooner—usually requires hospitalization. Viral infections should resolve within 10 days. For mild/mod. disease: Ask if recent antibiotic use (recent = in last month).		**Rx goals:** (1) Resolve infection, (2) prevent bacterial complications, e.g., subdural empyema, epidural abscess, brain abscess, meningitis and cavernous sinus thrombosis (LnID 7:62, 2007), (3) avoid chronic sinus disease, (4) avoid unnecessary antibiotic rx. 40-60% rate of spontaneous resolution. **For pts with pen/cephalosporin allergy, esp. severe IgE-mediated allergy, e.g., hives, anaphylaxis, treatment options: clarithro, azithro, TMP-SMX, doxy or FQs. Avoid FQs if under age 18. Do not use Clinda – no activity vs. Haemophilus or Moraxella sp.** ***Dosages in footnote***[38,39]***, page 48.*** If allergy just skin rash, po cephalosporin OK. *(Continued on next page)*

[37] Parapharyngeal space infection: **Ceftriaxone** 2 gm IV q24h; **cefotaxime** 2 gm IV q4–8h; **AM-SB** 3 gm IV q6h; **PIP-TZ** 3.375 gm IV q6h or 4-hr infusion of 3.375 gm q8h; **TC-CL** 3.1 gm IV q4–6h; **TMP-SMX** 8–10 mg per kg per day (based on TMP component) div q6h, q8h, or q12h.

Abbreviations on page 2. *NOTE: All dosage recommendations are for adults (unless otherwise indicated) and assume normal renal function.*

TABLE 1A (45)

ANATOMIC SITE/DIAGNOSIS/ MODIFYING CIRCUMSTANCES	ETIOLOGIES (usual)	SUGGESTED REGIMENS* PRIMARY	ALTERNATIVE§	ADJUNCT DIAGNOSTIC OR THERAPEUTIC MEASURES AND COMMENTS
SINUSES, PARANASAL/Sinusitis, acute; current terminology: acute rhinosinusitis *(continued)*				
Meta-analysis of 9 double-blind trials found no clinical signs/symptoms that justify treatment--even after 7-10 days of symptoms *(Ln 371:908, 2008)*.		**No Recent Antibiotic Use: Amox-HD** or **AM-CL-ER** or **cefdinir** or **cefpodoxime** or **cefprozil**	**Recent Antibiotic Use: AM-CL-ER** (adults) or resp. **FQ** (adults). For pen. allergy, *see Comments, previous page*. Use AM-CL susp. in peds.	**Usual rx 10 days**; but same efficacy with 3-7 days vs. 6-10 days *(LnID 8:543, 2008)*(meta-analysis). Watch for pts with fever & fascial erythema; ↑ risk of S. aureus infection, requires IV **nafcillin/oxacillin (antistaphylococcal penicillin, penicillinase-resistant for MSSA or vanco for MRSA).** NOTE: **Levo** 750 mg q24h x 5 days vs. **levo** 500 mg q24h x 10 days equivalent microbiologic and clinical efficacy *(Otolaryngol Head Neck Surg 134:10, 2006)*. **Complications:** From acute viral rhinosinusitis--transient hyposmia. From acute bacterial rhinosinusitis--orbital infections, meningitis, epidural abscess, brain abscess & cavernous sinus thrombosis. Adjunctive therapy for cavernous sinus thrombosis: topical decongestant (oxymetazoline) for < 5 d; nasal steroids of possible benefit; antihistamines (minor role); saline irrigation may help.
		In general, treat 10 days (see Comment); Adult and pediatric doses, footnote[38,39] and footnote[5], page 10 (Otitis). Adjunctive Rx, see Comment		
Clinical failure after 3 days	As above; consider diagnostic tap/aspirate	**Mild/Mod. Disease: AM-CL-ER** OR (**cefpodoxime**, **cefprozil**, or **cefdinir**) *Treat 5-10 days. Adult doses in footnote[39] & Comment*	**Severe Disease: Gati[NUS], Gemi, Levo, Moxi**	
Diabetes mellitus with acute keto-acidosis; neutropenia; deferox-amine rx: Mucormycosis	Rhizopus sp., (mucor), aspergillus	*See Table 11, pages 102 & 112.*		
Hospitalized + nasotracheal or nasogastric intubation	Gm-neg. bacilli 47% (pseu-domonas, acinetobacter, E. coli common), Gm+ (S. aureus) 35%, yeasts 18%. Polymicrobial in 80%	Remove nasotracheal tube: if fever persists and ENT available, recommend sinus aspiration for C/S prior to empiric therapy. **IMP** 0.5 gm IV q6h or **MER** 1 gm IV q8h. Add vanco for MRSA if Gram stain suggestive.	(**Ceftaz** 2 gm IV q8h + **vanco**) or (**CFP** 2 gm IV q12h + **vanco**).	After 7 days of nasotracheal or nasogastric tubes, 95% have x-ray "sinusitis" (fluid in sinuses), but on transnasal puncture only 38% culture + *(AJRCCM 150:776, 1994)*. For pts requiring mechanical ventilation with nasotracheal tube for ≥1 wk, bacterial sinusitis occurs in <10% *(CID 27:851, 1998)*. May need fluconazole if yeast on Gram stain of sinus aspirate.
Sinusitis, chronic Adults	Prevotella, anaerobic strep, & fusobacterium—common anaerobes. Strep sp., haemophilus, P. aeruginosa, S. aureus, & moraxella—aerobes. *(CID 35:428, 2002)*	Antibiotics usually not effective	Otolaryngology consultation. If acute exacerbation, treat as acute sinusitis.	Pathogenesis unclear and may be polyfactorial: damage to ostiomeatal complex during acute bacterial disease, allergy ± polyps, occult immunodeficiency, and/or odontogenic disease (periodontitis in maxillary teeth).
SKIN				
Acne vulgaris *(Med Lett 51:31, 2009; NEJM 352:1463, 2005; In the Clinic, AnIM, 149:ITC-1, 2008)*.				
Comedonal acne, "blackheads," "whiteheads," earliest form, no inflammation	Excessive sebum production & gland obstruction. No Propionibacterium acnes	Once-q24h: Topical **tretinoin** (cream 0.025 or 0.05%) or (gel 0.01 or 0.025%)	All once-q24h: Topical **adapalene** 0.1% gel OR **azelaic acid** 20% cream or **tazarotene** 0.1% cream	Goal is prevention, ↓ number of new comedones and create an environment unfavorable to P. acnes. Adapalene causes less irritation than tretinoin. Azelaic acid less potent but less irritating than retinoids. Expect 40–70% ↓ in comedones in 12 weeks.

[38] ***Pediatric doses for sinusitis (all oral):*** **Amox HD** high dose 90 mg per kg per day div. q8h or q12h, **AM-CL-ES** (extra strength) pediatric susp.: 90 mg **amox** component per kg per day div. q12h, **azithro** 10 mg per kg times 1, then 5 mg per kg per day times 3 days, **clarithro** 15 mg per kg per day div. q12h, **cefpodoxime** 10 mg per kg per day (max. 400 mg) div. q12–24h, **cefuroxime axetil** 30 mg per kg per day div. q12h, **cefdinir** 14 mg per kg per day once q24h or divided bid, **cefprozil** 15 mg/kg/day divided bid (max 1 gm/day); **TMP-SMX** 8–12 mg TMP/40–60 mg SMX per kg per day div. q12h.

[39] ***Adult doses for sinusitis (all oral):*** **AM-CL-ER** 2000/125 **mg** bid, **amox high-dose (HD)** 1 gm tid, **clarithro** 500 mg bid or **clarithro ext. release** 1 gm q24h, **doxy** 100 mg bid, **respiratory FQs** (**Gati** 400 mg q24hNUS due to hypo/hyperglycemia; **Gemi** 320 mg q24h *(not FDA indication but should work)*, **Levo** 750 mg q24h x 5 days, **Moxi** 400 mg q24h); **O Ceph** (**cefdinir** 300 mg q12h or 600 mg q24h, **cefpodoxime** 200 mg bid, **cefprozil** 250–500 mg bid, **cefuroxime** 250 mg bid), **TMP-SMX** 1 double-strength (TMP 160 mg) bid (results after 3- and 10-day rx similar).

 NOTE: All dosage recommendations are for adults (unless otherwise indicated) and assume normal renal function.

TABLE 1A (46)

ANATOMIC SITE/DIAGNOSIS/ MODIFYING CIRCUMSTANCES	ETIOLOGIES (usual)	SUGGESTED REGIMENS*		ADJUNCT DIAGNOSTIC OR THERAPEUTIC MEASURES AND COMMENTS
		PRIMARY	ALTERNATIVE[§]	
SKIN/Acne vulgaris *(continued)*				
Mild inflammatory acne: small papules or pustules	Proliferation of P. acnes + abnormal desquamation of follicular cells	Topical **erythro** 3% + **benzoyl peroxide** 5%, bid	Can substitute **clinda** 1% gel for erythro	In random. controlled trial, topical benzoyl peroxide + erythro of equal efficacy to oral minocycline & tetracycline and not affected by antibiotic resistance of propionibacteria *(Ln 364:2188, 2004)*.
Inflammatory acne: comedones, papules & pustules. Less common: deep nodules (cysts)	Progression of above events	(Topical **erythro** 3% + **benzoyl peroxide** 5% bid) ± oral antibiotic. *See Comment for mild acne*	Oral drugs: (**doxy** 100 mg bid) or (**minocycline** 50 mg bid). Others: **tetracycline**, **erythro**, **TMP-SMX**, **clinda**. Expensive extended release **once-daily minocycline** (Solodyn) 1 mg/kg/d *(Med Lett 48:95, 2006)*.	Systemic **isotretinoin** reserved for pts with severe widespread nodular cystic lesions that fail oral antibiotic rx; 4–5 mo. course of 0.1–1 mg per kg per day. Aggressive/violent behavior reported. **Tetracyclines** stain developing teeth. **Doxy** can cause photosensitivity. **Minocycline** side-effects: urticaria, vertigo, pigment deposition in skin or oral mucosa. Rare induced autoimmunity in children: fever; polyarthralgia, positive ANCA *(J Peds 153:314, 2008)*.
Acne rosacea Ref: *NEJM 352:793, 2005.*	Skin mite: Demadex folliculorum	**Azelaic acid gel** bid topical or **Metro** topical cream bid	Any of variety of low dose oral tetracycline regimens *(Med Lett 49:5, 2007)*.	
Anthrax, **cutaneous**, inhalation **To report bioterrorism event: 770-488-7100;** **For info: www.bt.cdc.gov** Refs.: *JAMA 281:1735, 1999, & MMWR 50:909, 2001*	B. anthracis Spores are introduced into/under the skin by contact with infected animals/animal products. *See Lung, page 40.*	**Adults (including pregnancy) and children >50 kg:** (**CIP** 500 mg po bid or **Levo** 500 mg IV/po q24h) x 60 days. **Children <50 kg:** (**CIP** 20–30 mg/kg day div q12h po (to max. 1 gm per day) or **levo** 8 mg/kg po q12h) x 60 days	**Adults (including pregnancy): Doxy** 100 mg po bid x 60 days. **Children: Doxy** >8 y/o & >45 kg: 100 mg po bid; >8 y/o & ≤45 kg: 2.2 mg/kg po bid; ≤8 y/o: 2.2 mg/kg po bid All for 60 days.	1. If penicillin susceptible, then: **Adults: Amox** 500 mg po q8h times 60 days. **Children: Amox** 80 mg per kg per day div. q8h (max. 500 mg q8h) 2. **Usual treatment of cutaneous anthrax is 7–10 days; 60 days in setting of bioterrorism with presumed aerosol exposure** 3. Other **FQs** (Levo, Moxi) should work based on in vitro susceptibility data 4. Intestinal anthrax can also occur *(NEJM 363:766, 2010)*.
Bacillary angiomatosis: For other Bartonella infections, see *Cat-scratch disease lymphadenitis, page 43, and Bartonella systemic infections, page 54*				
In immunocompromised (HIV-1, bone marrow transplant) patients *Also see* SANFORD GUIDE TO HIV/AIDS THERAPY	Bartonella henselae and quintana	**Clarithro** 500 mg po bid or ext. release 1 gm po q24h or **azithro** 250 mg po q24h or **CIP** 500–750 mg po bid *(see Comment)*	**Erythro** 500 mg po qid or **doxy** 100 mg po bid	In immunocompromised pts with severe disease, doxy 100 mg po/IV bid + RIF 300 mg po bid reported effective *(IDC No. Amer 12:37, 1998; Adv PID 11:1, 1996)*. Treat for 8 wks.
Bite: Remember tetanus prophylaxis— ***See Table 20B, page 198 for rabies prophylaxis.***				
Bat, raccoon, skunk	Strep & staph from skin; rabies	**AM-CL** 875/125 mg po bid or 500/125 mg po tid	**Doxy** 100 mg po bid	In Americas, **antirabies rx indicated:** rabies immune globulin + vaccine. *(See Table 20B, page **198**)*
Camel	S. aureus, P. aeruginosa, Other Gm-neg bacilli	**Diclox** 250-500 mg po q6h + **CIP** 750 mg po bid	**Cephalexin** 500 mg po qid + **CIP** 750 mg po bid	*See EJCMID 18:918, 1999.*
Cat: 80% get infected, culture & treat empirically. Cat-scratch disease: *page 43*	**Pasteurella multocida**, Staph. aureus	**AM-CL** 875/125 mg po bid or 500/125 mg po tid	**Cefuroxime axetil** 0.5 gm po q12h or **doxy** 100 mg po bid. **Do not use cephalexin.** Sens. to FQs in vitro.	**P. multocida resistant to dicloxacillin, cephalexin, clinda; many strains resistant to erythro** (most sensitive to azithro but no clinical data). P. multocida infection develops within 24 hrs. Observe for osteomyelitis. If culture + for only P. multocida, can switch to pen G IV or pen VK po. See Dog Bite
Catfish sting	Toxins	*See Comments*		Presents as immediate pain, erythema and edema. Resembles strep cellulitis. May become secondarily infected; AM-CL is reasonable choice for prophylaxis
Dog: Only 5% get infected; treat only if bite severe or bad co-morbidity (e.g. diabetes).	**Pasteurella canis**, S. aureus, Bacteroides sp., Fusobacterium sp., EF-4, Capnocytophaga	**AM-CL** 875/125 mg po bid or 500/125 mg po tid	**Clinda** 300 mg po qid + FQ (adults) or **clinda** + **TMP-SMX** (children)	Consider antirabies prophylaxis: rabies immune globulin + vaccine *(see Table 20B)*. Capnocytophaga in splenectomized pts may cause local eschar, sepsis with DIC. **P. canis resistant to diclox, cephalexin, clinda and erythro**; sensitive to ceftriaxone, cefuroxime, cefpodoxime and FQs.

Abbreviations on page 2. *NOTE: All dosage recommendations are for adults (unless otherwise indicated) and assume normal renal function.*

TABLE 1A (47)

ANATOMIC SITE/DIAGNOSIS/ MODIFYING CIRCUMSTANCES	ETIOLOGIES (usual)	SUGGESTED REGIMENS*		ADJUNCT DIAGNOSTIC OR THERAPEUTIC MEASURES AND COMMENTS
		PRIMARY	ALTERNATIVE[§]	
SKIN/Bite *(continued)*				
Human For bacteriology, *see CID 37:1481, 2003*	Viridans strep 100%, Staph epidermidis 53%, corynebacterium 41%, **Staph. aureus 29%, eikenella 15%**, bacteroides 82%, peptostrep 26%	**Early** (not yet infected): **AM-CL** 875/125 mg po bid times 5 days. **Later:** Signs of infection (usually in 3–24 hrs): (**AM-SB** 1.5 gm IV q6h or **cefoxitin** 2 gm IV q8h) or (**TC-CL** 3.1 gm IV q6h) or (**PIP-TZ** 3.375 gm IV q6h or 4.5 gm q8h or 4-hr infusion of 3.375 gm q8h). Pen allergy: **Clinda** + (either **CIP** or **TMP-SMX**)		**Cleaning, irrigation and debridement most important.** For clenched fist injuries, x-rays should be obtained. Bites inflicted by hospitalized pts, consider aerobic Gm-neg. bacilli. **Eikenella resistant to clinda, nafcillin/oxacillin, metro, P Ceph 1, and erythro; susceptible to FQs and TMP-SMX.**
Leech (Medicinal)	Aeromonas hydrophila	**CIP** (400 mg IV or 750 mg po) bid	**TMP-SMX DS** 1 tab po bid	Aeromonas found in GI tract of leeches. Some use prophylactic antibiotics when leeches used medicinally, but not universally accepted or necessary *(IDCP 10:211, 2001)*. Avoid Amp or 1st gen Cephalosporins *(CID 35:e1, 2002)*.
Pig (swine)	Polymicrobic: Gm+ cocci, Gm-neg. bacilli, anaerobes, Pasteurella sp.	**AM-CL** 875/125 mg po bid	**P Ceph 3** or **TC-CL** or **AM-SB** or **IMP**	Information limited but infection is common and serious *(Ln 348:888, 1996)*.
Prairie dog	Monkeypox	*See Table 14A, page 155.* No rx recommended		
Primate, non-human	Microbiology. Herpesvirus simiae	**Acyclovir**: *See Table 14B, page 158*		*CID 20:421, 1995*
Rat	Spirillum minus & Streptobacillus moniliformis	**AM-CL** 875/125 mg po bid	**Doxy**	Antirabies rx not indicated. Causes rat bite fever (Streptobacillus moniliformis): Pen G or doxy, alternatively erythro or clinda.
Seal	Marine mycoplasma	Tetracycline times 4 wks		Can take weeks to appear after bite *(Ln 364:448, 2004)*.
Snake: pit viper (Ref.: *NEJM 347:347, 2002*)	Pseudomonas sp., Enterobacteriaceae, Staph. epidermidis, Clostridium sp.		**Primary therapy is antivenom**. Penicillin generally used but would not be effective vs. organisms isolated. Ceftriaxone should be more effective. Tetanus prophylaxis indicated. Ref: *CID 43:1309, 2006*.	
Spider bite: Most necrotic ulcers attributed to spiders are probably due to another cause, e.g., cutaneous anthrax *(Ln 364:549, 2004)* or **MRSA infection** (spider bite painful; anthrax not painful.)				
Widow (Latrodectus)	Not infectious	None	May be confused with "acute abdomen." Diazepam or calcium gluconate helpful to control pain, muscle spasm. Tetanus prophylaxis.	
Brown recluse (Loxosceles) *NEJM 352:700, 2005*	Not infectious. Overdiagnosed! Spider distribution limited to S. Central & desert SW of US	Bite usually self-limited & self-healing. No therapy of proven efficacy.	**Dapsone** 50 mg po q24h often used despite marginal supportive data	Dapsone causes hemolysis (check for G6PD deficiency). Can cause hepatitis; baseline & weekly liver panels suggested.
Boils—Furunculosis—Subcutaneous abscesses in drug addicts ("skin poppers"). Carbuncles = multiple connecting furuncles; Emergency Dept Perspective *(IDC No Amer 22:89, 2008)*.				
Active lesions ***See Table 6, page 75*** Community-associated MRSA widespread. I&D mainstay of therapy. Ref: *CID 46:1032, 2008.* No difference between TMP/SMX and placebo in peds pts--most with abscess <5 cm: *An Emer Med (ePub, Apr 29), 2009*	Staph. aureus, both MSSA & MRSA—concern for community-associated MRSA *(See Comments)* *IDSA Guidelines: CID 52 (Feb 1):1, 2011.*	**If afebrile & abscess <5 cm in diameter: I&D**, culture, hot packs. No drugs. **If ≥5 cm in diameter: TMP-SMX-DS** 1-2 tabs po bid times 5–10 days. Alternatives (Adult dosage): **clinda** 300-600 mg po q6-8h or (**doxy** or **minocycline**) 100 mg po q12h **Incision and Drainage mainstay of therapy!**	**Febrile, large &/or multiple abscesses; outpatient care: I&D**, culture abscess & maybe blood, hot packs. (**TMP-SMX-DS** 1-2 tabs po bid ± **RIF** 300 mg bid) times 10 days. If no response after 2-3 days, look for complications and consider IV therapy.	Why 1-2 **TMP/SMX-DS**? *See discussion footnote 1 of Table 6 (MRSA)*. **TMP/SMX** activity vs. streptococci uncertain. Usually clear clinical separation of strep "cellulitis" (erysipelas) from *S. aureus* abscess. If unclear or strep, use **clinda** or **TMP/SMX** plus **beta-lactam**. Few days of **TMP/SMP** alone first. Other options: (1) **Linezolid** 600 mg po bid x 10 days; (2) **Fusidic acid**[NUS] 250-500 mg po q8-12h ± **RIF** *(CID 42:394, 2006)*; (3) **FQs** only if in vitro susceptibility known

 NOTE: All dosage recommendations are for adults (unless otherwise indicated) and assume normal renal function.

TABLE 1A (43)

ANATOMIC SITE/DIAGNOSIS/ MODIFYING CIRCUMSTANCES	ETIOLOGIES (usual)	SUGGESTED REGIMENS*		ADJUNCT DIAGNOSTIC OR THERAPEUTIC MEASURES AND COMMENTS
		PRIMARY	ALTERNATIVE[§]	
SKIN/Boils—Furunculosis—Subcutaneous abscesses in drug addicts *(continued)*				
To lessen number of furuncle recurrences --decolonization *For surgical prophylaxis, see Table 15B, page 177.*	MSSA & MRSA. *IDSA Guidelines, CID 52 (Feb 1):1, 2011.*	7-day therapy: **Chlorhexidine** (2%) washes daily; 2% **mupirocin ointment** anterior nares 2x daily + (**rifampin** 300 mg bid + **doxy** 100 mg bid).	**Mupirocin ointment** in anterior nares bid x 7 days + **chlorhexidine** (2%) washes daily x 7 days + (**TMP-SMX DS** 1 tab po bid + RIF 300 mg po bid) x 7 days	Optimal regimen uncertain. In randomized prospective study of combined topical & systemic therapy, negative MRSA cultures at 3 mos. in 74% of treated vs. 32% of not treated *(CID 44:178, 2007)*. Many mupirocin trials: *CID 48:922, 2009; JAC 64:9-15, 2009*. Since multiple sites of colonization are common, addition of chlorhexidine washes seem reasonable. Bacitracin oint inferior to Mupirocin *(ICHE 20:351, 1999)*.
Hidradenitis suppurativa	Lesions secondarily infected: S. aureus, Enterobacteriaceae, pseudomonas, anaerobes	Aspirate, base therapy on culture	Many pts ultimately require surgical excision	Caused by keratinous plugging of apocrine glands of axillary and/or inguinal areas.
Burns. For overall management: *NEJM 350:810, 2004—step-by-step case outlined & explained*				
Initial burn wound care *(CID 37:543, 2003& BMJ 332:649, 2006)*. Topical therapy options: *NEJM 359:1037, 2008.*	Not infected	Early excision & wound closure; Variety of skin grafts and skin substitutes: see *JAMA 283:717, 2000 & Adv Skin Wound Care 18:323, 2005;* shower hydrotherapy. Role of topical antimicrobics unclear	**Silver sulfadiazine** cream, 1%, apply 1–2 times per day or 0.5% **silver nitrate** solution or **mafenide acetate** cream. Apply bid.	Marrow-induced neutropenia can occur during 1st wk of sulfadiazine but resolves even if use is continued. Silver nitrate leaches electrolytes from wounds & stains everything. Mafenide inhibits carbonic anhydrase and can cause metabolic acidosis.
Burn wound sepsis	Strep. pyogenes, Enterobacter sp., S. aureus, S. epidermidis, E. faecalis E. coli, P. aeruginosa. Fungi rare. Herpesvirus rare.	(**Vanco** 1 gm IV q12h) + (**amikacin** 10 mg per kg loading dose then 7.5 mg per kg IV q12h) + [**PIP** 4 gm IV q4h (give ½ q24h dose of **piperacillin** into subeschar tissues with surgical eschar removal within 12 hours)]. Can use **PIP-TZ** if PIP not available.		**Monitor serum levels of Vanco and AMK as T½ of most antibiotics ↓.** Staph. aureus tend to remain localized to burn wound; if toxic, consider toxic shock syndrome. Candida sp. colonize but seldom invade. Pneumonia is the major non-burn infectious complication, often staph. Complications include septic thrombophlebitis at IV sites. Dapto (4 mg per kg IV q24h) alternative for vanco.
Cellulitis, erysipelas: Be wary of macrolide (erythro)-resistant Streptococcus sp.. Review: *NEJM 350:904, 2004* **NOTE:** Consider diseases that masquerade as cellulitis *(AnIM 142:47, 2005)*				
Extremities, non-diabetic *For diabetes, see below.* Practice guidelines: *CID 41:1373, 2005.*	Streptococcus sp., Groups A, B, C & G. Staph. aureus, including MRSA reported.	**Pen G** 1–2 million units IV q6h or (**Nafcillin** or **oxacillin** 2 gm IV q4h). If not severe, **dicloxacillin** 500 mg po q6h or **cefazolin** 1 gm IV q8h. *See Comment*	**Erythro** or **cefazolin** or **AM-CL** or **azithro** or **clarithro** or **tigecycline** or **dapto** 4 mg/kg/d IV *(Dosage, see Table 10C) See Comment*	**"Spontaneous" erysipelas of leg in non-diabetic is usually due to strep, Gps A,B,C or G.** Hence OK to **start with IV pen G 1–2 million units q6h** & observe for localized S. aureus infection. Look for tinea pedis with fissures, a common portal of entry; can often culture strep from between toes. Reports of CA-MRSA presenting as erysipelas rather than furunculosis. If MRSA is a concern, use empiric **vanco**, **dapto** or **linezolid**. Leg elevation is helpful.
Facial, adult (erysipelas)	Strep. sp. (Grp A, B, C & G), Staph. aureus (to include MRSA), S. pneumo	**Vanco** 1 gm IV q12h; if over 100 kg, 1.5 gm IV q12h	**Dapto** 4 mg/kg IV q 24h **or Linezolid** 600 mg IV q 12h	**Choice of empiric therapy must have activity vs. S. aureus**. S. aureus erysipelas of face can mimic streptococcal erysipelas of an extremity. Forced to treat empirically for MRSA until in vitro susceptibilities available.
Diabetes mellitus and erysipelas *(See Foot, "Diabetic", page 14)*	Strep. sp. (Grp A, B, C & G), Staph. aureus, Enterobacteriaceae; clostridia (rare)	**Early mild: TMP-SMX-DS** 1-2 tabs po bid + (**Pen VK** 500 mg po qid or **cephalexin** 500 mg po qid). **For severe disease: IMP** or **MER** or **ERTA** IV + (**linezolid** 600 mg IV/po bid or **vanco** IV or **dapto** 4 mg/kg IV q 24h). *Dosage, see page 14, Diabetic foot*		Prompt surgical debridement indicated to rule out necrotizing fasciitis and to obtain cultures. If septic, consider x-ray of extremity to demonstrate gas. **Prognosis dependent on blood supply: assess arteries.** *See diabetic foot, page 14.*
Erysipelas 2° to lymphedema (congenital = Milroy's disease); post-breast surgery with lymph node dissection	Streptococcus sp., Groups A, C, G	**Benzathine pen G** 1.2 million units IM q4 wks		Indicated only if pt is having frequent episodes of cellulitis. Pen V 250 mg po bid should be effective but not aware of clinical trials. In pen-allergic pts: erythro 500 mg po q24h, azithro 250 mg po q24h, or clarithro 500 mg po q24h.

TABLE 1A (49)

ANATOMIC SITE/DIAGNOSIS/ MODIFYING CIRCUMSTANCES	ETIOLOGIES (usual)	SUGGESTED REGIMENS*		ADJUNCT DIAGNOSTIC OR THERAPEUTIC MEASURES AND COMMENTS
		PRIMARY	ALTERNATIVE[§]	
SKIN *(continued)*				
Dandruff (seborrheic dermatitis)	Malassezia species	**Ketoconazole shampoo** 2% or **selenium sulfide** 2.5% *(see page 9, chronic external otitis)*		
Erythema multiforme	H. simplex type 1, mycoplasma, Strep. pyogenes, drugs (sulfonamides, phenytoin, penicillins)			**Rx: Acyclovir** if due to H. simplex
Erythema nodosum	Sarcoidosis, inflammatory bowel disease, M. tbc, coccidioidomycosis, yersinia, sulfonamides, Whipple's disease.			**Rx: NSAIDs; glucocorticoids** if refractory.
Erythrasma	Corynebacterium minutissimum	**Topical Clinda** 2-3 x daily x 7-14 days	**Clarithro** 500 mg po bid or **Erythro** 250 mg po bid) x 14 days	Dx: Coral red fluorescence with Wood's lamp.
Folliculitis	S. aureus, candida, P. aeruginosa common	Usually self-limited, no Rx needed. Could use topical mupirocin for Staph and topical antifungal for Candida.		
Furunculosis	Staph. aureus	*See Boils, page 50*		
Hemorrhagic bullous lesions				
Hx of sea water-contaminated abrasion or eating raw seafood.	**Vibrio vulnificus, V. damsela** *(CID 37:272, 2003)*	**Ceftazidime** 2 gm IV q8h + **doxy** 100 mg IV/po bid	Either **cefotaxime** 2 gm IV q8h or (**CIP** 750 mg po bid or 400 mg IV bid)	¾ pts have chronic liver disease with mortality of 50% *(NEJM 312:343, 1985)*. In Taiwan, the impression exists that ceftazidime is superior to tetracyclines *(CID 15:271, 1992)*, hence both.
Herpes zoster (shingles): *See Table 14*				
Impetigo—children, military				
"Honey-crust" lesions (non-bullous). Ecthyma is closely related. *See Comment.*	**Group A strep impetigo** (rarely Strept. sp. Groups B, C or G); crusted lesions can be Staph. aureus + streptococci. Staph. aureus may be secondary colonizer.	Mupirocin ointment 2% tid or fusidic acid cream[NUS] 2%, times 7–12 days or retapamulin ointment, 1% bid times 5 days	**Azithro** or **clarithro** or **erythro** or **O Ceph 2.** Watch out for macrolide resistance.	In meta-analysis that combined strep & staph impetigo, mupirocin had higher cure rates than placebo. Mupirocin superior to oral erythro. Penicillin inferior to erythro. Few placebo-controlled trials. Ref.: *Cochrane Database Systemic Reviews, 2004 (2): CD003261.* 46% of USA-300 CA-MRSA isolates carry gene encoding resistance to Mupirocin *(Ln 367:731, 2006)*. **Note**: While resistance to Mupirocin continues to evolve, over-the-counter triple antibiotic ointment (Neomycin, polymyxin B, Bacitracin) remains active in vitro *(DMID 54:63, 2006)*. **Ecthyma:** Infection deeper into epidermis than impetigo. May need parenteral penicillin. Military outbreaks reported: *CID 48: 1213 & 1220, 2009 (good images).*
		For dosages, see Table 10C for adults and Table 16, page 187 for children		
Bullous (if ruptured, thin "varnish-like" crust)	**Staph. aureus impetigo** MSSA & MRSA	**For MSSA:** po therapy with **dicloxacillin**, **oxacillin**, **cephalexin**, **AM-CL**, **azithro**, **clarithro**, or **mupirocin** ointment or **retapamulin** ointment	**For MRSA: Mupirocin** ointment or po therapy with, **TMP-SMX-DS, minocycline**, **doxy, clinda**	
		For dosages, see Table 10C		
Infected wound, extremity—Post-trauma *(for bites, see page 49; for post-operative, see below)*—**Gram stain negative**				
Mild to moderate; uncomplicated	Polymicrobic: S. aureus (MSSA & MRSA), aerobic & anaerobic strep, Enterobacteriaceae, Cl. Perfringens, Cl. tetani; if water exposure, Pseudomonas sp., Aeromonas sp. Acinetobacter in soldiers in Iraq *(see CID 47:444, 2008)*.	**TMP-SMX-DS** 1-2 tabs po bid or **clinda** 300–450 mg po tid ***(see Comment)***	**Minocycline** 100 mg po bid or **linezolid** 600 mg po bid ***(see Comment)***	**Culture & sensitivity, check Gram stain. Tetanus toxoid if indicated.** **Mild infection:** Suggested drugs focus on S. aureus & Strep species. If suspect Gm-neg. bacilli, add **AM-CL-ER** 1000/62.5 two tabs po bid. If MRSA is erythro-resistant, may have inducible resistance to clinda. **Fever—sepsis**: Another alternative is **linezolid** 600 mg IV/po q12h. If Gm-neg. bacilli & severe pen allergy, **CIP** 400 mg IV q12h (q8h if P. aeruginosa) or **Levo** 750 mg IV q24h. Why 1-2 **TMP/SMX-DS**? *See discussion in footnote 1 of Table 6 (MRSA)* **TMP/SMX** not predictably active vs. strep species.
Febrile with sepsis—hospitalized		[**TC-CL** or **PIP-TZ** or **DORI**[NAI] or **IMP** or **MER** or **ERTA** *(Dosage, page 23)*] + **vanco** 1 gm IV q12h (1.5 gm if > 100 kg)	(**Vanco** 1 gm IV q12h or **dapto** 6 mg/kg IV q 24h or **ceftaroline** 600 mg IV q12h or **telavancin** 10 mg/kg IV q24h) + (**CIP** or **Levo** IV—*dose in Comment)*	

 NOTE: All dosage recommendations are for adults (unless otherwise indicated) and assume normal renal function.

TABLE 1A (50)

ANATOMIC SITE/DIAGNOSIS/ MODIFYING CIRCUMSTANCES	ETIOLOGIES (usual)	SUGGESTED REGIMENS*		ADJUNCT DIAGNOSTIC OR THERAPEUTIC MEASURES AND COMMENTS
		PRIMARY	ALTERNATIVE[§]	
SKIN *(continued)*				
Infected wound, post-operative—Gram stain negative: for Gram stain positive cocci – see below				
Surgery not involving GI or female genital tract				
Without sepsis (mild)	Staph. aureus, Group A, B, C or G strept sp.	**TMP-SMX-DS** 1-2 tabs po bid	**Clinda** 300–450 mg po tid	Check Gram stain of exudate. If Gm-neg. bacilli, **add** β-lactam/β-lactamase inhibitor: **AM-CL-ER** po or (**ERTA** or **PIP-TZ** or **TC-CL**) IV. *Dosage on page 23.* Why 1-2 **TMP/SMX-DS**? *See discussion in footnote 1 of Table 6 (MRSA).* **TMP/SMX** not predictably active vs. strep species.
With sepsis (severe)		**Vanco** 1 gm IV q12h; if >100 kg, 1.5 gm q12h.	**Dapto** 6 mg per kg IV q24h or **ceftaroline** 600 mg IV q12h or **telavancin** 10 mg/kg IV q24h	
Surgery involving GI tract (includes oropharynx, esophagus) or female genital tract—fever, neutrophilia	MSSA/MRSA, coliforms, bacteroides & other anaerobes	[**PIP-TZ** or (**P Ceph 3** + **metro**) or **DORI** or **ERTA** or **IMP** or **MER**] + (**vanco** 1 gm IV q12h or **dapto** 6 mg/kg IV q 24h) **if severely ill.** **Mild infection: AM-CL-ER** 1000/62.5 mg 2 tabs po bid + **TMP-SMX-DS** 1-2 tabs po bid if Gm+ cocci on Gram stain. *Dosages Table 10C & footnote 41, page 58.*		For all treatment options, *see Peritonitis, page 44.* Most important: Drain wound & get cultures. Can sub **linezolid** for vanco. Can sub **CIP or Levo** for β-lactams. Why 2 **TMP/SMX-DS**? *See discussion in footnote 1 of Table 6 (MRSA)*
Meleney's synergistic gangrene	*See Necrotizing fasciitis, page 53*			
Infected wound, febrile patient—Gram stain: Gram-positive cocci in clusters	S. aureus, possibly MRSA	**Do culture & sensitivity; open & drain wound** **Oral: TMP-SMX-DS** 1-2 tabs po bid or **clinda** 300–450 mg po tid *(see Comment)*	**IV: Vanco** 1 gm IV q12h or **dapto** 4-6 mg/kg IV q24h or **ceftaroline** 600 mg IV q12h or **telavancin** 10 mg/kg IV q24h	Need culture & sensitivity to verify MRSA. Other po options for CA-MRSA include minocycline 100 mg po q12h or **Doxy** 100 mg po bid (inexpensive) & linezolid 600 mg po q12h (expensive). If MRSA clinda-sensitive but erythro-resistant, watch out for inducible clinda resistance.
Necrotizing fasciitis ("flesh-eating bacteria")				
Post-surgery, trauma, streptococcal skin infections *See Gas gangrene, page 43, & Toxic shock, page 60.* Refs: *CID 44:705, 2007; NEJM 360:281, 2009.*	**4 types:** (1) Strept sp., Grp A, C, G; (2) Clostridia sp.; (3) polymicrobic: aerobic + anaerobic (if S. aureus + anaerobic strep = Meleney's synergistic gangrene); (4) Community- associated MRSA	*For treatment of clostridia, see Muscle, gas gangrene, page 43.* The terminology of **polymicrobic** wound infections is not precise: Meleney's synergistic gangrene, Fournier's gangrene, necrotizing fasciitis have common pathophysiology. **All require prompt surgical debridement** + antibiotics. Dx of necrotizing fasciitis req incision & probing. If no resistance to probing subcut (fascial plane), diagnosis = necrotizing fasciitis. **Need Gram stain/culture** to determine if etiology is strep, clostridia, polymicrobial, or S. aureus. **Treatment: Pen G** if strep or clostridia; **DORI**[NAI], **IMP** or **MER** if polymicrobial, add **vanco OR dapto** if MRSA suspected. **NOTE:** If strep necrotizing fasciitis, reasonable to treat with penicillin & clinda; if clostridia ± gas gangrene, add clinda to penicillin *(see page 43)*. MRSA ref.: *NEJM 352:1445, 2005.* ***See toxic shock syndrome, streptococcal, page 60.***		
Puncture wound—nail	Through tennis shoe: P. aeruginosa	Local debridement to remove foreign body & tetanus prophylaxis; no antibiotic therapy.		Osteomyelitis evolves in only 1–2% of plantar puncture wounds.
Staphylococcal scalded skin syndrome Ref.: *PIDJ 19:819, 2000*	Toxin-producing S. aureus	**Nafcillin** or **oxacillin** 2 gm IV q4h (children: 150 mg/kg/ day div. q6h) x 5–7 days for MSSA; **vanco** 1 gm IV q12h (children 40–60 mg/kg/day div. q6h) for MRSA		Toxin causes **intraepidermal split** and positive Nikolsky sign. Biopsy differentiates: drugs cause epiderm/dermal split, **called toxic epidermal necrolysis**—more serious *(Ln 351:1417, 1998)*. Biopsy differentiates.
Ulcerated skin lesions: Differential Dx	Consider: anthrax, tularemia, P. aeruginosa (ecthyma gangrenosum), plague, blastomycosis, spider (rarely), mucormycosis, mycobacteria, leishmania, arterial insufficiency, venous stasis, and others.			
Ulcerated skin: venous/arterial insufficiency; pressure with secondary infection	Polymicrobic: Streptococcus sp. (Groups A, C, G), enterococci, anaerobic strep, Enterobacteriaceae, Pseudomonas sp., Bacteroides sp., Staph. aureus	Severe local or possible bacteremia: **IMP** or **MER** or **DORI** or **TC-CL** or **PIP-TZ** or **ERTA.** If Gm-pos cocci on gram stain, add **Vanco**.	[(**CIP** or **Levo**) + **Metro**] or [(**CFP** or **Ceftaz**) + **Metro**]. If Gm-pos cocci on gram stain, add **Vanco**.	If ulcer clinically inflamed, treat IV with no topical rx. If not clinically inflamed, consider debridement, removal of foreign body, lessening direct pressure for weight-bearing limbs & leg elevation (if no arterial insufficiency). Topical rx to reduce bacterial counts: silver sulfadiazine 1% or combination antibiotic ointment. Avoid chlorhexidine & povidone iodine.
		Dosages, see footnotes [6, 7, 8, 14, 19, 41]		

Abbreviations on page 2. *NOTE: All dosage recommendations are for adults (unless otherwise indicated) and assume normal renal function.*

TABLE 1A (51)

ANATOMIC SITE/DIAGNOSIS/ MODIFYING CIRCUMSTANCES	ETIOLOGIES (usual)	SUGGESTED REGIMENS* PRIMARY	SUGGESTED REGIMENS* ALTERNATIVE§	ADJUNCT DIAGNOSTIC OR THERAPEUTIC MEASURES AND COMMENTS
SKIN *(continued)*				
Whirlpool: (Hot Tub) folliculitis	Pseudomonas aeruginosa	Usually self-limited, treatment not indicated		Decontaminate hot tub: drain and chlorinate. Also associated with exfoliative beauty aids (loofah sponges).
Whirlpool: Nail Salon, soft tissue infection	Mycobacterium (fortuitum or chelonae)	Minocycline, doxy or CIP		Ref: *CID 38:38, 2004.*
SPLEEN. For post-splenectomy prophylaxis, *see Table 15B, page 177; for Septic Shock Post-Splenectomy, see Table 1, pg 60.*				
Splenic abscess				
Endocarditis, bacteremia	Staph. aureus, streptococci	**Nafcillin** or **oxacillin** 2 gm IV q4h if MSSA	**Vanco** 1 gm IV q12h if MRSA	Burkholderia (Pseudomonas) pseudomallei is common cause of splenic abscess in SE Asia.
Contiguous from intra-abdominal site	Polymicrobic	*Treat as Peritonitis, secondary, page 44*		
Immunocompromised	Candida sp.	**Amphotericin B** *(Dosage, see Table 11, page 104)*	**Fluconazole, caspofungin**	
SYSTEMIC SYNDROMES (FEBRILE/NON-FEBRILE)				
Spread by infected **TICK, FLEA, or LICE**: Epidemiologic history crucial. **Babesiosis, Lyme disease, & Anaplasma (Ehrlichiosis)** have same reservoir & tick vector.				
Babesiosis: *see CID 43:1089, 2006.* Do not treat if asymptomatic, young, has spleen, and immunocompetent; can be fatal in lymphoma pts *(CID 46:370, 2008).*	Etiol.: B. microti et al. Vector: Usually Ixodes ticks Host: White-footed mouse & others	[(**Atovaquone** 750 mg po q12h) + (**azithro** 500 mg po day 1, then 250 mg per day) times 7 days] OR [**clinda** 1.2 gm IV bid or 600 mg po tid times 7 days + **quinine** 650 mg po tid times 7 days. **Ped. dosage: Clinda** 20–40 mg per kg per day and **quinine** 25 mg per kg per day]. **Exchange transfusion**-- *See Comment*		**Seven diseases where pathogen visible in peripheral blood smear:** African/American trypanosomiasis; babesia; bartonellosis; filariasis; malaria; relapsing fever. **Dx:** Giemsa-stained blood smear; antibody test available. PCR under study. **Rx: Exchange transfusions successful adjunct, used early, in severe disease.** May need treatment for 6 or more wks if immunocompromised.
Bartonella infections: Review *EID 12:389, 2006*				
Bacteremia, asymptomatic	B. quintana, B. henselae	**Doxy** 100 mg po/IV times 15 days		Can lead to endocarditis &/or trench fever: found in homeless, alcoholics, esp. if lice/leg pain. Often missed since asymptomatic.
Cat-scratch disease	B. henselae	**Azithro** or symptomatic only—*see page 43:* usually lymphadenitis, can involve CNS, liver in immunocompetent pts		
Bacillary angiomatosis; Peliosis hepatis—pts with AIDS	B. henselae, B. quintana	(**Clarithro** 500 mg bid or **clarithro ER** 1 gm po q24h or **azithro** 250 mg po q24h or **CIP** 500–750 mg po bid) times 8 wks	(**Erythro** 500 mg po qid or **doxy** 100 mg po bid) times 8 wks or if severe, combination of **doxy** 100 mg po/IV bid + **RIF** 300 mg po bid	**Manifestations of Bartonella infections:** **HIV/AIDS Patient:** Bacillary angiomatosis; Bacillary peliosis; Bacteremia/endocarditis/FUO. **Immunocompetent Patient:** Bacteremia/endocarditis/FUO/ encephalitis; Cat scratch disease; Vertebral osteo; Trench fever; Parinaud's oculoglandular syndrome
Endocarditis *(see page 25) (Circ 111:3167, 2005)*	B. henselae, B. quintana	Surgical removal of infected valve. [**Ceftriaxone** 2 gm IV once daily x 6 wks +**Gentamicin** 1 mg/kg IV q8h x 14 days] with or without **doxy** 100 mg IV/po bid x 6 wks.		Presents as SBE. Diagnosis: ECHO, serology & PCR of resected heart valve.
Oroya fever (acute) & Verruga peruana (chronic)	B. bacilliformis	Oroya fever: (**Chloro** 500 mg IV/po x 14 d + beta lactam) or **Doxy** 100 mg po bid x 14 d.	Verruga peruana: **RIF** 10 mg/kg po once daily x 14 d or **Streptomycin** 15-20 mg/kg IM/IV once daily x 10 d.	Oroya fever transmitted by sandfly bite in Andes Mtns. Related Bartonella (B. rochalimae) caused bacteremia, fever and splenomegaly *(NEJM 356:2346 & 2381, 2007).*
Trench fever (FUO)	B. quintana	No endocarditis: **Doxy** 100 mg po bid x 4 wks ; If endocarditis: **Doxy** + **Gentamicin** 3 mg/kg once daily for 1st 2 wks of therapy *(AAC 48:1921, 2004).*		

Abbreviations on page 2. *NOTE: All dosage recommendations are for adults (unless otherwise indicated) and assume normal renal function.*

TABLE 1A (52)

ANATOMIC SITE/DIAGNOSIS/ MODIFYING CIRCUMSTANCES	ETIOLOGIES (usual)	SUGGESTED REGIMENS*		ADJUNCT DIAGNOSTIC OR THERAPEUTIC MEASURES AND COMMENTS
		PRIMARY	ALTERNATIVE[§]	
SYSTEMIC SYNDROMES (FEBRILE/NON-FEBRILE)/Spread by infected TICK, FLEA, or LICE/Ehrlichiosis *(continued)*				
Ehrlichiosis[40]. CDC def. is one of: (1) 4x ↑ IFA antibody, (2) detection of Ehrlichia DNA in blood or CSF by PCR, (3) visible morulae in WBC and IFA ≥1:64				
Human monocytic ehrlichiosis (HME) *(MMWR 55(RR-4), 2006; CID 43:1089, 2006)*	Ehrlichia chaffeensis (Lone Star tick is vector)	**Doxy** 100 mg po/IV bid times 7–14 days	**Tetracycline** 500 mg po qid x 7–14d. No current rec. for children or pregnancy	30 states: mostly SE of line from NJ to Ill. to Missouri to Oklahoma to Texas. History of outdoor activity and tick exposure. April-Sept. Fever, rash (36%), leukopenia and thrombocytopenia. Blood smears no help. PCR for early dx.
Human Anaplasmosis (formerly known as Human granulocytic ehrlichiosis)	Anaplasma (Ehrlichia) phagocytophilum (Ixodes sp. ticks are vector). Dog variant is Ehrlichia ewingii *(NEJM 341:148 & 195, 1999)*	**Doxy** 100 mg bid po or IV times 7–14 days	**Tetracycline** 500 mg po qid times 7–14 days. Not in children or pregnancy. *See Comment*	Upper Midwest, NE, West Coast & Europe. H/O tick exposure. April-Sept. Febrile flu-like illness after outdoor activity. No rash. Leukopenia/ thrombocytopenia common. **Dx:** Up to 80% have + blood smear. Antibody test for confirmation. **Rx:** RIF successful in pregnancy *(CID 27:213, 1998)* but worry about resistance developing. Based on in vitro studies, no clear alternative rx—Levo activity marginal *(AAC 47:413, 2003)*.
Lyme Disease NOTE: Think about concomitant tick-borne disease—e.g., babesiosis and ehrlichiosis. **Guidelines: *CID 43:1089, 2006; CID 51:1, 2010; Med Lett 52:53, 2010.***				
Bite by ixodes-infected tick in an endemic area -- Post-exposure prophylaxis	Borrelia burgdorferi **ISDA guidelines: *CID 43:1089, 2006; CID 51:1, 2010***	**If endemic area**, if nymphal partially engorged deer tick: **doxy** 200 mg po times 1 dose with food	**If not endemic area**, not engorged, not deer tick: No treatment	Prophylaxis study in endemic area: erythema migrans developed in 3% of the control group and 0.4% doxy group *(NEJM 345:79 & 133, 2001)*.
Early (erythema migrans) *See Comment*	Western blot diagnostic criteria: **IgM**—Need 2 of 3 positive of kilodaltons (KD): 23, 39, 41	**Doxy** 100 mg po bid. or **amoxicillin** 500 mg po tid or **cefuroxime axetil** 500 mg po bid or **erythro** 250 mg po qid. All regimens for 14–21 days. (10 days as good as 20: *AnIM 138:697, 2003*) *See Comment for peds doses*		High rate of clinical failure with azithro & erythro *(Drugs 57:157, 1999)*. **Peds** (all po for 14–21 days): **Amox** 50 mg per kg per day in 3 div. doses or **cefuroxime axetil** 30 mg per kg per day in 2 div. doses or **erythro** 30 mg per kg per day in 3 div. doses. Lesions usually homogenous—not target-like *(AnIM 136:423, 2002)*.
Carditis *See Comment*	**IgG**—Need 5 of 10 positive of KD: 18, 21, 28, 30, 39, 41, 45, 58, 66, 93	(**Ceftriaxone** 2 gm IV q24h) or (**cefotaxime** 2 gm IV q4h) or (**Pen G** 3 million units IV q4h) times 14–21 days	**Doxy** *(see Comments)* 100 mg po bid times 14–21 days or **amoxicillin** 500 mg po tid times 14–21 days.	First degree AV block: Oral regimen. Generally self-limited. High degree AV block (PR >0.3 sec.): IV therapy—permanent pacemaker not necessary.
Facial nerve paralysis (isolated finding, early)	For chronic lyme disease discussion see: *CID 51:1, 2010.*	(**Doxy** 100 mg po bid) or (**amoxicillin** 500 mg po) tid times 14–21 days	**Ceftriaxone** 2 gm IV q24h times 14–21 days	LP suggested to exclude central neurologic disease. If LP neg., oral regimen OK. If abnormal or not done, suggest parenteral Ceftriaxone.
Meningitis, encephalitis *For encephalopathy, see Comment*		**Ceftriaxone** 2 gm IV q24h times 14–28 days	(**Pen G** 20 million units IV q24h in div. dose) or (**cefotaxime** 2 gm IV q8h) times 14–28 days	Encephalopathy: memory difficulty, depression, somnolence, or headache, CSF abnormalities. 89% had objective CSF abnormalities. 18/18 pts improved with ceftriaxone 2 gm per day times 30 days *(JID 180:377, 1999)*. No compelling evidence that prolonged treatment has any benefit in post-Lyme syndrome *(Neurology 69:91, 2007)*.
Arthritis		(**Doxy** 100 mg po bid) or (**amoxicillin** 500 mg po tid), both times 30–60 days	(**Ceftriaxone** 2 gm IV q24h) or (**pen G** 20–24 million units per day IV) times 14–28 days	Start with 1 mo of therapy; if only partial response, treat for a second mo.
Pregnant women		Choice should **not** include doxy; **amoxicillin** 500 mg po tid times 21 days.	**If pen. allergic:** (**azithro** 500 mg po q24h times 7–10 days) or (**erythro** 500 mg po qid times 14–21 days)	
Post-Lyme Disease Syndromes		None indicated		No benefit from treatment *(CID 51:1, 2010; NEJM 345:85, 2001)*.

[40] In endemic area (New York), high % of both adult ticks and nymphs were jointly infected with both Anaplasma (HGE) and B. burgdorferi *(NEJM 337:49, 1997)*.

Abbreviations on page 2. *NOTE: All dosage recommendations are for adults (unless otherwise indicated) and assume normal renal function.*

TABLE 1A (53)

ANATOMIC SITE/DIAGNOSIS/ MODIFYING CIRCUMSTANCES	ETIOLOGIES (usual)	SUGGESTED REGIMENS*		ADJUNCT DIAGNOSTIC OR THERAPEUTIC MEASURES AND COMMENTS
		PRIMARY	ALTERNATIVE§	
SYSTEMIC SYNDROMES (FEBRILE/NON-FEBRILE)/Spread by infected TICK, FLEA, or LICE/Ehrlichiosis *(continued)*				
Relapsing fever *ID Clin No Amer 22:449, 2008.*	No. Amer: Borrelia hermsii & tunicate E. Africa: B. duttoni Elsewhere: B. recurrentis	**Doxy** 100 mg po bid x 7-10 days	**Erythro** 500 mg po qid x 7-10 days	Jarisch-Herxheimer (fever, ↑ pulse, ↑ resp., ↓ blood pressure) in most patients (occurs in ~2 hrs). Not prevented by prior steroids. **Dx: Examine peripheral blood smear during fever for spirochetes.** Can relapse up to 10 times. Post-exposure **doxy** pre-emptive therapy highly effective *(NEJM 355:148, 2006)*
Rickettsial diseases. Review—Disease in travelers *(CID 39:1493, 2004)*				
Spotted fevers (NOTE: Rickettsial pox not included)				
Rocky Mountain spotted fever (RMSF) *(LnID 8:143, 2008 and MMWR 55 (RR-4), 2007)* NOTE: Can mimic ehrlichiosis. Pattern of rash important—*see Comment*	R. rickettsii (Dermacentor ticks)	**Doxy** 100 mg po/IV bid times 7 days or for 2 days after temp. normal. Do not use in pregnancy.	**Chloro** 50 mg/kg/day in 4 div doses. Use in pregnancy.	Fever, rash (95%), petechiae 40–50%. **Rash spreads from distal extremities to trunk.** Dx: Immunohistology on skin biopsy; confirmation with antibody titers. Highest incidence in Mid-Atlantic states; also seen in Oklahoma, S. Dakota, Montana. **NOTE: Only 3–18% of pts present with fever, rash, and hx of tick exposure; esp. in children many early deaths & empiric doxy reasonable** *(MMWR 49: 885, 2000)*.
Other spotted fevers, e.g., Rickettsial pox, African tick bite fever	At least 8 species on 6 continents *(CID 45 (Suppl 1) S39, 2007)*.	**Doxy** 100 mg po bid times 7 days	**Chloro** 500 mg po/IV qid times 7 days Children <8 y.o.: **azithro** or **clarithro** *(if mild disease)*	Clinical diagnosis suggested by: 1) fever, intense myalgia, headache; 2) exposure to mites or ticks; 3) localized eschar (tache noire) or rash. Definitive Dx: PCR of blood, skin biopsy or sequential antibody tests.
Typhus group—Consider in returning travelers with fever				
Louse-borne: epidemic typhus Ref: *LnID 8:417, 2008.*	R. prowazekii (vector is body or head louse)	**Doxy** 100 mg IV/po bid times 7 days	**Chloro** 500 mg IV/po qid times 7 days	**Brill-Zinsser disease** *(Ln 357:1198, 2001)* is a relapse of typhus acquired during WWII. Truncal rash (64%) spreads centrifugally—opposite of RMSF. Louse borne typhus is a winter disease. Diagnosis by serology.
Murine typhus (cat flea typhus): *EID 14:1019, 2008.*	R. typhi (rat reservoir and flea vector): *CID 46:913, 2008*	**Doxy** 100 mg IV/po bid times 7 days	**Chloro** 500 mg IV/po qid times 7 days	Rash in 20-54%, not diagnostic. Without treatment most pts recover in 2 wks. Faster recovery with treatment. Dx based on suspicion; confirmed serologically.
Scrub typhus	O. tsutsugamushi [rodent reservoir; vector is larval stage of mites (chiggers)]	**Doxy** 100 mg po/IV bid x 7 days. In pregnancy: **Azithro** 500 mg po x one dose	**Chloro** 500 mg po/IV qid x 7 days	Asian rim of Pacific. Suspect Dx in endemic area. Confirm with serology. If Doxy resistance suspected, suggest **Doxy** + **RIF** 900 or 600 mg once daily *(Ln 356:1057, 2000)*.
Tularemia, typhoidal type Ref. **bioterrorism**: *see JAMA 285:2763, 2001*	Francisella tularensis. (Vector depends on geography: ticks, biting flies, mosquitoes identified)	[(**Gentamicin** or **tobra** 5 mg per kg per day div. q8h IV) or (**Streptomycin** 10 mg/kg IV/IM q12h)] x 10 days	[**CIP** 400 mg IV (or 750 mg po) bid or **Doxy** 100 mg IV/po bid] x 14-21 days	Diagnosis: Culture on cysteine-enriched media & serology. Dangerous in the lab. Hematogenous meningitis is a complication: treatment is **Streptomycin** + **Chloro** 50-100 mg/kg/day IV in 4 divided doses *(Arch Neurol 66:523, 2009)*.
Other Zoonotic Systemic Bacterial Febrile Illnesses: Obtain careful epidemiologic history				
Brucellosis *Review: NEJM 352:2325, 2005; Ref on vertebral osteo due to Brucella: CID 46:426, 2008.* **Treat osteomyelitis for 3 months.**				
Adult or child >8 years CDC: All positive rapid serologies require confirmation with Brucella-specific agglutination *(MMWR 57:603, 2008).*	Brucella sp. B. abortus—cattle B. suis—pigs B. melitensis—goats B. canis—dogs	[**Doxy** 100 mg po bid times 6 wks + **gentamicin** times 7 days *(see Table 10D, page 101)*] or [**doxy** times 6 wks + **streptomycin** 1 gm IM q24h times 2-3 wks] *See Comment*	[**Doxy** + **RIF** 600–900 mg po q24h, both times 6 wks] or [**TMP-SMX** 1 DS tab (160 mg TMP) po qid times 6 wks + **gentamicin** times 2 wks] or [(**doxy** + **RIF**) + **gentamicin**] *(BMJ 336:701, 2008)*.	**Clinical disease:** Protean. Fever in 91%. **Malodorous perspiration almost pathognomic.** Osteoarticular disease in approx. 20%; epididymitis/orchitis 6%. **Lab:** Mild hepatitis. Leukopenia & relative lymphocytosis. **Diagnosis:** Serology, bone marrow culture, real-time PCR if available. **Treatment:** Drugs must penetrate macrophages & act in acidic milieu. **Pregnancy:** TMP-SMX-DS + RIF reasonable. Prospective random. Study documents **doxy** + 7 days of **gent** as effective as **doxy + streptomycin** x 14 days *(CID 42:1075, 2006)*. Review of **FQs** (in combination) as alternative therapy *(AAC 50:22, 2006)*.
Child <8 years		**TMP-SMX** 5 mg per kg TMP po q12h times 6 wks + **gentamicin** 2 mg per kg IV/IM q8h times 2 wks		

Abbreviations on page 2. *NOTE: All dosage recommendations are for adults (unless otherwise indicated) and assume normal renal function.*

TABLE 1A (54)

ANATOMIC SITE/DIAGNOSIS/ MODIFYING CIRCUMSTANCES	ETIOLOGIES (usual)	SUGGESTED REGIMENS* PRIMARY	ALTERNATIVE[§]	ADJUNCT DIAGNOSTIC OR THERAPEUTIC MEASURES AND COMMENTS
SYSTEMIC SYNDROMES (FEBRILE/NON-FEBRILE)/Other Zoonotic Systemic Bacterial Febrile Illnesses *(continued)*				
Leptospirosis *(CID 36:1507 & 1514, 2003; LnID 3:757, 2003)*	Leptospira—in urine of domestic livestock, dogs, small rodents	**Pen G** 1.5 million units IV q6h or **ceftriaxone** 1 gm q24h. Duration: 7 days	(**Doxy** 100 mg IV/po q12h or **AMP** 0.5–1 gm IV q6h) x 7 days	**Severity varies**. Two-stage mild anicteric illness to severe icteric disease (Weil's disease) with renal failure and myocarditis. **Rx:** Azithro 1 gm once, then 500 mg daily x 2 days: non-inferior to, and fewer side effects than, doxy in standard dose *(AAC 51:3259, 2007)*.
Salmonella bacteremia (enteric fever most often caused by S. typhi). Look for extraintestinal infections.	Salmonella enteritidis—a variety of serotypes	(**CIP** 400 mg IV q12h or **Levo** 750 mg po once daily) x 14 days *(See Comment)*	**Ceftriaxone** 2 gm IV q24h *(See Comment)*	In vitro resistance to nalidixic acid indicates relative resistance to FQs. Bacteremia can infect any organ/tissue: look for infection of atherosclerotic aorta, osteomyelitis in sickle cell pts. Rx duration range 14 days (immunocompetent) to ≥6 wks if mycotic aneurism or endocarditis.
Miscellaneous Systemic Febrile Syndromes				
Fever in Returning Travelers *(NEJM 354:119, 2006; COID 20:449, 2007)*.	Dengue	Flavivirus	Supportive care; *see Table 14A, page 145*	Average incubation period 4 days; serodiagnosis.
	Malaria	Plasmodia sp.	Diagnosis: peripheral blood smear	See Table 13A, beginning at page 127
	Typhoid fever	Salmonella sp.	*See Table 1A, page 57.*	Average incubation 7-14 days; diarrhea in 45%.
Kawasaki syndrome 6 weeks to 12 yrs of age, peak at 1 yr of age; 85% below age 5. Ref: *Pediatrics 124:1, 2009.*	Acute self-limited vasculitis with ↑ temp., rash, conjunctivitis, stomatitis, cervical adenitis, red hands/feet & coronary artery aneurysms (25% if untreated)	**IVIG** 2 gm per kg over 8-12 hrs + **ASA** 20-25 mg per kg qid THEN **ASA** 3–5 mg per kg per day po q24h times 6–8 wks	If still febrile after 1st dose of IVIG, some give 2nd dose.	IV gamma globulin (2 gm per kg over 10 hrs) in pts rx before 10th day of illness ↓ coronary artery lesions *(Ln 347:1128, 1996)*. See *Table 14A, page 156* for IVIG adverse effects. Pulsed steroids of NO value: *NEJM 356:659 & 663, 2007.*
Rheumatic Fever, acute Ref.: *Ln 366:155, 2005*	Post-Group A strep pharyngitis (not Group B, C, or G)	(1) Symptom relief: **ASA** 80–100 mg per kg per day in children; 4–8 gm per day in adults. (2) Eradicate Group A strep: **Pen** times 10 days *(see Pharyngitis, page 46)*. (3) Start prophylaxis: *see below*		
Prophylaxis				
Primary prophylaxis: Treat S. pyogenes pharyngitis	**Benzathine pen G** 1.2 million units IM *(see Pharyngitis, p. 46)*		**Penicillin** for 10 days, prevents rheumatic fever even when started 7–9 days after onset of illness *(see page 46)*. **Alternative**: **Penicillin V** 250 mg po bid or **sulfadiazine (sulfisoxazole)** 1 gm po q24h or **erythro** 250 mg po bid.	
Secondary prophylaxis (previous documented rheumatic fever)	**Benzathine pen G** 1.2 million units IM q3–4 wks		**Duration?** No carditis: 5 yr or age 21, whichever is longer; carditis without residual heart disease: 10 yr; carditis with residual valvular disease: 10 yr since last episode & at least age 40 *(PEDS 96:758, 1995)*.	
Typhoidal syndrome (typhoid fever, enteric fever) *(Ln 366:749, 2005; LnID 5:623, 2005)* Decreased CIP susceptibility in S. paratyphi isolates from S.E. Asia *(CID 46:1656, 2008)*.	Salmonella typhi, S. paratyphi NOTE: In vitro resistance to nalidixic acid often predicts clinical failure of CIP (FQs) *(Ln 366:749, 2005)*	(**CIP** 400 mg IV q24h or **Levo** 750 mg po/IV q24h) x 7-10 d. If SE Asian pt, do not treat until in vitro data available. *(See Comment)* In children, CIP superior to ceftriaxone *(LnID 3:537, 2003)*	(**Ceftriaxone** 2 gm IV daily x 7-14 d) or (**Azithro** 1 gm po x 1 dose, then 500 mg po daily x 5-7 d) or (**Chloro** 500 mg po/IV q6h x 14 d) *(See Comment)*	**Dexamethasone:** In controlled trial, mortality lower than in pts given Chloro + dex vs. Chloro alone *(NEJM 310:82, 1984)*. No data on dex + FQs or Ceftriaxone. Use in severely ill pts. 1st dose just prior to antibiotic, 3 mg/kg IV, then 1 mg/kg q6h x 8 doses. **Complications:** perforation of terminal ileum &/or cecum, osteo, septic arthritis, **mycotic aneurysm** (approx. 10% over age 50, *AJM 110:62, 2001*), meningitis.

TABLE 1A (55)

ANATOMIC SITE/DIAGNOSIS/ MODIFYING CIRCUMSTANCES	ETIOLOGIES (usual)	SUGGESTED REGIMENS*		ADJUNCT DIAGNOSTIC OR THERAPEUTIC MEASURES AND COMMENTS
		PRIMARY	ALTERNATIVE[§]	
SYSTEMIC SYNDROMES (FEBRILE/NON-FEBRILE) *(continued)*				
Sepsis: Following suggested **empiric** therapy assumes pt is bacteremic; mimicked by viral, fungal, rickettsial infections and pancreatitis *(Intensive Care Medicine 34:17, 2008; IDC No Amer 22:1, 2008)*.				
Neonatal—early onset <1 week old	Group B strep, E. coli, klebsiella, enterobacter, Staph. aureus (uncommon), listeria (rare in U.S.)	**AMP** 25 mg per kg IV q8h + **cefotaxime** 50 mg per kg q12h	(**AMP** + **gent** 2.5 mg per kg IV/IM q12h) or (**AMP** + **ceftriaxone** 50 mg per kg IV/IM q24h)	Blood cultures are key but only 5–10% +. Discontinue antibiotics after 72 hrs if cultures and course do not support diagnosis. In Spain, listeria predominates; in S. America, salmonella.
Neonatal—late onset 1–4 weeks old	As above + H. influenzae & S. epidermidis	(**AMP** 25 mg per kg IV q6h + **cefotaxime** 50 mg per kg q8h) or (**AMP** + **ceftriaxone** 75 mg per kg IV q24h)	**AMP** + **gent** 2.5 mg per kg q8h IV or IM	**If MSSA/MRSA a concern, add vanco.**
Child; not neutropenic	Strep. pneumoniae, meningococci, Staph. aureus (MSSA & MRSA), H. influenzae now rare	(**Cefotaxime** 50 mg per kg IV q8h or **ceftriaxone** 100 mg per kg IV q24h) + **vanco** 15 mg per kg IV q6h	**Aztreonam** 7.5 mg per kg IV q6h + **linezolid** *(see Table 16, page 187 for dose)*	Major concerns are S. pneumoniae & community-associated MRSA. Coverage for Gm-neg. bacilli included but H. influenzae infection now rare. Meningococcemia mortality remains high *(Ln 356:961, 2000)*.
Adult; not neutropenic; NO HYPOTENSION but LIFE-THREATENING!—*For Septic shock, see page 60*				Systemic inflammatory response syndrome **(SIRS):** 2 or more of the following: 1. Temperature >38°C or <36°C 2. Heart rate >90 beats per min. 3. Respiratory rate >20 breaths per min. 4. WBC >12,000 per mcL or >10% bands **Sepsis:** SIRS + a documented infection (+ culture) **Severe sepsis:** Sepsis + organ dysfunction: hypotension or hypoperfusion abnormalities (lactic acidosis, oliguria, ↓ mental status) **Septic shock:** Sepsis-induced hypotension (systolic BP <90 mmHg) not responsive to 500 mL IV fluid challenge + peripheral hypoperfusion.
Source unclear—consider primary bacteremia, intra-abdominal or skin source. May be **Life-threatening**. Survival greater with quicker, effective empiric antibiotic Rx *(CCM 38:1045 & 1211, 2010)*.	Aerobic Gm-neg. bacilli; S. aureus; streptococci; others	(**ERTA** or **IMP** or **MER**) + **vanco** Could substitute linezolid for vanco or dapto; however, linezolid bacteriostatic vs. S. aureus. *Dosages in footnote[41]*	(**Dapto** 6 mg per kg IV q24h) + (**cefepime** or **PIP-TZ** or **TC-CL**)	
If suspect biliary source *(see p.11)*	Enterococci + aerobic Gm-neg. bacilli	**PIP-TZ** or **TC-CL**	**Ceftriaxone** + **metro;** (**CIP** or **Levo**) + **metro.** *Dosages–footnote[41]*	
If community-acquired pneumonia *(see page 36 and following pages)*	**S. pneumoniae; MRSA, Legionella, Gm-neg. bacillus**	(**Levo** or **moxi**) + (**PIP-TZ**) + **Vanco**	**Aztreonam** + (**Levo** or **moxi**) + **linezolid**	Many categories of CAP, *see material beginning at page 36*. Suggestions based on most severe CAP, e.g., MRSA after influenza or Klebsiella pneumonia in an alcoholic.
If illicit use IV drugs	S. aureus	**Vanco if high prevalence of MRSA. Do NOT use empiric vanco + oxacillin pending organism ID.** In vitro nafcillin increased production of toxins by CA-MRSA *(JID 195:202, 2007)*. ***Dosages—footnote [41], page 58***		
If suspect intra-abdominal source	Mixture aerobic & anaerobic Gm-neg. bacilli	*See secondary peritonitis, page 45.*		
If petechial rash	Meningococcemia	**Ceftriaxone** 2 gm IV q12h (until sure no meningitis); consider Rocky Mountain spotted fever—*see page 56*		
If suspect urinary source, e.g. pyelonephritis	Aerobic Gm-neg. bacilli & enterococci	*See pyelonephritis, page 31*		

[41] **P Ceph 3** (**cefotaxime** 2 gm IV q8h, use q4h if life-threatening; **ceftizoxime** 2 gm IV q4h; **ceftriaxone** 2 gm IV q12h), **AP Pen** (**piperacillin** 3 gm IV q4h, **ticarcillin** 3 gm IV q4h), **TC-CL** 3.1 gm IV q4h, **PIP-TZ** 3.375 gm IV q4h or 4-hr infusion of 3.375 gm q8h, **Aminoglycosides** *(see Table 10D, page 101)*, **AMP** 200 mg/kg/day divided q6h, **clinda** 900 mg IV q8h, **IMP** 0.5 gm IV q6h, **MER** 1 gm IV q8h, **ERTA** 1 gm IV q24h, **DORI** 500 mg IV q8h (1-hr infusion), **Nafcillin** or **oxacillin** 2 gm IV q4h, **aztreonam** 2 gm IV q8h, **metro** 1 gm loading dose then 0.5 gm q6h or 1 gm IV q12h, **vanco** 1 gm IV q12h, **ceftazidime** 2 gm IV q8h, [**Cefepime** 2 gm IV q12h (q8h if neutropenic), **cefpirome**[NUS] 2 gm IV q12h], **CIP** 400 mg IV q12h, **levo** 750 mg IV q24h, **linezolid** 600 mg IV q12h.

Abbreviations on page 2. *NOTE: All dosage recommendations are for adults (unless otherwise indicated) and assume normal renal function.*

TABLE 1A (56)

ANATOMIC SITE/DIAGNOSIS/ MODIFYING CIRCUMSTANCES	ETIOLOGIES (usual)	SUGGESTED REGIMENS*		ADJUNCT DIAGNOSTIC OR THERAPEUTIC MEASURES AND COMMENTS
		PRIMARY	ALTERNATIVE[§]	
SYSTEMIC SYNDROMES (FEBRILE/NON-FEBRILE)/Sepsis *(continued)*				
Neutropenia: Child or Adult (absolute PMN count <500 per mm3) in cancer and transplant patients. Guideline: ***CID 34:730, 2002***				
Prophylaxis *(LnID 9:97, 2009)*.				
Post-chemotherapy—impending neutropenia	Aerobic Gm-neg. bacilli, pneumocystis (PCP), Viridans strep	Meta-analysis demonstrates substantive reduction in mortality with **CIP** 500 mg po bid *(AnIM 142:979, 2005)*. Similar results in observational study using **Levo** 500 mg po q24h *(CID 40:1087 & 1094, 2005)*. Also *NEJM 353:977, 988 & 1052, 2005*.		
Post-chemotherapy in AIDS patient	↑ risk pneumocystis, aerobic Gm-neg bacilli	**TMP-SMX-DS** 1 tab po once daily—adults 10 mg per kg per day div bid po—children		TMP-SMX DS has prophylactic efficacy vs. PCP and E. coli.
Post-marrow ablation, bone marrow transplant	Aerobic Gm-neg bacilli, ↑ risk pneumocystis, herpes viruses, candida	**TMP-SMX** as above + [either **acyclovir** or **ganciclovir**] + **fluconazole]**		Combined regimen justified by combined effect of neutropenia and immuno-suppression.
Empiric therapy—febrile neutropenia (≥38.3°C for > 1 hr or sustained >38°C and absolute neutrophil count <500 cells/µL)				
Low-risk adults *(Low risk defined in Comment)*	Aerobic Gm-neg bacilli, Viridans strep	**CIP** 750 mg po bid + **AM-CL** 875 /125 mg po bid. Treat until absolute neutrophil count >1000 cells/µL	**Treat as outpatients with 24/7 access to inpatient care if: no focal findings, no hypotension, no COPD, no fungal infection, no dehydration, age range 16-60 yrs; motivated and compliant pts & family**	
High-risk adults and children Oral "mucositis" can falsely elevate oral temperature readings *(CID 46:1859, 2008)*.	**Aerobic Gm-neg. bacilli; to include P. aeruginosa; cephalosporin-resistant viridans strep; MRSA**	**Monotherapy: ceftaz or IMP** *(see Comment)* **or MER or CFP or PIP-TZ** *Dosages: Footnote[41] and Table 10* **Include empiric vanco** if: suspect IV access infected; colonized with drug-resistant S. pneumo or MRSA; blood culture pos. for Gm.-pos. cocci; pt hypotensive	**Combination therapy: (Gent** or **tobra) + (TC-CL** or **PIP-TZ)**	Increasing resistance of viridans streptococci to penicillins, cephalosporins & FQs *(CID 34:1469 & 1524, 2002)*. **What if severe IgE-mediated β-lactam allergy?** No formal trials, but [aminoglycoside (or CIP) + aztreonam] ± vanco should work. **IMP:** 0.5 gm q6h achieved MIC90 coverage in only 53%. If GFR OK, dose of 500 mg q4h or 750 mg (over 2 hrs) q6h may be better *(AAC 53:785, 2009)*.
Persistent fever and neutropenia after 5 days of empiric antibacterial therapy—see ***CID 34:730, 2002*****—General guidelines**				
	Candida species, aspergillus	Add either (**caspofungin** 70 mg IV day 1, then 50 mg IV q24h or **Micafungin** 100 mg IV q24h or **Anidulafungin** 200 mg IV x 1 dose then 100 mg IV q24h) **OR voriconazole** 6 mg per kg IV q12h times 2 doses, then 3 mg per kg IV q12h		Conventional **ampho B** causes more fever & nephrotoxicity & lower efficacy than lipid-based ampho B; both **caspofungin** & **voriconazole** better tolerated & perhaps more efficacious than lipid-based ampho B *(NEJM 346:225, 2002 & 351:1391 & 1445, 2005)*.

NOTE: All dosage recommendations are for adults (unless otherwise indicated) and assume normal renal function.

TABLE 1A (57)

ANATOMIC SITE/DIAGNOSIS/ MODIFYING CIRCUMSTANCES	ETIOLOGIES (usual)	SUGGESTED REGIMENS* PRIMARY	SUGGESTED REGIMENS* ALTERNATIVE[§]	ADJUNCT DIAGNOSTIC OR THERAPEUTIC MEASURES AND COMMENTS
SYSTEMIC FEBRILE SYNDROMES *(continued)*				
Shock syndromes				
Septic shock: Fever & hypotension **Bacteremic shock, endotoxin shock** Antimicrobial therapy: *CCM 32 (Suppl):S495, 2004 & Surviving Sepsis Campaign: CCM 36:296, 2008 & Intensive Care Med 34:17, 2008.* A polymyxin B fiber column reduced 28 day mortality in pts with intra-abdominal gram-negative infections (not available in U.S.): *JAMA 301:2445, 2009; JAMA 302:1968, 2009*	Bacteremia with aerobic Gm-neg. bacteria or Gm+ cocci	**Proven Therapies**: - Replete intravascular vol with IV saline; goal is CVP >8 cm within 6 hr of admission. - Attempt to correct source of bacteremia. - Blood cultures, then antibiotics appropriate for clinical syndrome. Time to 1st dose crucial *(Chest 136:1237, 2009; CCM 38:1045 & 1211, 2010)*. - If still hypotensive & lactate > 36 mg/dL either nor-epinephrine or dopamine *(NEJM 362:779 & 841, 2010)*.		- Low dose glucocorticoids: data controversial. Currently, consider use if pt still hypotensive & vasopressor dependent after 2+ days of fluids, antibiotics & success w/source control *(JAMA 301:2362, 2009; CID 49:93, 2009)*. Hard to interp ACTH stim. data. - Insulin Rx: Current target is glucose level of 150 mg/dL. Attempts at tight control (80-110 mg/dL) resulted in excessive hypoglycemia *(NEJM 360:1283 & 1346, 2009; JAMA 303:341, 2010)*. - Activated Protein C (Drotrecogin): Only consider use in pts with APACHE score > 25, multiorgan failure and no bleeding risk factors *(NEJM 361:2646, 2009)*. Dose: 24 μg/kg/hr over 96h. DC 2 hr prior to surgery; restart 12 hr post-surgery.
Septic shock: post-splenectomy or functional asplenia	S. pneumoniae, N. meningitidis, H. influenzae, Capnocytophaga (DF-2)	**Ceftriaxone** 2 gm IV q24h (↑ to 2 gm q12h if meningitis) Other management as per Septic shock, above	(**Levo** 750 mg or **Moxi** 400 mg) once IV q24h	Howell-Jolly bodies in peripheral blood smear confirm absence of functional spleen. Often results in **symmetrical peripheral gangrene of digits** due to severe DIC. For prophylaxis, *see Table 15A, page176*.
Toxic shock syndrome, Clostridium sordellii				
Post-partum, post-abortion, post-mifepristone, IUD *CID 43:1436 & 1447, 2006 (See comment)*	Clostridium sordellii Mortality 69%!	Fluids, aq. **penicillin G** 18–20 million units per day div. q4–6h + **clindamycin** 900 mg IV q8h. Surgical debridement.	Several deaths reported after use of abortifacient regimen of mifepristone (RU486) & misoprostol. Clinically: often afebrile, rapid progression, hypotension, hemoconcentration (high Hct), neutrophilia (WBC >50,000). 2001-2006 standard medical abortion: po mifepristone & then vaginal misoprostol. Since 2006, switch to buccal, instead of vaginal misoprostol, plus prophylactic Doxy resulted in dramatic decrease in TSS *(NEJM 361:145, 2009)*.	
Toxic shock syndrome, staphylococcal. Review: *LnID 2: 9:392, 2009*				
Colonization by toxin-producing Staph. aureus of: vagina (tampon-assoc.), surgical/traumatic wounds, endometrium, burns	Staph. aureus (toxic shock toxin-mediated)	(**Nafcillin** or **oxacillin** 2 gm IV q4h) or (if MRSA, **vanco** 1 gm IV q12h) + **IVIG**	(**Cefazolin** 1–2 gm IV q8h) or (if MRSA, **vanco** 1 gm IV q12h OR **dapto** 6 mg/kg IV q24h) + **IVIG**	**IVIG reasonable** *(see Streptococcal TSS)*— dose 1 gm per kg on day 1, then 0.5 gm per kg days 2 & 3—antitoxin antibodies present. If suspect TSS, "turn off" toxin production with clinda; report of success with **linezolid** *(JID 195:202, 2007)*. *Exposure of MRSA to nafcillin increased toxin production in vitro: JID 195:202, 2007.*
Toxic shock syndrome, streptococcal. NOTE: For Necrotizing fasciitis without toxic shock, *see page 53*. Ref: *LnID 9:281, 2009.*				
Associated with invasive disease, i.e., erysipelas, necrotizing fasciitis; secondary strep infection of varicella. Secondary TSS cases reported *(NEJM 335:547 & 590, 1996; CID 27:150, 1998)*.	Group A, B, C, & G Strep. pyogenes, Group B strept ref: *EID 15:223, 2009.*	(**Pen G** 24 million units per day IV in div. doses) + (**clinda** 900 mg IV q8h) **IVIG** associated with ↓ in sepsis-related organ failure *(CID 37:333 & 341, 2003)*. IVIG dose: 1 gm per kg day 1, then 0.5 gm per kg days 2 & 3. IVIG preps vary in neutralizing antibody content *(CID 43:743, 2006)*. In multicenter retrospect study, no benefit from IVIG-controversial *(CID 1369 & 1377, 2009)*.	**Ceftriaxone** 2 gm IV q24h + **clinda** 900 mg IV q8h	**Definition:** Isolation of Group A strep, hypotension and ≥2 of: renal impairment, coagulopathy, liver involvement, ARDS, generalized rash, soft tissue necrosis. Associated with invasive disease. **Surgery usually required.** Mortality with fasciitis 30–50%, myositis 80% even with early rx *(CID 14:2, 1992)*. Clinda ↓ toxin production. Use of NSAID may predispose to TSS. For reasons pen G may fail in fulminant S. pyogenes infections *(see JID 167:1401, 1993)*.

 NOTE: All dosage recommendations are for adults (unless otherwise indicated) and assume normal renal function.

TABLE 1A (58)

ANATOMIC SITE/DIAGNOSIS/ MODIFYING CIRCUMSTANCES	ETIOLOGIES (usual)	SUGGESTED REGIMENS*		ADJUNCT DIAGNOSTIC OR THERAPEUTIC MEASURES AND COMMENTS
		PRIMARY	ALTERNATIVE§	
SYSTEMIC FEBRILE SYNDROMES *(continued)*				
Toxin-Mediated Syndromes—no fever unless complicated				
Botulism *(CID 41:1167, 2005. As* **biologic weapon:** *JAMA 285:1059, 2001; www.bt.cdc.gov)*				
	Clostridium botulinum	For all types: Follow vital capacity; other supportive care		**Equine antitoxin:** Heptavalent currently only antitoxin available (U.S) for non-infant botulism: *CDC (+1 404-639-2206 M-F OR +1 404-639-2888 evenings/weekends).* For infants, *use Baby BIG (human botulism immune globulin): California Infant Botulism Treat & Prevent Program.* **Antimicrobials:** May make infant botulism worse. Untested in wound botulism. When used, pen G 10–20 million units per day usual dose. If complications (pneumonia, UTI) occur, avoid antimicrobials with assoc. neuromuscular blockade, i.e., aminoglycosides, tetracycline, polymyxins. **Differential dx:** Guillain-Barré, myasthenia gravis, tick paralysis, organophosphate toxicity, West Nile virus
Food-borne Dyspnea at presentation bad sign *(CID 43:1247, 2006)*		If no ileus, purge GI tract	Heptavalent equine serum antitoxin—CDC *(see Comment)*	
Infant		Human botulinum immunoglobulin (BIG) IV, single dose. Call (+1) 510-540-2646. Do not use equine antitoxin.	No antibiotics; may lyse C. botulinum in gut and ↑ load of toxin	
Wound		Debridement & anaerobic cultures. No proven value of local antitoxin. Role of antibiotics untested	Trivalent equine antitoxin *(see Comment)*	Wound botulism can result from spore contamination of tar heroin. Ref: *CID 31:1018, 2000.* Mouse bioassay failed to detect toxin in 1/3 of patients *(CID 48:1669, 2009)*.
Tetanus	C. tetani	(**Pen G** 3 million units q4h in div. dose or **doxy** 100 mg IV q12h) times 7–10 days	**Metro** 500 mg po q6h or 1 gm IV q12h times 7–10 days *(See Comment)*	Multifaceted treatment: Wound debridement, tetanus immunoglobulin (250–500 units IM), antimicrobics, & tetanus toxoid (tetanus does not confer immunity). Options for control of muscle spasms: continuous infusion of midazolam, IV propofol, and/or intrathecal baclofen *(CID 38:321, 2004)*.
VASCULAR				
IV line infection *(see LnID 7:645, 2007)*: **Treatment:** *(For Prevention, see below).* ***Diagnosis of infected line*** *without removal of IV catheter? See CID 44:820 & 827, 2007.*				
Heparin lock, midline catheter, **non-tunneled** central venous catheter (subclavian, internal jugular), peripherally inserted central catheter (PICC) Avoid femoral vein if possible: ↑ risk of infection and/or thrombosis *(JAMA 286:700, 2001)*--especially if BMI >28.4 *(JAMA 299:2413, 2008)*.	Staph. epidermidis, Staph. aureus (MSSA/MRSA)	**Vanco** 1 gm IV q12h. **Other alternatives—see Comment.** Other rx and duration: **(1) If S. aureus,** remove catheter. Can use TEE result to determine if 2 or 4 wks of therapy *(JAC 57:1172, 2006)*. **(2) If S. epidermidis,** can try to "save" catheter. 80% cure after 7–10 days of therapy. With only systemic antibiotics, high rate of recurrence *(CID 49:1187, 2009)*. If **leuconostoc** or **lactobacillus**, need **Pen G**, **Amp** or **Clinda**.		If no response to, or intolerant of, **vanco**: switch to **daptomycin** 6 mg per kg IV q24h. **Quinupristin-dalfopristin** an option: 7.5 mg per kg IV q8h via central line. Culture removed catheter. With "roll" method, >15 colonies *(NEJM 312:1142, 1985)* suggests infection. Lines do not require "routine" changing when not infected. When infected, do not insert new catheter over a wire. Antimicrobial-impregnated catheters may ↓ infection risk; the debate is lively *(CID 37:65, 2003 & 38:1287, 2004 & 39:1829, 2004)*.
Tunnel type indwelling venous catheters and ports (Broviac, Hickman, Groshong, Quinton), dual lumen hemodialysis catheters (Permacath). *For prevention, see below.*	Staph. epidermidis, Staph. aureus, (Candida sp.). Rarely: leuconostoc or lactobacillus—both resistant to vanco *(see Table 2, page 63)*			If subcutaneous tunnel infected, very low cure rates; need to remove catheter.

Abbreviations on page 2. *NOTE: All dosage recommendations are for adults (unless otherwise indicated) and assume normal renal function.*

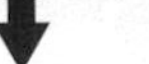

TABLE 1A (59)

ANATOMIC SITE/DIAGNOSIS/ MODIFYING CIRCUMSTANCES	ETIOLOGIES (usual)	SUGGESTED REGIMENS*		ADJUNCT DIAGNOSTIC OR THERAPEUTIC MEASURES AND COMMENTS
		PRIMARY	ALTERNATIVE[§]	
VASCULAR/IV line infection *(continued)*				
Impaired host (burn, neutropenic)	As above + Pseudomonas sp., Enterobacteriaceae, Corynebacterium jeikeium, aspergillus, rhizopus	[**Vanco** + (**Cefepime** or **Ceftaz**) or (**Vanco** + **Pip-Tazo**) or **IMP** or [(**Cefepime** or **Ceftaz**) + **Aminoglycoside**]. *(Dosage in footnotes[34,41], pages 44 and 58)*		Usually have associated septic thrombophlebitis: biopsy of vein to rule out fungi. If fungal, surgical excision + amphotericin B. Surgical drainage, ligation or removal often indicated.
Hyperalimentation	As with tunnel, Candida sp. common *(see Table 11, resistant Candida species)*	If candida, **voriconazole or an echinocandin** (**anidulafungin**, **micafungin**, **caspofungin**) if clinically stable. Dosage: *see Table 11B, page 114.*		Remove venous catheter and discontinue antimicrobial agents if possible. Ophthalmologic consultation recommended. **Rx all patients with + blood cultures.** *See Table 11A, Candidiasis, page 104*
Intravenous lipid emulsion	Staph. epidermidis	**Vanco** 1 gm IV q12h		Discontinue intralipid
	Malassezia furfur	**Fluconazole** 400 mg IV q24h		
Prevention of Infection of Long-Term IV Lines *NEJM 355:2725 & 2781, 2006; LnID 7:645, 2007*	To minimize risk of infection: **Hand washing and** **1.** Maximal sterile barrier precautions during catheter insertion **2.** Use 2% chlorhexidine for skin antisepsis **3.** If infection rate high despite #1 & 2, use either chlorhexidine/silver sulfadiazine or minocycline/rifampin-impregnated catheters or "lock" solutions *(see Comment)*. **4.** If possible, use subclavian vein, avoid femoral vessels. Lower infection risk in jugular than femoral if BMI >28.4 *(JAMA 299:2413, 2008)*.			**IV line "lock" solutions under study. No FDA-approved product.**
Suppurative pelvic thrombophlebitis (with or without septic pulmonary emboli) Postpartum or postabortion or postpelvic surgery	Streptococci, bacteroides, Enterobacteriaceae	**Metro** + **P Ceph 3**; **cefoxitin**; **TC-CL**; **PIP-TZ** *Dosages: Table 10C, page 92*	**IMP** or **MER** or **ERTA** or [**clinda** + (**aztreonam** or **gent**)]	Use heparin during antibiotic regimen. Duration unclear; one study shows benefit of anticoagulation *(Am J Obstet Gyn 181:143, 1999)*. Cefotetan less active than cefoxitin vs. non-fragilis bacteroides. Cefotetan has methyltetrazole side-chain which is associated with hypoprothrombinemia (prevent with vitamin K).
Suppurative Cavernous sinus thrombosis	Staph. aureus, Streptococcus sp., H. influenzae, aspergillus/mucor/rhizopus	**Vanco** 1 gm IV q12h + **ceftriaxone** 2 gm IV q12h	(**Dapto** 6 mg per kg IV q24h[NAI] or **linezolid** 600 mg IV q12h) + **ceftriaxone** 2 gm IV q12h	CT or MRI scan for diagnosis. **Heparin** usually used.
Other Suppurative phlebitis: femoral, saphenous, internal jugular, subclavian	S. aureus, S. pyogenes, Strept sp. (Group B), Fusobacterium necrophorum (Lemierre's Syndrome)	**Vancomycin** 15 mg/kg IV q12h (normal weight) + **ceftriaxone** 1 gm IV q24h	**Daptomycin** 6 mg/kg IV q12h + **ceftriaxone** 1 gm IV q24h	Retrospective study: 2-3 weeks IV therapy + 2 weeks po therapy *(CID 49:741, 2008)*. If involved vein accessible, surgical I&D or excision may help, esp. if bacteremic pt.

NOTE: All dosage recommendations are for adults (unless otherwise indicated) and assume normal renal function.

TABLE 2 – RECOMMENDED ANTIMICROBIAL AGENTS AGAINST SELECTED BACTERIA

BACTERIAL SPECIES	ANTIMICROBIAL AGENT (See page 2 for abbreviations)		
	RECOMMENDED	ALTERNATIVE	ALSO EFFECTIVE[1] (COMMENTS)
Alcaligenes xylosoxidans (Achromobacter xylosoxidans)	IMP, MER, AP Pen	TMP-SMX. Some strains susc. to ceftaz *(AAC 32: 276, 1988)*	Resistant to APAG; P Ceph 1, 2, 3, 4; aztreonam; FQ *(AAC 40:772, 1996)*
Acinetobacter calcoaceticus—baumannii complex	IMP or MER or Dori or [FQ + (amikacin or ceftaz)]	AM-SB *(CID 24:932, 1997; CID 34:1425, 2002)*. Sulbactam[NUS] also effective *(JAC 42:793, 1998)*; colistin *(CID 36:1111, 2003)*	Up to 10% isolates resistant to IMP, MER; resistance to FQs, amikacin increasing. Doxy + amikacin effective in animal model *(JAC 45: 493, 2000)*. Minocycline, tigecycline also effective against many strains *(IDCP 16:16, 2008; JAC 62:45, 2008)* *(See Table 5, pg 74)*
Actinomyces israelii	AMP or Pen G	Doxy, ceftriaxone	Clindamycin, erythro
Aeromonas hydrophila	FQ	TMP-SMX or (P Ceph 3, 4)	APAG; ERTA; IMP; MER; tetracycline (some resistant to carbapenems)
Arcanobacterium (C.) haemolyticum	Erythro	Benzathine Pen G	Sensitive to most drugs, resistant to TMP-SMX *(AAC 38:142, 1994)*
Bacillus anthracis (anthrax): inhalation	*See Table 1A, page 40*		
Bacillus cereus, B. subtilis	Vancomycin, clinda	FQ, IMP	
Bacteroides fragilis (ssp. fragilis)	Metronidazole	Cefoxitin, Dori, ERTA, IMP, MER, TC-CL, PIP-TZ, AM-SB, cefotetan, AM-CL	Resist to clindamycin, cefotetan limit utility against B.frag. *(JAC 53(Suppl2):29, 2004; CID 35:5126, 2002)*.
"DOT" group of bacteroides			(not cefotetan)
Bartonella (Rochalimaea) henselae, quintana *See Table 1A, pages 43, 49, 54*	Azithro, clarithro, CIP (bacillary angiomatosis), azithro (cat-scratch) *(PIDJ 17:447, 1998; AAC 48:1921, 2004)*	Erythro or doxy	Other drugs: TMP-SMX *(IDC N Amer 12: 137, 1998)*. Consider doxy + RIF for severe bacillary angiomatosis *(IDC N.Amer 12: 137, 1998)*; doxy + gentamicin optimal for endocarditis *(AAC 47:2204, 2003)*
Bordetella pertussis	Erythro	TMP-SMX	An erythro-resistant strain reported in Arizona *(MMWR 43:807, 1994)*
Borrelia burgdorferi, B. afzelii, B. garinii	Ceftriaxone, cefuroxime axetil, doxy, amox *(See Comments)*	Penicillin G (HD), cefotaxime	Clarithro. Choice depends on stage of disease, *Table 1A, pg 55*
Borrelia sp.	Doxy	Erythro	Penicillin G
Brucella sp.	Doxy + either gent or SM *(IDCP 7, 2004; CID 42:1075, 2006)*	(Doxy + RIF) or (TMP-SMX + gentamicin)	FQ + RIF *(AAC 41:80,1997; EID 3: 213, 1997; CID 21:283,1995)*. Mino + RIF *(J Chemother 15:248, 2003)*.
Burkholderia (Pseudomonas) cepacia	TMP-SMX or MER or CIP	Minocycline or chloramphenicol	(Usually resist to APAG, AG, polymyxins) *(AAC 37: 123, 1993 & 43:213, 1999; Inf Med 18:49, 2001)* (Some resist to carbapenems). May need combo rx *(AJRCCM 161:1206, 2000)*.
Burkholderia (Pseudomonas) pseudomallei *See Table 1A, pg 38, & Ln 361:1715, 2003*	Initially, IV ceftaz or IMP *(CID 29:381, 1999; CID 41:1105, 2005)*	Then po TMP-SMX + doxy x 3 mo ± chloro *(AAC 49:4020, 2005)*	(Thai, 12–80% strains resist to TMP-SMX). FQ active in vitro. Combo chloro, TMP-SMX, doxy ↑ effective than doxy alone for maintenance *(CID 29:375, 1999)*. MER also effective *(AAC 48: 1763, 2004)*
Campylobacter jejuni	Erythro	FQ (↑ resistance, *NEJM 340:1525,1999)*	Clindamycin, doxy, azithro, clarithro *(see Table 5, pg 74)*
Campylobacter fetus	Gentamicin	P Ceph 3	AMP, chloramphenicol
Capnocytophaga ochracea (DF-1) and	Clinda or AM-CL	CIP, Pen G	P Ceph 3, IMP, cefoxitin, FQ, (resist to APAG, TMP-SMX). C. haemolytica & C. granulosa oft resist to β-lactams & aminoglycosides *[CID 35 (Suppl.1): S17, 2002]*
canimorsus (DF 2)	AM-CL		
Chlamydophila pneumoniae	Doxy	Erythro, FQ	Azithro, clarithro
Chlamydia trachomatis	Doxy or azithro	Erythro	
Chryseobacterium meningosepticum (now Elizabethkingia meningoseptica)	Vancomycin ± RIF *(CID 26:1169, 1998)*	CIP, levofloxacin	In vitro susceptibilities may not correlate with clinical efficacy *(AAC 41:1301, 1997; CID 26:1169, 1998)*
Citrobacter diversus (koseri), C. freundii	AP Pen	FQ	APAG
Clostridium difficile	Metronidazole (po)	Vancomycin (po)	Bacitracin (po); nitazoxanide *(CID 43:421, 2006; JAC 59:705, 2007)*. Rifaximin *(CID 44:846, 2007). See also Table 1A re severity of disease.*
Clostridium perfringens	Pen G ± clindamycin	Doxy	Erythro, chloramphenicol, cefazolin, cefoxitin, AP Pen, CARB
Clostridium tetani	Metronidazole or Pen G	Doxy	AP Pen
Corynebacterium jeikeium	Vancomycin	Pen G + APAG	
C. diphtheriae	Erythro	Clindamycin	RIF. Penicillin reported effective *(CID 27:845, 1998)*
Coxiella burnetii (Q fever) acute disease	Doxy *(see Table 1A, page 28)*	Erythro	In meningitis consider FQ *(CID 20: 489, 1995)*. Endocarditis: doxy + hydroxychloroquine *(JID 188:1322, 2003; LnID 3:709, 2003)*.
chronic disease	(CIP or doxy) + RIF	FQ + doxy x 3 yrs *(CID 20:489, 1995)*	CQ + doxy *(AAC 37:1773, 1993)*. ? gamma interferon *(Ln 20:546, 2001)*

TABLE 2 (2)

BACTERIAL SPECIES	ANTIMICROBIAL AGENT *(See page 2 for abbreviations)*		
	RECOMMENDED	**ALTERNATIVE**	**ALSO EFFECTIVE[1] (COMMENTS)**
Ehrlichia chaffeensis, Ehrlichia ewubguum Anaplasma (Ehrlichia) phagocytophillium	Doxy	Tetracycline, RIF *(CID 27:213, 1998)*	CIP, oflox, chloramphenicol also active in vitro. Resist to clinda, TMP-SMX, IMP, AMP, erythro, & azithro *(AAC 41:76, 1997)*.
Eikenella corrodens	Penicillin G or AMP or AM-CL	TMP-SMX, FQ	Doxy, cefoxitin, cefotaxime, IMP (Resistant to clinda, cephalexin, erythro, & metro)
Enterobacter species	Recommended agents vary with clinical setting. *See Table 1A & Table 5*		
Enterococcus faecalis	*See Table 5, pg 73*		
Enterococcus faecium, β-lactamase +, high-level aminoglycoside resist., vancomycin resist.: *See Table 5, pg 73*			
Erysipelothrix rhusiopathiae	Penicillin G or AMP	P Ceph 3, FQ	IMP, AP Pen (vancomycin, APAG, TMP-SMX resistant)
Escherichia coli	Recommended agents vary with clinical setting. *See Table 1A & 4; Table 5 for ESBL-producers*		
Francisella tularensis (tularemia) *See Table 1A, page 42*	Gentamicin, tobramycin, or streptomycin	Doxy or CIP	Chloramphenicol, RIF. Doxy/chloro bacteriostatic → relapses
Gardnerella vaginalis (bacterial vaginosis)	Metronidazole or Tinidazole	Clindamycin	*See Table 1A, pg 24 for dosage*
Hafnia alvei	*Same as Enterobacter spp.*		
Helicobacter pylori	*See Table 1A, pg 19*		Drugs effective in vitro often fail in vivo.
Haemophilus aphrophilus	[(Penicillin or AMP) ± gentamicin] or [AM-SB ± gentamicin]	P Ceph 2, 3 ± gentamicin	(Resistant to vancomycin, clindamycin, methicillin)
Haemophilus ducreyi (chancroid)	Azithro or ceftriaxone	Erythro, CIP	Most strains resistant to tetracycline, amox, TMP-SMX
Haemophilus influenzae Meningitis, epiglottitis & other life-threatening illness	Cefotaxime, ceftriaxone	TMP-SMX, AP Pen, FQs (AMP if ß-lactamase neg) (US 25–30% AMP resist, Japan 35%)	Chloramphenicol (downgrade from 1st choice due to hematotoxicity). 9% US strains resist to TMP-SMX *(AAC 41:292, 1997)*
non-life threatening illness	AM-CL, O Ceph 2/3, TMP-SMX, AM-SB		Azithro, clarithro, telithro
Klebsiella ozaenae/ rhinoscleromatis	FQ	RIF + TMP-SMX	*(Ln 342:122, 1993)*
Klebsiella species	Recommended agents vary with clinical setting. *See Table 1A & Table 5*		
Lactobacillus species	(Pen G or AMP) ± gentamicin	Clindamycin, erythro	**May be resistant to vancomycin**
Legionella sp. *(42 species & 60 serotypes recognized) (Sem Resp Inf 13:90, 1998)*	FQ, or azithro, or (erythro ± RIF)	Clarithro	TMP-SMX, doxy. Most active FQs in vitro: Gemi, Levo, Moxi. *See AnIM 129:328, 1998.* Telithro active in vitro.
Leptospira interrogans	Penicillin G	Doxy	Ceftriaxone *(CID 36:1507, 2003)*, cefotaxime *(CID 39:1417, 2004)*.
Leuconostoc	Pen G or AMP	Clinda, erythro, minocycline	APAG **NOTE: Resistant to vancomycin**
Listeria monocytogenes	AMP	TMP-SMX	Erythro, penicillin G (high dose), APAG may be synergistic with β-lactams. Meropenem active in vitro. **Cephalosporin-resistant!**
Moraxella (Branhamella) catarrhalis	AM-CL or O Ceph 2/3, TMP-SMX	Azithro, clarithro, dirithromycin, telithro	Erythro, doxy, FQs
Morganella species	Recommended agents vary with clinical setting. *See Table 1A & Table 4*		
Mycoplasma pneumoniae	Erythro, azithro, clarithro, FQ	Doxy	(Clindamycin & ß lactams NOT effective)
Neisseria gonorrhoeae (gonococcus)	Ceftriaxone, cefixime, cefpodoxime	Spectinomycin, azithro	High prevalence of FQ resistance in Asia. FQ resistance now so high in U.S. that FQs are no longer recommended *(MMWR 56:332, 2007; AIM 148:606, 2008)*.
Neisseria meningitidis (meningococcus)	Penicillin G	Ceftriaxone, cefuroxime, cefotaxime	Sulfonamide (some strains), chloramphenicol. Chloro-resist strains in SE Asia *(NEJM 339:868, 1998) (Prophylaxis: pg 9)*
Nocardia asteroides	TMP-SMX, sulfonamides (high dose),	Minocycline	Amikacin + (IMP or ceftriaxone or cefuroxime) for brain abscess
Nocardia brasiliensis	TMP-SMX, sulfonamides (high dose)	AM-CL	Amikacin + ceftriaxone
Pasteurella multocida	Pen G, AMP, amox	Doxy, AM-CL	Ceftriaxone, cefpodoxime, FQ (active in vitro), azithro (active in vitro) *(DMID 30:99, 1998; AAC 43:1475, 1999); resistant to cephalexin, oxacillin, clindamycin.*
Plesiomonas shigelloides	CIP	TMP-SMX	AM-CL, P Ceph 1,2,3,4, IMP, MER, tetracycline, aztreonam
Propionibacterium acnes	Penicillin, Ceftriaxone	Vanco, Dapto, Linezolid	Resistant to Metronidazole
Proteus mirabilis (indole–)	AMP	TMP-SMX	Most agents except nafcillin/oxacillin. β-lactamase (including ESBL) production now being described in P. mirabilis *(J Clin Micro 40:1549, 2002)*
vulgaris (indole +)	P Ceph 3 or FQ	APAG	Aztreonam, BL/BLI, AP-Pen
Providencia sp.	Amikacin, P Ceph 3, FQ	TMP-SMX	AP-Pen + amikacin, IMP

TABLE 2 (3)

BACTERIAL SPECIES	ANTIMICROBIAL AGENT (See page 2 for abbreviations)		
	RECOMMENDED	ALTERNATIVE	ALSO EFFECTIVE[1] (COMMENTS)
Pseudomonas aeruginosa	AP Pen, AP Ceph 3, Dori, IMP, MER, tobramycin, CIP, aztreonam. For serious inf., use AP β-lactam + tobramycin or CIP *(LnID 4:519, 2004)*	For UTI, single drugs usually effective: AP Pen, AP Ceph 3, cefepime, IMP, MER, APAG, CIP, aztreonam	Resistance to β-lactams (IMP, ceftaz) may emerge during rx. β-lactam inhibitor adds nothing to activity of TC or PIP against P. aeruginosa. Clavulanic acid antag TC in vitro *(AAC 43:882, 1999). (See also Table 5).* Recommend combination therapy for serious infections, but value of combos controversial *(LnID 5:192, 2005).*
Rhodococcus (C. equi)	IMP, APAG, erythro, vanco, or RIF (Consider 2 agents)	CIP (variable)[resistant strains in SE Asia *(CID 27:370, 1998)*], TMP-SMX, tetra, or clinda	Vancomycin active in vitro but intracellular location of R. equi may impair efficacy *(Sem Resp Inf 12:57, 1997; CID 34:1379, 2002)*
Rickettsiae species	Doxy	Chloramphenicol	FQ; clari, azithro effective for Mediterranean spotted fever in children *(CID 34:154, 2002).*
Salmonella typhi	FQ, ceftriaxone	Chloramphenicol, amox, TMP-SMX, azithro (for uncomplicated disease: *AAC 43:1441, 1999)*	Multi drug resistant strains (chloramphenicol, AMP, TMP-SMX) common in many developing countries, seen in immigrants. FQ resistance now being reported *(AJTMH 61:163, 1999).*
Serratia marcescens	P Ceph 3, ERTA, IMP, MER, FQ	Aztreonam, gentamicin	TC-CL, PIP-TZ
Shigella sp.	FQ or azithro	TMP-SMX and AMP (resistance common in Middle East, Latin America). Azithro ref.: *AnIM 126:697, 1997.* Cefixime, ceftriaxone.	
Staph. aureus, methicillin-susceptible	Oxacillin/nafcillin	P Ceph 1, vanco, teicoplanin[NUS], clinda, ceftaroline	ERTA, IMP, MER, BL/BLI, FQ, erythro, clarithro, azithro, telithro, quinu-dalfo, linezolid, dapto, telavancin.
Staph. aureus, methicillin-resistant (health-care associated) *IDSA Guidelines: CID 52 (Feb 1):1, 2011.*	Vancomycin	Teicoplanin[NUS], TMP-SMX (some strains resistant), quinu-dalfo, linezolid, daptomycin, telavancin, ceftaroline	Fusidic acid[NUS]. >60% CIP-resistant in U.S. (Fosfomycin + RIF), novobiocin. Partially vancomycin-resistant strains (GISA, VISA) & highly resistant strains now described—*see Table 6, pg 75.*
Staph. aureus, methicillin-resistant [community- associated (CA-MRSA)]			CA-MRSA usually not multiply-resistant *(Ln 359: 1819, 2002; JAMA 286: 1201, 2001).* Oft resist to erythro & variably to FQ. Vanco, teico[NUS], telavancin or daptomycin can be used in pts requiring hospitalization *(see Table 6, pg 75).* Also, ceftaroline.
Mild-moderate infection	(TMP-SMX or doxy or mino) ± RIF *(CID 52 (Feb 1):1, 2011)*	Clinda (if D-test neg—*see Table 5 & 6)*	
Severe infection	Vanco or teico[NUS]	Linezolid or daptomycin	
Staph. epidermidis	Vancomycin ± RIF	RIF + (TMP-SMX or FQ), daptomycin *(AAC 51:3420, 2007)*	Cephalothin or nafcillin/oxacillin if sensitive to nafcillin/oxacillin but 75% are resistant. FQs. *(See Table 5).*
Staph. haemolyticus	TMP-SMX, FQ, nitrofurantoin	Oral cephalosporin	Recommendations apply to UTI only.
Staph. lugdunensis	Oxacillin/nafcillin or penicillin G (if β-lactamase neg.) *(Inf Dis Alert 22:193, 2003)*	P Ceph 1 or vancomycin or teico[NUS]	Approx. 75% are penicillin-susceptible. Usually susceptible to gentamicin, RIF *(Clin Micro Rev 21:111, 2008).*
Staph. saprophyticus (UTI)	Oral cephalosporin or AM-CL	FQ	Suscept to most agents used for UTI; occ. failure of sulfonamides, nitrofurantoin reported *(JID 155:170, 1987).* Resist to fosfomycin.
Stenotrophomonas (Xanthomonas, Pseudomonas) maltophilia	TMP-SMX	TC-CL or (aztreonam + TC-CL) *(AAC 41:2612, 1997)*	Minocycline, doxy, tigecycline, CIP, Ceftriaxone, moxifloxacin, ceftaz *(LnID 9:312, 2009; JAC 62:889, 2008).* [In vitro synergy (TC-CL + TMP-SMX) & (TC-CL + CIP), *JAC 62:889, 2008].*
Streptobacillus moniliformis	Penicillin G or doxy	Erythro, clindamycin	
Streptococcus, anaerobic (Peptostreptococcus)	Penicillin G	Clindamycin	Erythro, doxy, vancomycin
Streptococcus pneumoniae penicillin-susceptible	Penicillin G	Multiple agents effective, e.g., amox	*See footnote Drugs & peds dosage on Table 1A, page 10.*
penicillin-resistant (MIC ≥2.0)	(Vancomycin + RIF) or (Gemi, Gati, Levo, or Moxi). *See footnote[2] pg 7 and Table 5, pg 74*		For non-meningeal infec: P Ceph 3/4, AP Pen, quinu-dalfo, linezolid, telithro, ceftaroline
Streptococcus pyogenes, Groups A, B, C, G, F, Strep. milleri (constellatus, intermedius, anginosus)	Penicillin G or V (some add gent for serious Group B infec & some add clinda for serious invasive Group A) *(SMJ 96:968, 2003)*	All β lactams, erythro, azithro, clarithro, telithro	Macrolide resistance increasing.
Vibrio cholerae	Doxy, FQ	TMP-SMX	Strain 0139 is resistant to TMP-SMX
Vibrio parahaemolyticus	Antibiotic rx does not ↓ course		Sensitive in vitro to FQ, doxy
Vibrio vulnificus, alginolyticus, damsela	Doxy + ceftaz	Cefotaxime, FQ (eg, levo, *AAC 46:3580, 2002)*	APAG often used in combo with ceftaz
Yersinia enterocolitica	TMP-SMX or FQ	P Ceph 3 or APAG	*CID 19:655, 1994*
Yersinia pestis (plague)	*See Table 1A, pg 39*		

[1] Agents are more variable in effectiveness than "Recommended" or "Alternative." Selection of "Alternative" or "Also Effective" based on in vitro susceptibility testing, pharmacokinetics, host factors such as auditory, renal, hepatic function, & cost.

TABLE 3 – SUGGESTED DURATION OF ANTIBIOTIC THERAPY IN IMMUNOCOMPETENT PATIENTS[1,2]

CLINICAL SITUATION		DURATION OF THERAPY (Days)
SITE	**CLINICAL DIAGNOSIS**	
Bacteremia	Bacteremia with removable focus (no endocarditis)	10–14 *(CID 14:75, 1992) (See Table 1A)*
Bone	Osteomyelitis, adult; acute	42
	adult; chronic	Until ESR normal (often > 3 months)
	child; acute; staph. and enterobacteriaceae[3]	21
	child; acute; strep, meningococci, haemophilus[3]	14
Ear	Otitis media with effusion	<2 yr: 10 (or 1 dose ceftriaxone).; ≥2 yr: 5–7
	Recent meta-analysis suggests 3 days of azithro *(JAC 52:469, 2003)* or 5 days of "short-acting" antibiotics effective for uncomplicated otitis media *(JAMA 279:1736, 1998)*, but may be inadequate for severe disease *(NEJM 347:1169, 2002)*.	
Endo-cardium	Infective endocarditis, native valve	
	Viridans strep	14 or 28 *(See Table 1A, page 25)*
	Enterococci	28 or 42 *(See Table 1A, page 26)*
	Staph. aureus	14 (R-sided only) or 28 *(See Table 1A, page 27)*
GI *Also see Table 1A*	Bacillary dysentery (shigellosis)/traveler's diarrhea	3
	Typhoid fever (S. typhi): Azithro	5 (children/adolescents)
	Ceftriaxone	14 [Short course ↑ effective *(AAC 44:450, 2000)*]
	FQ	5–7
	Chloramphenicol	14
	Helicobacter pylori	10–14. For triple-drug regimens, 7 days probably adequate *(AIM 147:553, 2007)*.
	Pseudomembranous enterocolitis (C. difficile)	10
Genital	Non-gonococcal urethritis or mucopurulent cervicitis	7 days doxy or single dose azithro
	Pelvic inflammatory disease	14
Heart	Pericarditis (purulent)	28
Joint	Septic arthritis (non-gonococcal) Adult	14–28 *(Ln 351:197, 1998)*
	Infant/child	Rx as osteomyelitis above. Recent study suggests 10-14 days of therapy sufficient *(CID 48:1201, 2009)*, but not complete agreement on this *(CID 48:1211, 2009)*.
	Gonococcal arthritis/disseminated GC infection	7 *(See Table 1A, page 21)*
Kidney	Cystitis (bladder bacteriuria)	3 (Single dose extended-release cipro also effective) *(AAC 49:4137, 2005)*
	Pyelonephritis	14 (7 days if CIP used; 5 days if levo 750 mg)
	Recurrent (failure after 14 days rx)	42
Lung	Pneumonia, pneumococcal	Until afebrile 3–5 days (minimum 5 days).
	Community-acquired pneumonia	Minimum 5 days and afebrile for 2-3 days *(CID 44:S55, 2007; AJM 120:783, 2007)*.
	Pneumonia, enterobacteriaceae or pseudomonal	21, often up to 42
	Pneumonia, staphylococcal	21–28
	Pneumocystis carinii, in AIDS;	21
	other immunocompromised	14
	Legionella, mycoplasma, chlamydia	7–14
	Lung abscess	Usually 28–42[4]
Meninges[5] *(CID 39:1267, 2004)*	N. meningitidis	7
	H. influenzae	7
	S. pneumoniae	10–14
	Listeria meningoencephalitis, gp B strep, coliforms	21 (longer in immunocompromised)
Multiple systems	Brucellosis *(See Table 1A, page 56)*	42 (add SM or gent for 1st 7–14 days) *(JAC 65:1028, 2010)*
	Tularemia *(See Table 1A, pages 42, 56)*	7–14
Muscle	Gas gangrene (clostridial)	10
Pharynx	Group A strep pharyngitis Also see Pharyngitis, *Table 1A, page 46*	10 O Ceph 2/3, azithromycin effective at 5 days *(JAC 45, Topic TI 23, 2000; JIC 14:213, 2008)*. 3 days less effective *(Inf Med 18:515, 2001). Single dose extended rel Azithro (2 gm) as effective as 3 days of immediate rel Azithro (CMI 15:1103, 2009). See also 2009 Cochrane Review (www.thecochranelibrary.com).*
	Diphtheria (membranous)	7–14
	Carrier	7
Prostate	Chronic prostatitis (TMP/SMX)	30–90
	(FQ)	28–42
Sinuses	Acute sinusitis	5–14[6]
Skin	Cellulitis	Until 3 days after acute inflamm disappears
Systemic	Lyme disease	*See Table 1A, page 55*
	Rocky Mountain spotted fever *(See Table 1A, page 56)*	Until afebrile 2 days

[1] Early change from IV to po regimens (about 72 hrs) is cost-effective with many infections, i.e., intra-abdominal *(AJM 91:462, 1991)*. There is emerging evidence that serum **procalcitonin** level determination (a measure of bacterial or fungal infection) may allow early stopping of empiric therapy *(JCM 48:2325, 2010)*.

[2] The recommended duration is a minimum or average time and should not be construed as absolute.

[3] These times are with proviso: sx & signs resolve within 7 days and ESR is normalized *(J.D. Nelson, APID 6:59, 1991)*.

[4] After patient afebrile 4-5 days, change to oral therapy.

[5] In children relapses seldom occur until 3 days or more after termination of rx. For meningitis in children, *see Table 1A, page 7*.

[6] Duration of therapy dependent upon agent used and severity of infection. Longer duration (10-14 days) optimal for beta-lactams and patients with severe disease. For sinusitis of mild-moderate severity shorter courses of therapy (5-7 days) effective with "respiratory FQs" (including gemifloxacin, levofloxacin 750 mg), azithromycin. Courses as short as 3 days reported effective for TMP-SMX and azithro and one study reports effectiveness of single dose extended-release azithro. Authors feel such "super-short" courses should be restricted to patients with mild-mod disease *(JAMA 273:1015, 1995; AAC 47:2770, 2003; Otolaryngol-Head Neck Surg 133:194, 2005; Otolaryngol-Head Neck Surg 127:1, 2002; Otolaryngol-Head Neck Surg 134:10, 2006)*.

TABLE 4 – COMPARISON OF ANTIBACTERIAL SPECTRA

Editorial Note: Choice of antibacterial agent must be made in consideration of local/institutional patterns of organism susceptibility and drug resistance. Patterns vary considerably based on geography and temporal changes in patterns are continuous. These data are intended to convey a generalized image of susceptibility/resistance to provide a basis for making decisions concerning initial empiric as well as specific antibacterial therapy.

Organisms	Penicillins		Antistaphylo-coccal Penicillins			Amino-Penicillins			Anti-Pseudomonal Penicillins				Carbapenems					Fluoroquinolones						
	Penicillin G	Penicillin V	Methicillin	Nafcillin/Oxacillin	Cloxacillin[NUS]/Diclox.	AMP/Amox	Amox/Clav	AMP-Sulb	Ticarcillin	Ticar-Clav	Pip-Tazo	Piperacillin	Doripenem	Ertapenem	Imipenem	Meropenem	Aztreonam	Ciprofloxacin	Ofloxacin	Pefloxacin[NUS]	Levofloxacin	Moxifloxacin	Gemifloxacin	Gatifloxacin
GRAM-POSITIVE:																								
Strep, Group A, B, C, G	+	+	+	−	+	+	+	+	+	+	−	+	+	+	+	+	0	±	±	0	+	+	+	+
Strep. pneumoniae	+	+	+	−	+	+	+	+	+	+	−	+	+	+	+	+	0	±	±	0	+	+	+	+
Viridans strep	±	±	±	±	±	±	±	±	±	±	±	±	−	+	+	+	0	0	0		+	+	+	+
Strep. milleri	+	+	+	+	+	+	+	+	+	+	+	+	−	+	+	+	0	0	0		+	+	+	+
Enterococcus faecalis	+	+	0	0	0	+	+	+	±	±	+	+	±	0	+	±	0	**	**	0	+	+	+	+
Enterococcus faecium	±	±	0	0	0	+	+	+	±	±	±	±	0	0	±	0	0	0	0	0	0	±	±	±
Staph. aureus (MSSA)	**0**	**0**	**+**	**+**	**+**	**0**	**+**	**+**	**0**	**+**	**+**	**0**	**+**	**+**	**+**	**+**	**0**	**+**	**+**	**+**	**+**	**+**	**+**	**+**
Staph. aureus (MRSA)	**0**	**0**	**0**	**0**	**0**	**0**	**0**	**0**	**0**	**0**	**0**	**0**	**0**	**0**	**0**	**0**	**0**	**0**	**0**	**0**	**0**	**±**	**±**	**±**
Staph. aureus (CA-MRSA)	**0**	**0**	**0**	**0**	**0**	**0**	**0**	**0**	**0**	**0**	**0**	**0**	**0**	**0**	**0**	**0**	**0**	**±**			**±**	**±**	**±**	**±**
Staph. epidermidis	0	0	−	+	+	0	0	0	±	±	+	0	+	+	+	+	0	+	+	+	+	+	+	+
C. jeikeium	0	0	0	0	0	0	0	0	0	0		0		0	0		0	0	0					
L. monocytogenes	**+**	**0**	**0**	**0**	**0**	**+**		**+**	**+**			**+**	**+**	**±**	**+**	**+**	**0**	**+**	**0**	**0**	**+**	**+**	**+**	**+**
GRAM-NEGATIVE:																								
N. gonorrhoeae	0	0	0	0	0	0	+	+	+	+	+	+	+	+	+	+	+	+[1]	+[1]	+[1]	+[1]	+[1]		+[1]
N. meningitidis	**+**	**0**	**0**	**0**	**0**	**+**	**+**	**+**	**+**	**+**	**+**	**+**	**+**	**+**	**+**	**+**	**+**	**+**	**+**	**+**	**+**	**+**		**+**
M. catarrhalis	0	0	0	0	0	0	+	+	0	+	+	±	+	+	+	+	+	+	+	+	+	+	+	+
H. influenzae	0	0	0	0	0	±	+	+	±	+	+	±	+	+	+	+	+	+	+	+	+	+	+	+
E. coli	**0**	**0**	**0**	**0**	**0**	**±**	**+**	**+**	**±**	**+**	**+**	**+**	**+**	**+**	**+**	**+**	**+**	**+**	**+**	**+**	**+**	**+**	**+**	**+**
Klebsiella sp.	0	0	0	0	0	0	+	+	0	+	+	+	+	+	+	+	+	+	+	+	+	+	+	+
E. coli/Klebs sp ESBL+	0	0	0	0	0	0	0	0	0	±	±	0	+	+	+	+	0	+	+	+	+	+	+	+
E. coli/Klebs sp KPC+	0	0	0	0	0	0	0	0	0	0	0	0	0	0	0	0	0							
Enterobacter sp.	0	0	0	0	0	0	0	0	+	+	+	+	+	+	+	+	+	+	+	+	+	+		+

[1] Prevalence of quinolone-resistant GC varies worldwide from <1% to 30.9% in Europe and >90% in Taiwan. In US in 2006 it was 6.7% overall and as a result, CDC no longer recommends FQs for first line therapy of GC (*MMWR 56:332, 2007; JAC 58:587, 2006; CID 40:188, 2005; AnIM 147:81, 2007*).

+ = **usually susceptible;** ± = **variably susceptible/resistant;** 0 = **usually resistant;** blank = **no data**
** Most strains ±, can be used in UTI, not in systemic infection

TABLE 4 (2)

Organisms	Penicillins		Antistaphylococcal Penicillins			Amino-Penicillins			Anti-Pseudomonal Penicillins				Carbapenems					Fluoroquinolones						
	Penicillin G	Penicillin V	Methicillin	Nafcillin/Oxacillin	Cloxacillin[NUS]/Diclox.	AMP/Amox	Amox/Clav	AMP-Sulb	Ticarcillin	Ticar-Clav	Pip-Tazo	Piperacillin	Doripenem	Ertapenem	Imipenem	Meropenem	Aztreonam	Ciprofloxacin	Ofloxacin	Pefloxacin[NUS]	Levofloxacin	Moxifloxacin	Gemifloxacin	Gatifloxacin
Serratia sp.	0	0	0	0	0	0	0	0	+	+	+	0	+	+	+	+	+	+	+	+	+	+		+
Salmonella sp.	0	0	0	0	0	±	+	+	+	+	+	+	+	+	+	+		+	+	+	+	+		+
Shigella sp.	0	0	0	0	0	±	+	+	+	+	+	+	+	+	+	+	+	+	+	+	+	+		+
Proteus mirabilis	0	0	0	0	0	+	+	+	+	+	+	+	+	+	+	+	+	+	+	+	+	+		+
Proteus vulgaris	0	0	0	0	0	0	+	+	+	+	+	+	+	+	+	+	+	+	+	+	+	+	+	+
Providencia sp.	0	0	0	0	0	0	+	+	+	+	+	+	+	+	+	+	+	+	+	+	+	+		+
Morganella sp.	0	0	0	0	0	0	±	+	+	+	+	+	+	+	+	+	+	+	+	+	+	+		+
Citrobacter sp.	0	0	0	0	0	0	0	0	+	+	+	+	+	+	+	+	+	+	+	+	+	+		+
Aeromonas sp.	0	0	0	0	0	0	+	+	+	+	+	+	+	+	+	+	+	+	+		+	+		+
Acinetobacter sp.	0	0	0	0	0	0	0	+	0	±	±	0	±	0	±	±	0	±	±		±	±	±	±
Ps. aeruginosa	**0**	**0**	**0**	**0**	**0**	**0**	**0**	**0**	**+**	**+**	**+**	**+**	**+**	**0**	**+**	**+**	**+**	**+**	**±**		**±**	**±**		**±**
B. (Ps.) cepacia	0	0	0	0	0	0	0	0	0				±	0	0	+	0	0	0			0		0
S. (X.) maltophilia	0	0	0	0	0	0	0	0		±	±	±	0	0	0	0	0	0	0	0	±	+		
Y. enterocolitica	0	0	0	0	0	0	±	±	±	+		+	+		+		+	+	+	+	+	+		+
Legionella sp.	**0**	**0**	**0**	**0**	**0**	**0**	**0**	**0**	**0**	**0**	**0**	**0**	**0**	**0**	**0**	**0**	**0**	**+**	**+**	**+**	**+**	**+**	**+**	**+**
P. multocida	+	+	0	0	0	+	+	+	+	+		+	+	+	+		+	+	+	+	+	+		+
H. ducreyi	+					0	+	+																
MISC.:																								
Chlamydophila sp	0	0	0	0	0	0	0	0	0	0	0	0	0	0	0	0	0	+	+	+	+	+	+	+
M. pneumoniae	**0**	**0**	**0**	**0**	**0**	**0**	**0**	**0**	**0**	**0**	**0**	**0**	**0**	**0**	**0**	**0**	**0**	**+**	**+**	**+**	**+**	**+**	**+**	**+**
ANAEROBES:																								
Actinomyces	+	±	0	0	0	+	+	+				+		+	+		0	0	±			+		+
Bacteroides fragilis	**0**	**±**	**0**	**0**	**0**	**0**	**+**	**+**	**0**	**+**	**+**	**0**	**+**	**+**	**+**	**+**	**0**	**0**	**0**	**0**	**0**	**+**		**±**
P. melaninogenica	+	0	0	0	0	+	+	+	+	+	+	+	+	+	+	+	0	0	±		+	+		+
Clostridium difficile	**+**[2]							**+**[1]				**+**[2]	**+**	**+**	**+**	**+**	**0**	**0**			**0**	**0**		**0**
Clostridium *(not difficile)*	**+**	**+**				**+**	**+**	**+**	**+**	**+**	**+**	**+**	**+**	**+**	**+**	**+**	**0**	**±**	**±**		**+**	**+**		**+**
Peptostreptococcus sp.	+	+	+	+	+	+	+	+	+	+	+	+	+	+	+	+	0	±	±		+	+		+

[2] No clinical evidence that penicillins or fluoroquinolones are effective for *C. difficile* enterocolitis (but they may cover this organism in mixed intra-abdominal and pelvic infections).

+ =usually susceptible; ± = **variably susceptible/resistant;** 0 = **usually resistant;** blank = **no data**

* A 1-carbacephem best classified as a cephalosporin

TABLE 4 (3)

Organisms	CEPHALOSPORINS: 1st Generation	2nd Generation			3rd/4th Generation (including anti-MRSA)							Oral Agents: 1st Generation		2nd Generation			3rd Generation		
	Cefazolin	Cefotetan	Cefoxitin	Cefuroxime	Cefotaxime	Ceftizoxime	Ceftriaxone	Ceftobiprole	Ceftaroline	Ceftazidime	Cefepime	Cefadroxil	Cephalexin	Cefaclor/Loracarbef*	Cefprozil	Cefuroxime axetil	Cefixime	Ceftibuten	Cefpodox/Cefdinir/Cefditoren
GRAM-POSITIVE:																			
Strep, Group A, B, C, G	+	+	+	+	+	+	−	+	+	+	+	+	+	+	+	+	+	+	+
Strep. pneumoniae[3]	+	+	+	+	+	+	−	+	+	+[3]	+	+	+	+	+	+	+	±	+
Viridans strep	+	+	+	+	+	+	+	+	+	±[3]	+	+	+	+	0	+	+	0	+
Enterococcus faecalis	0	0	0	0	0	0	0	+	+	0	0	0	0	0	0	0	0	0	0
Staph. aureus (MSSA)	**+**	**+**	**+**	**+**	**+**	**+**	**+**	**+**	**+**	**±**	**+**	**+**	**+**	**+**	**+**	**+**	**0**	**0**	**+**
Staph. aureus (MRSA)	**0**	**0**	**0**	**0**	**0**	**0**	**0**	**+**	**+**	**0**	**0**	**0**	**0**	**0**	**0**	**0**	**0**	**0**	**0**
Staph. aureus (CA-MRSA)	**0**	**0**	**0**	**0**	**0**	**0**	**0**	**+**	**−**	**0**	**0**	**0**	**0**	**0**	**0**	**0**	**0**	**0**	**0**
Staph. epidermidis	±	±	±	±	±	±	±	+	−	±	±	±	±	±	±	±	0	0	±
C. jeikeium	0	0	0	0	0	0	0			0		0	0	0	0	0	0	0	
L. monocytogenes	**0**	**0**	**0**	**0**	**0**	**0**	**0**			**0**	**0**	**0**	**0**	**0**	**0**	**0**	**0**	**0**	**0**
GRAM-NEGATIVE																			
N. gonorrhoeae	+	±	±	±	±	±	+	+	+	±	+	0	0	±	±	±	+	±	+
N. meningitidis	**0**	**±**	**±**	**+**	**+**	**±**	**+**	**+**	**+**	**±**	**+**	**0**	**0**	**±**	**±**	**±**	**±**	**±**	
M. catarrhalis	±	+	+	+	+	+	+	+	+	+	+	0	0	±	+	+	+	+	+
H. influenzae	+	+	+	+	+	+	+	+	+	+	+		0	+	+	+	+	+	+
E. coli	**+**	**+**	**+**	**+**	**+**	**+**	**+**	**+**	**+**	**+**	**+**	**+**	**+**	**+**	**+**	**+**	**+**	**+**	**+**
Klebsiella sp.	+	+	+	+	+	+	+	+	+	+	+	+	+	+	+	+	+	+	+
E. coli/Klebs sp ESBL+	0	0	0	0	0	0	0	0	0	0	0	0	0	0	0	0	0	0	0
E. coli/Klebs sp KPC+	0	0	0	0	0	0	0	0	0	0	0	0	0	0	0	0	0	0	0
Enterobacter sp.	0	±	0	±	+	−	+	+	+	+	+	0	0	0	0	0	0	±	0
Serratia sp.	0	+	0	0	+	−	+	+	+	+	+	0	0	0	0	0	±	±	0
Salmonella sp.					+	−	+	+	+	+	+	0	0				+	+	+
Shigella sp.					+	−	+			+	+	0	0				+	+	+
Proteus mirabilis	+	+	+	+	+	−	+	+	+	+	+	+	+	+	+	+	+	+	+
Proteus vulgaris	0	+	+	+	+	−	+	+	+	+	+	0	0	0	0	0	+	+	±
Providencia sp.	0	+	+	0	+	−	+	+	+	−	+	0	0	0	0	+	+	+	
Morganella sp.	0	+	+	±	+	+	+	+	+	−	+	0	0	0	0	±	0	0	0

[3] Ceftaz 8–16 times less active than cefotax/ceftriax, effective only vs Pen-sens. strains (*AAC 39:2193, 1995*). Oral cefuroxime, cefprozil, cefpodoxime most active in vitro vs resistant S. pneumo (*PIDJ 14:1037, 1995*).

+ = usually susceptible; ± = variably susceptible/resistant; 0 = **usually resistant;** blank = **no data**

* A 1-carbacephem best classified as a cephalosporin

TABLE 4 (4)

Organisms	CEPHALOSPORINS																		
												Oral Agents							
	1st Generation	2nd Generation			3rd/4th Generation (including anti-MRSA)							1st Generation		2nd Generation			3rd Generation		
	Cefazolin	Cefotetan	Cefoxitin	Cefuroxime	Cefotaxime	Ceftizoxime	Ceftriaxone	Ceftobiprole	Ceftaroline	Ceftazidime	Cefepime	Cefadroxil	Cephalexin	Cefaclor/Loracarbef*	Cefprozil	Cefuroxime axetil	Cefixime	Ceftibuten	Cefpodox/Cefdinir/Cefditoren
C. freundii	0	0	0	0	+	0	+			0	+	0	0	0	0	0	0	0	0
C. diversus	0	±	±	±	+	+	+	+	+	+	+	0	0	0	0			+	
Citrobacter sp.	0	±	±	±	+	+	+	+	+	+	+		0	±	0	±	+	+	+
Aeromonas sp.	0	+	±	+	+	+	+	+	+	+	+						+	+	
Acinetobacter sp.	0	0	0	0	0	0	0	±		±	±	0	0	0	0	0	0	0	
Ps. aeruginosa	0	0	0	0	±	±	±	+	±	+	+	0	0	0	0	0	0	0	0
B. (Ps.) cepacia	0	0	0	0	±	±	±	0	0	+	±	0	0	0	0	0	0	+	
S. (X.) maltophilia	0	0	0	0	0	0	0	0	0	±	0	0	0	0	0	0	0	0	
Y. enterocolitica	0	±	±	±	+	+	+			±	+						+	+	
Legionella sp.	0	0	0	0	0	0	0	0	0	0	0	0	0	0	0	0	0	0	0
P. multocida		+		+	+	+	+				+		0				+		+
H. ducreyi			+		+	+	+			+							+		
ANAEROBES:																			
Actinomyces						+	+												
Bacteroides fragilis	0	±[4]	+	0	0	±	0	0	0	0	0		0	0	0	0	0	0	
P. melaninogenica		+	+	+	+	+	±	±		+	0			+	+	+	+		
Clostridium difficile			0		0	0		0			0								
Clostridium *(not difficile)*		+	+	+	+	+	+	+		+					+	+	0		
Peptostreptococcus sp.		+	+	+	+	+	+	+		+	+		+	+	+	+	+		

[4] Cefotetan is less active against B. ovatus, B. distasonis, B. thetaiotaomicron.

+ =usually susceptible; ± = variably susceptible/resistant; 0 = **usually resistant;** blank = **no data**

* A 1-carbacephem best classified as a cephalosporin

TABLE 4 (5)

Organisms	AMINO-GLYCOSIDES					MACROLIDES			KETOLIDE	TETRA-CYCLINES		GLYCYL-CYCLINE	GLYCO-/LIPOGLYCO-PEPTIDES						AGENTS URINARY TRACT		MISCELLANEOUS					
	Gentamicin	Tobramycin	Amikacin	Chloramphenicol	Clindamycin	Erythro	Azithromycin	Clarithromycin	Telithromycin	Doxycycline	Minocycline	Tigecycline	Vancomycin	Teicoplanin[NUS]	Telavancin	Fusidic Acid[NUS]	Trimethoprim	TMP-SMX	Nitrofurantoin	Fosfomycin	Rifampin	Metronidazole	Quinupristin-dalfopristin	Linezolid	Daptomycin	Colistimethate (Colistin)
GRAM-POSITIVE:																										
Strep Group A, B, C, G	0	0	0	+	+	±	±	±	+	±	+	+	+	+	+	±	+	+[5]	+		+	0	+	+	+	0
Strep. pneumoniae	0	0	0	+	+	±	±	±	+	+	+	+	+	+	+	±	±	+	+		+	0	+	+	+[6]	0
Enterococcus faecalis	S	S	S	±	0	0	0	0	±	0	0	+	+	+	+	+	+	+[5]	+	+	±	0	0	+	+	0
Enterococcus faecium	S	0	0	±	0	0	0	0	0	0	0	+	±	±	+		0	0	+	±	0	0	+	+	+	0
Staph. aureus (MSSA)	**+**	**+**	**+**	**±**	**+**	**±**	**+**	**+**	**+**	**±**	**+**	**+**	**+**	**+**	**+**	**+**	**±**	**+**	**+**		**+**	**0**	**+**	**+**	**+**	**0**
Staph. aureus (MRSA)	**0**	**0**	**0**	**0**	**0**	**0**	**0**	**0**	**0**	**±**	**±**	**+**	**+**	**+**	**+**	**+**	**±**	**+**	**+**		**+**	**0**	**+**	**+**	**+**	**0**
Staph. aureus (CA-MRSA)					**±**	**±**	**±**	**±**	**±**	**+**	**+**	**+**	**+**	**+**	**+**	**+**	**+**	**+**	**+**		**+**	**0**	**+**	**+**	**+**	**0**
Staph. epidermidis	±	±	±	0	0	±	0	0	0	0	0	+	+	±	+	+	+	±			+	0	+	+	+	0
C. jeikeium	0	0	0	0	0	0	0	0	0	0	0	+	+	+	+	+	0	0	0		+	0	+	+	+	0
L. monocytogenes	**S**	**S**	**S**	**+**		**+**	**+**	**+**	**+**	**+**	**+**	**+**	**+**	**+**	**+**		**+**	**+**			**+**	**0**	**+**	**+**	**±**	**0**
GRAM-NEGATIVE:																										
N. gonorrhoeae	0	0	0	+	0	±	±	±	+	±	±	+	0	0	0	+	0	±	+	+	+	0	+		0	0
N. meningitidis	**0**	**0**	**0**	**+**	**0**	**+**	**+**		**+**	**+**	**+**		**0**	**0**	**0**	**+**	**±**	**+**			**+**	**0**	**0**	**0**	**0**	**0**
M. catarrhalis	+	+	+	+	0	+	+	+	+	+	+	+						+			+	0	+	±	0	
H. influenzae	+	+	+	+	0	±	+	+	+	+	+	+					±	±			+	0	±	±	0	
Aeromonas	0			+						+	+	+	0	0	0			+			0	0			0	
E. coli	**+**	**+**	**+**	**+**	**0**	**0**	**0**	**0**	**0**	**+**	**+**	**+**	**0**	**0**	**0**	**0**	**+**	**±**	**+**	**+**	**0**	**0**	**0**	**0**	**0**	**+**
Klebsiella sp.	+	+	+	±	0	0	0	0	0	±	±	+	0	0	0	0	±	±	±	±	0	0	0	0	0	+
E. coli/Klebs sp ESBL+	+	+	+	±	0	0	0	0	0	±	±	+	0	0	0	0	±	±			0	0	0	0	0	+
E. coli/Klebs sp KPC+													0	0	0	0							0	0	0	+
Enterobacter sp.	+	+	+	0	0	0	0	0	0	0	0	+	0	0	0	0	±		±	±	0	0	0	0	0	+
Salmonella sp.				+	0	0	±	0	0	±	±	+	0	0	0	0	±	±	+		0	0	0	0	0	
Shigella sp.	+	+	+	+	0	0	±	0	0	±	±	+	0	0	0	0	±	±	+		0	0	0	0	0	

[5] Although active in vitro, TMP-SMX is not clinically effective for Group A strep pharyngitis or for infections due to E. faecalis.
[6] Although active in vitro, daptomycin is not clinically effective for pneumonia caused by strep pneumonia.

+ =usually susceptible; ± = variably susceptible/resistant; 0 = usually resistant; blank = **no data**
Antimicrobials such as azithromycin have high tissue penetration & some such as clarithromycin are metabolized to more active compounds, hence in vivo activity may exceed in vitro activity.
** Vancomycin, metronidazole given po active vs C. difficile; IV vancomycin not effective. S = Synergistic with cell wall-active antibiotics.

TABLE 4 (6)

Organisms	AMINO-GLYCOSIDES					MACROLIDES			KETOLIDE	TETRA-CYCLINES		GLYCYL-CYCLINE	GLYCO-/LIPOGLYCO-PEPTIDES						AGENTS URINARY TRACT		MISCELLANEOUS					
	Gentamicin	Tobramycin	Amikacin	Chloramphenicol	Clindamycin	Erythro	Azithromycin	Clarithromycin	Telithromycin	Doxycycline	Minocycline	Tigecycline	Vancomycin	Teicoplanin[NUS]	Telavancin	Fusidic Acid[NUS]	Trimethoprim	TMP-SMX	Nitrofurantoin	Fosfomycin	Rifampin	Metronidazole	Quinupristin-dalfopristin	Linezolid	Daptomycin	Colistimethate (Colistin)
Serratia marcescens	+	+	+	0	0	0	0	0	0	0	0	+	0	0	0	0	0	±	0	±	0	0		0	0	0
Proteus vulgaris	+	+	+	±	0	0	0	0	0	0	0	±	0	0	0	0	0	0	0	±	0	0		0	0	0
Acinetobacter sp.	0	0	±	0	0	0	0	0	0	0	0	±	0	0	0	0	0	±			0	0		0	0	+
Ps. aeruginosa	+	+	+	0	0	0	0	0	0	0	0	0	0	0	0	0	0	0	0		0	0	0	0	0	+
B. (Ps.) cepacia	0	0	0	+	0	0	0	0	0	0	±	±	0	0	0	0	+	+	0		0	0		0	0	0
S. (X.) maltophilia	0	0	0	+	0	0	0	0	0	0	0	+	0	0	0	0	0	+	0			0		0	0	±
Y. enterocolitica	+	+	+	+	0	0	0	0	0	0	0					0		+				0		0	0	
F. tularensis	+			+						+								+			+	0		0	0	
Brucella sp.	+			+	0	0	0	0	0	+	+		0	0	0		+	+			+	0		0	0	
Legionella sp.						+	+	+	+	+	+	+				±	+	+				0			0	
H. ducreyi				+	+	+	+						0					±				0			0	
V. vulnificus	±	±	±	+						+	+					0						0			0	
MISC.:																										
Chlamydophila sp.	0	0	0	+	±	+	+	+	+	+	+	+				0	0		0		+	0	+	+		
M. pneumoniae	0	0	0	+	0	+	+	+	+	+	+	+				0						0	+	0		
Rickettsia sp.	0	0	0	+		±			+	+	+		0	0	0	0						0				
Mycobacterium avium			+				+	+		0	0	0										0	0	0		
ANAEROBES:																										
Actinomyces	0	0	0	+	+	+	+	+		+	+		+		+	+						0				
Bacteroides fragilis	0	0	0	+	±	0	0	0		±	±	+	0		0		+	0				+		±		
P. melaninogenica	0	0	0	+	+		+	+		+	+	+	0		0	+						+	+			
Clostridium difficile	0	0	0	±									+	+	+							+	±	±		
Clostridium *(not difficile)***				+		±	+	+		+	+	+	+	+	+	+						+	+	+		
Peptostreptococcus sp.	0	0	0	+	+	±	+	±	+	+	+	+	+	+	+	+						+		+		

+ =usually susceptible; ± = variably susceptible/resistant; 0 = usually resistant; blank = **no data**
Antimicrobials such as azithromycin have high tissue penetration & some such as clarithromycin are metabolized to more active compounds, hence in vivo activity may exceed in vitro activity.
****** Vancomycin, metronidazole given po active vs C. difficile; IV vancomycin not effective. S = Synergistic with cell wall-active antibiotics.

TABLE 5 – TREATMENT OPTIONS FOR SELECTED HIGHLY RESISTANT BACTERIA

(See page 2 for abbreviations)

ORGANISM/RESISTANCE	THERAPEUTIC OPTIONS	COMMENT[1]
E. faecalis. Resistant to:		
Vanco + strep/gentamicin (MIC >500 mcg per mL); β-lactamase neg. *(JAC 40:161, 1997)*.	**Penicillin G** or **AMP** (systemic infections); **Nitrofurantoin**, **fosfomycin** (UTI only). Usually resistant to **quinu-dalfo**.	AMP + ceftriaxone effective for endocarditis due to E. faecalis with high level AG resistance (no comparator treated with AMP alone) but no data for therapy of VRE *(AnIM 146:574, 2007)*. Non BL+ strains of E. faecalis resistant to penicillin and AMP described in Spain, but unknown (except BL+ strains) in U.S. and elsewhere *(AAC 40:2420, 1996)*. Linezolid effective in 60–70% of cases *(AnIM 138:135, 2003)*. Daptomycin, tigecycline, ceftaroline, ceftobiprole active in vitro *(JAC 52:123, 2003)*.
Penicillin (β-lactamase producers)	**Vanco**, **AM-SB**	Appear susceptible to AMP and penicillin by standard in vitro methods. Must use direct test for β-lactamase with chromogenic cephalosporin (nitrocefin) to identify. Rare since early 1990s. Ceftobiprole active in vitro *(AAC 51:2043, 2007)*.
E. faecium. Resistant to:		
Vanco and high levels (MIC >500 mcg per mL) of streptomycin and gentamicin	**Penicillin G** or **AMP** (systemic infections) **fosfomycin, nitrofurantoin** (UTI only)	For strains with pen/AMP MICs of >8 ≤64 mcg per mL, anecdotal evidence that high-dose (300 mg per kg per day) AMP rx may be effective. Daptomycin, tigecycline active in vitro *(JAC 52:123, 2003)*.
Penicillin, AMP, vanco, & high-level resist. to streptomycin and gentamicin *(NEJM 342:710, 2000)*	**Linezolid** 600 mg po or IV q12h and **quinu-dalfo** 7.5 mg per kg IV q8h are bacteriostatic against most strains of E. faecium. Can try combinations of cell wall-active antibiotics with other agents (including FQ, chloramphenicol, RIF, or **doxy**). Chloramphenicol alone effective in some cases of bacteremia *(Clin Micro Inf 7:17, 2001)*. **Nitrofurantoin** or **fosfomycin** may work for UTI.	For strains with Van B phenotype (vanco R, teico S), teicoplanin[NUS], preferably in combination with streptomycin or gentamicin (if not highly AG resistant), may be effective. Synercid roughly 70% effective in clinical trials *(CID 30:790, 2000, & 33:1816, 2001)*. Linezolid shows similar efficacy. Comparable but somewhat lower (58% linezolid, 43% QD) response rates in cancer pts *(JAC 53:646, 2004)*. Emergence of resistance with therapeutic failure has occurred during monotherapy with either quinu-dalfo or linezolid *(CID 30:790, 2000; Ln 357:1179, 2001)*. Nosocomial spread of linezolid-resistant E. faecium possible *(NEJM 346:867, 2002)*. Daptomycin active in vitro against most strains *(JAC 52:123, 2003)* but therapeutic failure with or without development of resistance reported *(CID 45:1343, 2007)*. Tigecycline also active in vitro *(Circulation 111:e394, 2005)*. **Infectious disease consultation imperative!** For review of therapeutic options, see *CMI 16:555, 2010*.
S. aureus. Resistant to:		
Methicillin (health-care associated) For community-associated MRSA infections, see *Table 6* *IDSA Guidelines: CID 52 (Feb 1):1, 2011.*	**Vanco** [For persistent bacteremia (≥7 days) on vanco or teicoplanin[NUS], *see Table 6*]	Alternatives: teicoplanin[NUS], daptomycin *(AAC 49:770, 2005; NEJM 355:653, 2006)*, telavancin *(CID 46:1683, 2008)*, linezolid *(Chest 124:1789, 2003)*, TMP-SMX (test susceptibility first), minocycline & doxy (some strains)*(NEJM 357:380, 2007)*, tigecycline *[CID 41(Suppl 5):S303, 2005]*, or quinu-dalfo *(CID 34:1481, 2002)*. Fusidic acid[NUS], fosfomycin, RIF may be active; use only in combination to prevent in vivo emergence of resistance. Staphylococci (incl. CA-MRSA) with inducible MLS_B resistance may appear susceptible to clindamycin in vitro. Clinda therapy may result in therapeutic failure *(CID 37:1257, 2003)*. Test for inducible resistance [double-disc ("D test")] before treating with clinda *(J Clin Micro 42:2777, 2004)*. Ceftaroline also effective for skin and soft tissue infection caused by MRSA *(CID 51:641, 2010)*.
Vanco, methicillin (VISA & VRSA) *(CID 32:108, 2001; MMWR 51:902, 2002; NEJM 348:1342, 2003; CID 46:668, 2008) IDSA Guidelines: CID 52 (Feb 1):1, 2011.*	Unknown, but even high-dose vanco may fail. **Linezolid**, **quinu-dalfo**, **daptomycin**, **telavancin** active in vitro.	VISA/GISA: Vanco-intermediate resistance of MRSA with MICs of ≤16 mcg/mL; Anecdotal data on treatment regimens. Most susceptible to TMP-SMX, minocycline, doxycycline, RIF and AGs *(CID 32:108, 2001)*. RIF should always be combined with a 2nd therapeutic agent to prevent emergence of RIF resistance during therapy. VRSA: only 6 clinical isolates of truly vancomycin-resistant (MIC >64) MRSA described. Organisms still susceptible to TMP-SMX, chloro, linezolid, minocycline, quinu-dalfo, ceftobiprole, ceftaroline *(MMWR 51:902, 2002; NEJM 348:1342, 2003)*.
S. epidermidis. Resistant to:		
Methicillin	**Vanco** (+ **RIF** and **gentamicin** for prosthetic valve endocarditis)	
Methicillin, glycopeptides *(AAC 49: 770, 2005)*	**Quinu-dalfo** *(see comments on E. faecium)* generally active in vitro as are **linezolid** & **daptomycin**.	Vanco more active than teicoplanin[NUS] *(Clin Micro Rev 8:585, 1995)*. New FQs (levofloxacin, gatifloxacin, moxifloxacin) active in vitro, but development of resistance is a potential problem.

[1] Guideline on prevention of resistance: *CID 25:584, 1997*

TABLE 5 (2)

ORGANISM/RESISTANCE	THERAPEUTIC OPTIONS	COMMENT[1]
S. pneumoniae. Resistant to: Penicillin G (MIC >0.1 ≤2.0)	**Ceftriaxone** or **cefotaxime**. High-dose penicillin (≥10 million units per day) or **AMP** (**amox**) likely effective for nonmeningeal sites of infection (e.g., pneumonia), **telithro**	IMP, ERTA, cefepime, cefpodoxime, cefuroxime also active *(IDCP 3:75, 1994)*. MER less active than IMP *(AAC 38:898, 1994)*. Gemi, moxi, levo also have good activity *(AAC 38:898, 1994; DMID 31:45, 1998; Exp Opin Invest Drugs 8:123, 1999)*. High-dose cefotaxime (300 mg per kg per day, max. 24 gm per day) effective in meningitis due to strains with cefotaxime MICs as high as 2 mcg per mL *(AAC 40:218, 1996)*. Review: *IDCP 6 (Suppl 2):S21, 1997*.
Penicillin G (MIC ≥4.0)	(**Vanco** ± **RIF**). Alternatives if non-meningeal infection: **ceftriax/cefotax**, **high-dose AMP**, **ERTA**, **IMP**, **MER**, or an active FQ: (**Gemi**, **moxi**, **levo**), **telithro**	Note new CLSI breakpoints for penicillin susceptibilities. Meningeal isolates ≤0.06 = S; 0.12-1.0 = I; ≥2.0= R. For non-meningeal isolates ≤2.0 = S; 4.0 = I; ≥8.0 = R.
Penicillin, erythro, tetracycline, chloramphenicol, TMP-SMX	**Vanco** ± **RIF**; (**Gemi**, **moxi**, or **levo**); **telithro** (non-meningeal infections)	60–80% of strains susceptible to clindamycin *(DMID 25:201, 1996)*.
Acinetobacter baumannii. Resistant to: IMP, P Ceph 3 AP, AP Pen, APAG, FQ *(see page 2 for abbreviations)*	**AM-SB** *(CID 34:1425, 2002)*. Sulbactam alone is active against some A. baumannii *(JAC 42:793, 1998)*. **Colistin** effective most multi-resistant strains *(CID 36:1111, 2003; JAC 54:1085, 2004; CID 43:S89, 2006)*. May be given intrathecally for meningitis *(CMI 16:888, 2010)*. AM-SB appears more effective than colistin *(JAC 61:1369, 2008)*.	6/8 patients with A. baumannii meningitis (7 organisms resistant to IMP) cured with AM/SB *(CID 24: 932, 1997)*. Various combinations of FQs and AGs, IMP and AGs or RIF, or AP Pens or P Ceph 3 APs with AGs or RIF + colistin may show activity against **some** multiresistant strains *(CID 36:1268, 2003; JAC 61:417, 2008; AAC 54:1165, 2010)*. MER + sulbactam active in vitro & in vivo *(JAC 53:393, 2004)*. Active in vitro: triple drug combinations of polymyxin B, IMP, & RIF *(AAC 48:753, 2004)*, *other colistin-containing combination regimens (CID 43:S95, 2006; AAC 51:1621, 2007)* & tigecycline *(CID 41:S315, 2005)*, but several studies document borderline activity of tigecycline against acinetobacter and emergence of resistance during therapy *(JAC 59:772, 2007; AAC 51: 376, 2007; CID 46:567, 2008)*. Definitive data concerning its effectiveness not yet available *(JAC 62:45, 2008)*. Amikacin-tigecycline synergistic in vitro *(AAC 52:2940, 2008)*. Minocycline effective in traumatic wound infections *(IDCP 16:16, 2008)*. Arbekacin[NUS] active in vitro against strains from traumatic wounds *(AAC 54:3015, 2010)*. For extensive review of current treatment options, *see CID 51:79, 2010*.
Campylobacter jejuni. Resistant to: FQs	**Erythro**, **azithro**, **clarithro**, **doxy**, **clindamycin**	Resistance to **both** FQs & macrolides reported *(CID 22:868, 1996; EID 7:24, 2002; AAC 47:2358, 2003)*.
E. coli (producing CTX-M ESBLs) **Resistant to:** Oral cephalosporins, TMP/SMX, fluoroquinolones	For UTI (most common infection caused by these organisms): **fosfomycin**, **nitrofurantoin**, **ertapenem** *(AAC 53:1278, 2009)*.	Resistant to cefdinir but combination of cefdinir with amox/clav active in vitro *(AAC 53:1278, 2009)*.
Klebsiella pneumoniae (producing ESBL) **Resistant to:** Ceftazidime & other 3rd generation cephalosporins *(see Table 10C)*, aztreonam	**DORI**, **IMP**, **MER**, *(CID 39:31, 2004)* *(See Comment)*	P Ceph 4, TC-CL, PIP-TZ show in vitro activity, but not proven entirely effective in animal models *(IJAA 8:37, 1997)*; some strains which hyperproduce ESBLs are primarily resistant to TC-CL and PIP-TZ *(J Clin Micro 34:358, 1996)*. Note: there are strains of ESBL-producing klebsiella sensitive in vitro to P Ceph 2, 3 but resistant to ceftazidime; infections with such strains do not respond to P Ceph 2 or 3 *(J Clin Micro 39:2206, 2001)*. FQ may be effective if susceptible but many strains resistant. Note Klebsiella sp. with carbapenem resistance due to class A carbapenemase. Some of these organisms resistant to all antimicrobials except colistin *(CID 39:55, 2004)*. Tigecycline active in vitro *(AAC 50:3166, 2006)*. Ertapenem active against ESBL-producing E. coli in pharmacodynamic model *(JAC 61:643, 2008)*.
Resistant to: Carbapenems, 2nd & 3rd generation cephalosporins due to KPC enzymes	**Colistin** *(AAC 48:4793, 2004)*	
Pseudomonas aeruginosa. **Resistant to:** **IMP, MER**	**CIP** (check susceptibility), **APAG** (check susceptibility). **Colistin** effective for multiresistant strains *(CID 28:1008, 1999; CMI 13:560, 2007)*.	Many strains remain susceptible to aztreonam & ceftazidime or AP Pens *(JAC 36:1037, 1995)*. Combinations of (AP Pen & APAG) or (AP Ceph 3 + APAG) may show in vitro activity *(AAC 39:2411, 1995)*. Combinations of Dori, Polymyxin B and RIF show bactericidal activity against multi-resistant strains *(AAC 54:2732, 2010)* and Fosfomycin synergistic with aminoglycosides against some strains in vitro and in vivo *(JAC 64:563, 2009)*. Doripenem + tobramycin reported effective in one case of P. aeruginosa ventriculitis *(JAC 63:1297, 2009)*.

TABLE 6 – SUGGESTED MANAGEMENT OF SUSPECTED OR CULTURE-POSITIVE COMMUNITY-ASSOCIATED METHICILLIN-RESISTANT S. AUREUS (CA-MRSA) INFECTIONS

(See footnote[1] for doses)

IDSA Guidelines: *CID 52 (Feb 1):1, 2011.* With the magnitude of the clinical problem and a number of new drugs, it is likely new data will require frequent revisions of the regimens suggested. *(See page 2 for abbreviations).*
NOTE: Distinction between community and hospital strains of MRSA blurring.

CLINICAL ILLNESS	ABSCESS, AFEBRILE; & IMMUNOCOMPETENT: OUTPATIENT CARE	ABSCESS(ES) WITH FEVER; OUTPATIENT CARE	PNEUMONIA	BACTEREMIA OR POSSIBLE ENDOCARDITIS OR BACTEREMIC SHOCK	TREATMENT FAILURE *(See footnote[2])*
Management ***Drug doses in footnote.***	**TMP-SMX-DS** or **doxycycline or minocycline** or **clindamycin** *(CID 40:1429, 2005 & AAC 51:2628, 2007).* **NOTE: I&D** alone may be sufficient *(PIDJ 23:123, 2004; AAC 51:4044, 2007; NEJM 357:380, 2007; Ann Emerg Med Apr 29, 2009, Epub)*	**TMP-SMX-DS** or **clindamycin** or **doxycycline** plus **incision and drainage.**	**Vanco** IV or **linezolid** IV	**Vanco or dapto IV. Dapto** not inferior to **vanco** in bacteremia trial *(NEJM 355:653, 2006).* No apparent benefit of adding RIF, maybe harm *(AAC 52:2463, 2008).*	Confirm adequate vanco troughs of 15-20 μg/ml and vancomycin susceptibility; search for deep focus of infection. Switch to alternative regimen if vanco MIC ≥ 2 μg/ml. **Dapto** resistance reported after **vanco** exposure & prior to **dapto** therapy *(CID 45:601, 2007).* **Dapto appears safe at doses of up to** 12 mg/kg/d *(AAC 50:3245, 2006).*
Comments continue on next page		Culture abscess & maybe blood **I&D.** Hot packs. Close follow-up.		**Vanco** MICs ↑; disproportionate ↑ in MBCs *(CID 42:513, 2006 & 44:1208, 2007).* Ideal **vanco** trough level unclear. More nephrotoxicity with higher troughs *(Clin Ther 29:107, 2007).* If **vanco** MIC≥2 μg/mL, consider alternative therapy; ID consultation suggested.	Data extremely limited concerning salvage regimens for treatment failures. Addition of aminoglycoside or rifampin to vancomycin not effective in one retrospective study (0% success), whereas linezolid with or without a carbapenem was effective (88% success in patients with bacteremia due to pneumonia, vascular catheter or graft infection; no patient had endocarditis) *(CID 49:395, 2009).* **Options:** For endocarditis or complicated bacteremia **dapto** 10 mg/kg IV once daily plus **gentamicin** 1 mg/kg IV every 8 hours or **RIF** 300-450 mg twice daily; **linezolid** + a second agent *(JAC 58:273, 2006 & JAC 56:923, 2005);* **quinupristin-dalfopristin** (Q-D) ± with **vanco**.

[1] **Clindamycin:** 300 mg po tid. **Daptomycin:** 6 mg/kg IV q24h is the standard dose; higher doses (10 mg/kg) and use of combination therapy recommended for vancomycin treatment failures. **Doxycycline or minocycline:** 100 mg po bid. **Linezolid:** 600 mg po/IV bid. **Quinupristin-dalfopristin (Q-D):** 7.5 mg per /kg IV q8h via central line. **Rifampin:** Long serum half-life justifies dosing 600 mg po q24h; however, frequency of nausea less with 300 mg po bid. **TMP-SMX-DS:** Standard dose 8–10 mg per kg per day. For 70 kg person = 700 mg TMP component per day. **TMP-SMX** contains 160 mg TMP and 800 mg SMX. The dose for treatment of CA-MRSA skin and soft tissue infections (SSTI) is not established. In one small study 1 DS tablet twice daily was effective, although 3/14 subjects failed therapy *(AAC 51:2628, 2007);* therefore 2 DS tablets twice daily is recommended for treatment of patients with fever or complicated SSTI. **Vancomycin:** 1 gm IV q12h; up to 45-60 mg/kg/day in divided doses may be required to achieve target trough concentrations of 15-20 mcg/mL recommended for serious infections.

[2] The median duration of bacteremia in endocarditis is 7-9 days in patients treated with vancomycin *(AnIM 115:674, 1991).* Longer duration of bacteremia, greater likelihood of endocarditis *(JID 190:1140, 2004).* Definition of failure unclear. Clinical response should be factored in. **Unsatisfactory clinical response especially if blood cultures remain positive beyond 5-7 days is an indication for change in therapy.**

TABLE 6 (2)

CLINICAL ILLNESS	ABSCESS, AFEBRILE; & IMMUNOCOMPETENT: OUTPATIENT CARE	ABSCESS(ES) WITH FEVER; OUTPATIENT CARE	PNEUMONIA	BACTEREMIA OR POSSIBLE ENDOCARDITIS OR BACTEREMIC SHOCK	TREATMENT FAILURE (*See footnote*[2])
Comments	Effective dose of **TMP-SMX-DS** is unclear. IV dose is 8-10 mg/kg/d; roughly equivalent to 2 tabs po bid. Anecdotally, most pts respond to I&D and 1 tab bid although failures may occur *(see footnote*[1]*)*. **Fusidic acid** 500 mg tid (not available in the US) **+ rifampin** also an option *(J Antimicrob Chemother 61: 976, 2008 and Can J Infect Dis Med Microbiol; 17(Suppl C): 4C, 2006)*; do not use rifampin alone as resistance rapidly emerges. One retrospective study *(Peds 123: e959, 2009)* in children reports increased risk of treatment failure with TMP-SMX compared to other agents for undrained, uncultured skin and soft tissue infections; presumably these were mainly cellulitis, which could reflect less activity of this agent against Group A streptococcus.	Note: Increasing frequency of strains with inducible resistance to clindamycin. Some authorities recommend addition of rifampin to TMP/SMX; do not use rifampin alone as resistance rapidly emerges. Patients not responding after 2-3 days should be evaluated for complicated infection and switched to **vancomycin**.	**Linezolid** superior to **vanco** in retrospective subset analysis; prospective study in progress.	Efficacy of IV **TMP-SMX** vs CA-MRSA uncertain. IV **TMP-SMX** was inferior to **vanco** vs bacteremic MSSA *(AnIM 117:390, 1992)*. **Dapto** failures associated with development of **dapto** resistance *(NEJM 355:653, 2006)*	If MRSA resistant to **erythro**, likely that Q-D will have bacteriostatic & not bactericidal activity. Interest in Q-D + vanco, but no data. Do not add **linezolid** to **vanco**; no benefit & may be antagonistic *(AAC 47:3002, 2003)*. Linezolid successful in compassionate use *(JAC 50:1017, 2002)* & in pts with reduced vanco in vitro suscept. *(CID 38:521, 2004)*. New drugs likely available: ceftobiprole and ceftaroline.

TABLE 7 – METHODS FOR DRUG DESENSITIZATION

I. Penicillin Desensitization

(CID 35:26, 2002; AJM 121:572, 2008)

Perform in ICU setting. Discontinue all β-adrenergic antagonists. Have IV line, ECG and spirometer *(CCTID 13:131, 1993)*. Once desensitized, rx must not lapse or risk of allergic reactions ↑. A history of Stevens-Johnson syndrome, exfoliative dermatitis, erythroderma are nearly absolute contraindications to desensitization (use only as an approach to IgE sensitivity).

Oral Route: If oral prep available and pt has functional GI tract, oral route is preferred. 1/3 pts will develop transient reaction during desensitization or treatment, usually mild.

Step *	**1**	**2**	**3**	**4**	**5**	**6**	**7**	**8**	**9**	**10**	**11**	**12**	**13**	**14**
Drug (mg per mL)	0.5	0.5	0.5	0.5	0.5	0.5	0.5	5.0	5.0	5.0	50	50	50	50
Amount (mL)	0.1	0.2	0.4	0.8	1.6	3.2	6.4	1.2	2.4	4.8	1	2	4	8

* Interval between doses: 15 min. After Step 14, observe for 30 minutes, then 1 gm IV.

Parenteral Route:

Step **	**1**	**2**	**3**	**4**	**5**	**6**	**7**	**8**	**9**	**10**	**11**	**12**	**13**	**14**	**15**	**16**	**17**
Drug (mg per mL)	0.1	0.1	0.1	0.1	1.0	1.0	1.0	10	10	10	100	100	100	100	1000	1000	1000
Amount (mL)	0.1	0.2	0.4	0.8	0.16	0.32	0.64	0.12	0.24	0.48	0.1	0.2	0.4	0.8	0.16	0.32	0.64

** Interval between doses: 15 min. After Step 17, observe for 30 minutes, then 1 gm IV. *[Adapted from Sullivan, TJ, in Allergy: Principles and Practice, C.V. Mosby, 1993, p. 1726, with permission.]*

II. Ceftriaxone Desensitization

(Allergol Immunopathol (Modr) 37:105, 2009)

Infuse ceftriaxone IV, 20 minutes between doses:
Day 1: 0.001, 0.01, 0.1 and 1 mg
Day 2: 1, 5, 10, 50 mg
Day 3: 100, 250, 500 mg
Day 4 & thereafter: 1000 mg

III. Rapid Oral TMP-SMX Desensitization

Comment: Perform in hospital or clinic. Use oral suspension [40 mg TMP/ 200 mg SMX per 5 mL (tsp)]. Take 6 oz water after each dose. Corticosteroids, anti-histaminics NOT used.
Refs.: *CID 20:849, 1995; AIDS 5:311, 1991*

Hour	**Dose (TMP/SMX)**	**Hour**	**Dose (TMP/SMX)**
0	0.004/0.02	3	4/20
1	0.04/0.2	4	40/200
2	0.4/2	5	160/800

TABLE 8 – RISK CATEGORIES OF ANTIMICROBICS IN PREGNANCY

DRUG	FDA CATEGORIES*	DRUG	FDA CATEGORIES	DRUG	FDA CATEGORIES	DRUG	FDA CATEGORIES
Antibacterial Agents		**Antibacterial Agents** *(continued)*		**Antimycobacterial Agents:**		**Antiviral Agents:** *(continued)*	
Aminoglycosides:		Tetracyclines, tigecycline	**D**	Quinine	**X**	Fosamprenavir	C
Amikacin, gentamicin, isepamicin[NUS],		Tinidazole	C	Capreomycin	C	Foscarnet	C
netilmicin[NUS], streptomycin & tobramycin	**D**	Vancomycin	C	Clofazimine/cycloserine	"avoid"	Ganciclovir	C
Beta Lactams		**Antifungal Agents:** *(CID 27:1151, 1998)*		Dapsone	C	Indinavir	C
Penicillins; pens + BLI;		Amphotericin B preparations	B	Ethambutol	"safe"	Interferons	C
cephalosporins; aztreonam	B	Anidulafungin	C	Ethionamide	"do not use"	Lamivudine	C
Imipenem/cilastatin	C	Caspofungin	C	INH, pyrazinamide	C	Lopinavir/ritonavir	C
Meropenem, ertapenem, doripenem	B	Fluconazole, itraconazole, ketoconazole,		Rifabutin	B	Maraviroc	B
Chloramphenicol	C	flucytosine	C	Rifampin	C	Nelfinavir	B
Ciprofloxacin, oflox, levo, gati,		Micafungin	C	Thalidomide	**X**	Nevirapine	C
gemi, moxi	C	Posaconazole	C	**Antiviral Agents:**		Oseltamivir	C
Clindamycin	B	Terbinafine	B	Abacavir	C	Raltegravir	C
Colistin	C	Voriconazole	**D**	Acyclovir	B	Ribavirin	**X**
Daptomycin	B	**Antiparasitic Agents:**		Adefovir	C	Rimantadine	C
Fosfomycin	B	Albendazole/mebendazole	C	Amantadine	C	Ritonavir	B
Fusidic acid[1]	*See Footnote* [1]	Artemether/lumefantrine	C	Atazanavir	B	Saquinavir	B
Linezolid	C	Atovaquone/proguanil; atovaquone alone	C	Cidofovir	C	Stavudine	C
Macrolides:		Chloroquine	C	Darunavir	B	Telbivudine	B
Erythromycins/azithromycin	B	Dapsone	C	Delavirdine	C	Tenofovir	B
Clarithromycin	C	Eflornithine	C	Didanosine (ddI)	B	Tipranavir	C
Metronidazole	B	Ivermectin	C	Efavirenz	**D**	Valacyclovir	B
Nitrofurantoin	B	Mefloquine	C	Emtricitabine	B	Valganciclovir	C
Polymyxin B	B	Miltefosine	**X**	Enfuvirtide	B	Zalcitabine	C
Quinupristin-Dalfopristin	B	Nitazoxanide	B	Entecavir	C	Zanamivir	C
Rifaximin	C	Pentamidine	C	Etravirine	B	Zidovudine	C
Sulfonamides/trimethoprim	C	Praziquantel	B	Famciclovir	B		
Telavancin	C	Proguanil	C				
Telithromycin	C	Pyrimethamine/pyrisulfadoxine	C				
		Quinidine	C				

* **FDA Pregnancy Categories: A**—studies in pregnant women, no risk; **B**—animal studies no risk, but human not adequate or animal toxicity but human studies no risk; **C**—animal studies show toxicity, human studies inadequate but benefit of use may exceed risk; **D**—evidence of human risk, but benefits may outweigh; **X**—fetal abnormalities in humans, risk > benefit

[1] **Fusidic acid**: no problems reported

TABLE 9A – SELECTED PHARMACOLOGIC FEATURES OF ANTIMICROBIAL AGENTS

For pharmacodynamics, see Table 9B; for Cytochrome P450 interactions, see Table 9C. Table terminology key at bottom of each page. Additional footnotes at end of Table 9A, page 85.

DRUG	REFERENCE DOSE/ROUTE	PREG RISK	FOOD EFFECT (PO Prep)[1]	ORAL %AB	PEAK SERUM LEVEL (µg/mL)	PROTEIN BINDING (%)	VOLUME OF DISTR B (Vd)	AVER SERUM T½, hrs[2]	BILIARY PENETRATION (%)[3]	CSF[4]/BLOOD (%)	CSF PENETRATION[5]	AUC (µg*hr/mL)
PENICILLINS: Natural												
Benz Pen G	1.2 million units IM	B			0.15 (SD)							
Penicillin G	2 million units IV	B			20 (SD)	65	0.35 L/kg		500	5-10	Yes: Pen-sens S. pneumo	
Penicillin V	500 mg po	B	Tab/soln no food	60-73	5–6 (SD)	65		0.5				
PEN'ASE-RESISTANT PENICILLINS												
Clox/Diclox	500 mg po	B	Cap no food	50	10–15 (SD)	95–98	0.1 L/kg	0.5				
Nafcillin/Oxacillin	500 mg IV	B		Erratic	30-40 (SD)	90–94	Naf: 27.1 L Vss	0.5	>100/25	9–20	Yes: high-dose IV Rx	Naf: 18.1
AMINOPENICILLINS												
Amoxicillin	500 mg po	B	Cap/tab/susp no food	80	5.5-7.5 (SD)	17	0.36 L/kg	1.2	100–3000	13–14	Yes	22
Amoxicillin ER	775 mg po	B	Tab + food		6.6 (SD)	20		1.2-1.5				29.8
AM-CL	875/125 mg po	B	Cap/tab/susp ± food		11.6/2.2 (SD)	20/30		1.4/1.1	100–3000			AM: 26.8 - CL: 5.1
AM-CL-ER	2 tabs [1000/62.5 mg]	B	Tab + food		17/2.1 (SD)	18/25		1.3/1.0				AM: 71.6 - CL: 5.3
Ampicillin	2 gm IV	B			47 (SD)	18–22	0.29 L/kg	1.2	100–3000	13–14	Yes	
AM-SB	3 gm IV	B			109-150/48-88 (SD)	28/38		1.2				AM: 120- SB: 71
ANTIPSEUDOMONAL PENICILLINS												
PIP-TZ	3/.375 gm IV	B			242/24 (SD)	16–48	PIP: 0.24 L/kg	1.0	>100			PIP: 242 - TZ: 25
TC-CL	3.1 gm IV	B			330/8 (SD)	45/25	TC 9.7 Vss	1.2/1.0				TC: 485 - CL: 8.2
CEPHALOSPORINS—1st Generation												
Cefadroxil	500 mg po	B	Cap/tab/susp ± food	90	16 (SD)	20	0.31 L/kg V/F	1.5	22			47.4
Cefazolin	1 gm IV	B			188 (SD)	73–87	0.19 L/kg	1.9	29–300	1–4	No	236
Cephalexin	500 mg po	B	Cap/tab/susp ±	90	18 (SD)	5–15	0.38 L/kg V/F	1.0	216			29
CEPHALOSPORINS—2nd Generation												
Cefaclor	500 mg po	B	Cap/susp ± food	93	13 (SD)	22–25	0.33 L/kg V/F	0.8	≥60			20.5
Cefaclor-CD	500 mg po	B	Tab + food		8.4 (SD)	22–25		0.8	≥60			18.1
Cefotetan	1 gm IV	B			158 (SD)	78–91	10.3 L	4.2	2–21			504

Preg Risk: FDA risk categories: A = no risk, **B** = No risk – human studies, **C** = toxicity in animals - inadequate human studies, **D** = human risk, but benefit may outweigh risk, **X** = fetal abnormalities – risk > benefit; **Food Effect (PO dosing): + food** = take with food, **no food** = take without food, **± food** = take with or without food; **Oral % AB** = % absorbed; **Peak Serum Level: SD** = after single dose, **SS** = steady state after multiple doses; **Volume of Distribution (Vd): V/F** = Vd/oral bioavailability, **Vss** = Vd at steady state, **Vss/F** = Vd at steady state/oral bioavailability; **CSF Penetration:** therapeutic efficacy comment based on dose, usual susceptibility or target organism & penetration into CSF; **AUC** = area under drug concentration curve; **24hr** = AUC 0-24.

TABLE 9A (2) *(Footnotes at the end of table)*

DRUG	REFERENCE DOSE/ROUTE	PREG RISK	FOOD EFFECT (PO Prep)[1]	ORAL %AB	PEAK SERUM LEVEL (μg/mL)	PROTEIN BINDING (%)	VOLUME OF DISTRIB (Vd)	AVER SERUM T½, hrs[2]	BILIARY PENETRATION (%)[3]	CSF[4]/ BLOOD (%)	CSF PENETRATION[5]	AUC (μg*hr/mL)
CEPHALOSPORINS—2nd Generation *(continued)*												
Cefoxitin	1 gm IV	B			110 (SD)	65–79	16.1 L Vss	0.8	280	3	No	
Cefprozil	500 mg po	B	Tab/susp ± food	95	10.5 (SD)	36	0.23 L/kg Vss/F	1.5				25.7
Cefuroxime	1.5 gm IV	B			100 (SD)	33–50	0.19 L/kg Vss	1.5	35–80	17–88	Marginal	150
Cefuroxime axetil	250 mg tabs po	B	Susp + food; Tab ± food	52	4.1 (SD)	50	0.66 L/kg V/F	1.5				12.9
CEPHALOSPORINS—3rd Generation												
Cefdinir	300 mg po	B	Cap/susp ± food	25	1.6 (SD)	60–70	0.35 L/kg V/F	1.7				7.1
Cefditoren pivoxil	400 mg po	B	Tab + food	16	4 (SD)	88	9.3 L Vss/F	1.6				20
Cefixime	400 mg tabs po	B	Tab/susp ± food	50	3–5 (SD)	65	0.93 L/kg V/F	3.1	800			25.8
Cefotaxime	1 gm IV	B			100	30–51	0.28 L/kg	1.5	15–75	10	Yes	70
Cefpodoxime proxetil	200 mg po	B	Tab + food Susp ± food	46	2.3 (SD)	40	0.7 L/kg V/F	2.3	115			14.5
Ceftazidime	1 gm IV	B			69 (SD)	<10	0.24 L/kg Vss	1.9	13–54	20–40	Yes	127
Ceftibuten	400 mg po	B	Cap/susp no food	80	15 (SD)	65	0.21 L/kg V/F	2.4				73.7
Ceftizoxime	1 gm IV	B			60 (SD)	30	0.34 L/kg	1.7	34–82			85
Ceftriaxone	1 gm IV	B			150 (SD), 172-204 (SS)	85–95	5.8-13.5 L	8	200–500	8–16	Yes	1006
CEPHALOSPORIN—4th Generation and Anti-MRSA												
Cefepime	2 gm IV	B			164 (SD)	20	18 L Vss	2.0	∝ 5	10	Yes	284.8
Ceftaroline	600 mg IV	B			21.3	20	20.3 Vss	2.7				56.3
Ceftobiprole	500 mg IV	B			33–34.2 (SD)	16	18 L Vss	2.9–3.3				116
CARBAPENEMS												
Doripenem	500 mg IV	B			23	8.1	16.8 L Vss	1	117 (0–611)			36.3
Ertapenem	1 gm IV	B			154	95	0.12 L Vss	4	10			572.1
Imipenem	500 mg IV	C			40	15–25	0.27 L/kg	1	minimal	8.5	+[6]	42.2
Meropenem	1 gm IV	B			49	2	0.29 L/kg	1	3–300	Approx. 2	+	72.5
MONOBACTAM												
Aztreonam	1 gm IV	B			90 (SD)	56	12.6 L Vss	2	115–405	3–52	±	271
AMINOGLYCOSIDES												
Amikacin, gentamicin, kanamycin, tobramycin—*see Table 10D, page 101, for dose & serum levels*		D				0–10	0.26 L/kg	2.5	10–60	0–30	No; intrathecal dose: 5–10 mg	
Neomycin	po	D	Tab/soln ± food	<3	0							

<u>**Preg Risk**</u>**: FDA risk categories: A** = no risk, **B** = No risk – human studies, **C** = toxicity in animals - inadequate human studies, **D** = human risk, but benefit may outweigh risk, **X** = fetal abnormalities – risk > benefit; <u>**Food Effect**</u> **(PO dosing): + food** = take with food, **no food** = take without food, **± food** = take with or without food; **Oral % AB** = % absorbed; <u>**Peak Serum Level**</u>**: SD** = after single dose, **SS** = steady state after multiple doses; <u>**Volume of Distribution (Vd)**</u>**: V/F** = Vd/oral bioavailability, **Vss** = Vd at steady state, **Vss/F** = Vd at steady state/oral bioavailability; <u>**CSF Penetration:**</u> therapeutic efficacy comment based on dose, usual susceptibility or target organism & penetration into CSF; **AUC** = area under drug concentration curve; **24hr** = AUC 0-24.

TABLE 9A (3) *(Footnotes at the end of table)*

DRUG	REFERENCE DOSE/ROUTE	PREG RISK	FOOD EFFECT (PO Prep)[1]	ORAL %AB	PEAK SERUM LEVEL (µg/mL)	PROTEIN BINDING (%)	VOLUME OF DISTRIB (Vd)	AVER SERUM T½, hrs[2]	BILIARY PENETRATION (%)[3]	CSF[4]/ BLOOD (%)	CSF PENETRATION[5]	AUC (µg*hr/mL)
FLUOROQUINOLONES[7]												
Ciprofloxacin	750 mg po q12h	C	Tab + food	70	3.6 (SS)	20–40	2.4 L/kg	4	2800–4500			31.6 (24 hr)
	400 mg IV q12h	C			4.6 (SS)	20–40		4	2800–4500	26	1 µg/mL: Inadequate for Strep. sp. *(CID 31:1131, 2000)*.	25.4 (24 hr)
	500 mg ER po q24h	C	Tab no food		1.6 (SS)	20–40		6.6				8 (24 hr)
	1000 mg ER po q24h	C	Tab no food		3.1 (SS)	20–40		6.3				16 (24 hr)
Gemifloxacin	320 mg po q24h	C	Tab ± food	71	1.6 (SS)	55–73	2-12 L/kg Vss/F	7				9.9 (24 hr)
Levofloxacin	500 mg po/IV q24h	C	Tab ± food	99	5.7/6.4 (SS)	24–38	74-112 L Vss	7		30–50		PO:47.5, IV 54.6 (24 hr)
	750 mg po/IV q24h	C	Tab ± food	99	8.6/12.1 (SS)	24–38		7				PO 90.7, IV 108 (24 hr)
Moxifloxacin	400 mg po/IV q24h	C	Tab ± food	89	4.2-4.6/4.5 (SS)	30–50	2.2 L/kg	10–14		>50	Yes *(CID 49:1080 2009)*	PO 48, IV 38 (24 hr)
Ofloxacin	400 mg po/IV q12h	C	Tab ± food	98	4.6/6.2 (SS)	32	1-2.5 L/kg	7				PO 82.4, IV 87 (24 hr)
MACROLIDES, AZALIDES, LINCOSAMIDES, KETOLIDES												
Azithromycin	500 mg po	B	Tab/Susp ± food	37	0.4 (SD)	7–51	31.1 L/kg Vss/F	68	High			4.3
	500 mg IV	B			3.6 (SD)	7–51		12/68				9.6 (24 hr, pre SS)
Azithromycin-ER	2 gm po	B	Susp no food	∝ 30	0.8 (SD)	7–50		59	High			20
Clarithromycin	500 mg po q12h	C	Tab/Susp ± food	50	3–4 (SS)	65–70	4 L/kg	5–7	7000			20 (24 hr)
	1000 mg ER po q24h	C	Tab + food	∝ 50	2–3 (SS)	65–70						
Erythromycin Oral (various)	500 mg po	B	Tab/Susp no food DR Caps ± food	13–45	0.1–2 (SD)	70–74	0.6 L/kg	2–4		2–13	No	
Lacto/glucep	500 mg IV	B			3–4 (SD)	70–74		2–4				
Telithromycin	800 mg po q24h	C	Tab ± food		2.3 (SS)	60–70	2.9 L/kg	10	7			12.5 (24 hr)
Clindamycin	150 mg po	B	Cap ± food	57	2.5 (SD)	85–94	1.1 L/kg	2.4	250–300		No	
	900 mg IV	B		90	14.1 (SS)	85–94		2.4	250–300		No	
MISCELLANEOUS ANTIBACTERIALS												
Chloramphenicol	1 gm po q6h	C	Cap ± food	High	18 (SS)	25–50	0.8 L/kg	4.1		45–89	Yes	
Colistin (Polymyxin E)	150 mg IV	C			5–7.5 (SD)		0.34 L/kg	2–3	0		No *(AAC 53:4907, 2009)*	

Preg Risk: FDA risk categories: A = no risk, **B** = No risk – human studies, **C** = toxicity in animals - inadequate human studies, **D** = human risk, but benefit may outweigh risk, **X** = fetal abnormalities – risk > benefit; **Food Effect (PO dosing): + food** = take with food, **no food** = take without food, **± food** = take with or without food; **Oral % AB** = % absorbed; **Peak Serum Level: SD** = after single dose, **SS** = steady state after multiple doses; **Volume of Distribution (Vd): V/F** = Vd/oral bioavailability, **Vss** = Vd at steady state, **Vss/F** = Vd at steady state/oral bioavailability; **CSF Penetration:** therapeutic efficacy comment based on dose, usual susceptibility or target organism & penetration into CSF; **AUC** = area under drug concentration curve; **24hr** = AUC 0-24.

TABLE 9A (4) *(Footnotes at the end of table)*

DRUG	REFERENCE DOSE/ROUTE	PREG RISK	FOOD EFFECT (PO Prep)[1]	ORAL %AB	PEAK SERUM LEVEL (μg/mL)	PROTEIN BINDING (%)	VOLUME OF DISTRIB (Vd)	AVER SERUM T½, hrs[2]	BILIARY PENETRATION (%)[3]	CSF[4]/ BLOOD (%)	CSF PENETRATION[5]	AUC (μg*hr/mL)
MISCELLANEOUS ANTIBACTERIALS *(continued)*												
Daptomycin	4–6 mg/kg IV q24h	B			58–99 (SS)	92	0.1 L/kg Vss	8–9				494-632 (24 hr)
Doxycycline	100 mg po	B	Tab/cap/susp ± food		1.5–2.1 (SD)	93	53-134 L Vss	18	200–3200		No (26%)	31.7
Fosfomycin	3 gm po	-	Sachet ± food		26 (SD)	<10	136.1 L Vss/F	5.7				150
Fusidic acid	500 mg po	C	Tab + food	91	30 (SD)	95-99	0.3 L/kg	5-15	100–200			315
Linezolid	600 mg po/IV q12h	C	Tab/susp ± food	100	15–20 (SS)	31	40-50 L Vss	5		60–70	Yes *(AAC 50:3971, 2006)*	PO: 276/IV: 179 (24 hr)
Metronidazole	500 mg po/IV q6h	B	ER tab no food, Tab/cap ± food		20–25 (SS)	20	0.6-0.85 L/kg	6–14	100	45–89		560 (24 hr)
Minocycline	200 mg po	D	Cap/tab ± food		2.0–3.5 (SD)	76	80-114 L Vss	16	200–3200			48.3
Polymyxin B	2 mg/kg IV	C			1–8 (SD)	78–92	0.07-0.2 L/kg	4.3–6			No	Dal: 31.8 (24 hr)
Quinu-Dalfo	7.5 mg/kg IV q8h	B			3.2/8 (SS)		0.45/0.24 L/kg Vss	1.5				58
Rifampin	600 mg po	C	Cap no food		4–32 (SD)	80	0.65 L/kg Vss	2–5	10,000			
Rifaximin	200 mg po	C	Tab ± food	<0.4	0.004–0.01 (SD)							
Tetracycline	250 mg po	D	Cap no food		1.5–2.2 (SD)		1.3 L/kg	6–12	200–3200		No (7%)	30
Telavancin	10 mg/kg/q24h	C			108 (SS)	90	0.13 L/kg	8.1	Low			780 (24 hr)
Tigecycline	50 mg IV q12h	D			0.63 (SS)	71–89	7-9 L/kg	42	138		No	4.7 (24 hr)
Trimethoprim (TMP)	100 mg po	C	Tab ± food	80	1 (SD)		100-120 V/F	8–15				
TMP-SMX-DS	160/800 mg po q12h	C	Tab/susp ± food	85	1–2/40–60 (SS)		TM: 100-120 L SM: 12-18 L		100–200	50/40		
	160/800 mg IV q8h	C			9/105 (SS)				40–70			
Vancomycin	1 gm IV q12h	C			20–50 (SS)	<10–55	0.7 L/kg	4–6	50	7–14		
ANTIFUNGALS												
Amphotericin B:												
Standard	0.4–0.7 mg/kg IV	B			0.5–3.5 (SS)		4 L/kg	24		0		17
Lipid (ABLC)	5 mg/kg IV	B			1–2.5 (SS)		131 L/kg	173				14 (24 hr)
Cholesteryl complex	4 mg/kg IV	B			2.9 (SS)		4.3 L/kg	39				36 (24 hr)
Liposomal	5 mg/kg IV	B			83 (SS)		0.1-0.4 L/kg Vss	6.8 ± 2.1				555 (24 hr)
Fluconazole	400 mg po/IV	C	Tab/susp ± food	90	6.7 (SD)	10	50 L V/F	20–50		50–94	Yes	
	800 mg po/IV	C	Tab/susp ± food	90	Approx. 14 (SD)			20–50				
Itraconazole	200 mg po soln	C	Soln no food	Low	0.3–0.7 (SD)	99.8	796 L	35		0		29.3 (24 hr)

Preg Risk: FDA risk categories: A = no risk, **B** = No risk – human studies, **C** = toxicity in animals - inadequate human studies, **D** = human risk, but benefit may outweigh risk, **X** = fetal abnormalities – risk > benefit; **Food Effect (PO dosing): + food** = take with food, **no food** = take without food, **± food** = take with or without food; **Oral % AB** = % absorbed; **Peak Serum Level: SD** = after single dose, **SS** = steady state after multiple doses; **Volume of Distribution (Vd): V/F** = Vd/oral bioavailability, **Vss** = Vd at steady state, **Vss/F** = Vd at steady state/oral bioavailability; **CSF Penetration:** therapeutic efficacy comment based on dose, usual susceptibility or target organism & penetration into CSF; **AUC** = area under drug concentration curve; **24hr** = AUC 0-24.

TABLE 9A (5) *(Footnotes at the end of table)*

DRUG	REFERENCE DOSE/ROUTE	PREG RISK	FOOD EFFECT (PO Prep)[1]	ORAL %AB	PEAK SERUM LEVEL (µg/mL)	PROTEIN BINDING (%)	VOLUME OF DISTRIB (Vd)	AVER SERUM T½, hrs[2]	BILIARY PENETRATION (%)[3]	CSF[4]/ BLOOD (%)	CSF PENETRATION[5]	AUC (µg*hr/mL)
ANTIFUNGALS *(continued)*												
Posaconazole	200 mg po	C	Susp + food		0.2-1.0 (SD)	98-99	1774 L	20-66			Yes (*JAC 56:745, 2005*)	15.1
Voriconazole	200 mg po q12h	D	Tab/susp no food	96	3 (SS)	58	4.6 L/kg Vss	6		22–100	Yes (*CID 37:728, 2003*)	39.8 (24 hr)
Anidulafungin	200 mg IV x 1, then 100 mg IV q24h	C			7.2 (SS)	>99	30-50 L	26.5			No	112 (24 hr)
Caspofungin	70 mg IV x 1, then 50 mg IV qd	C			9.9 (SD)	97	9.7 L Vss	9–11			No	87.3 (24 hr)
Flucytosine	2.5 gm po	C	Cap ± food	78–90	30–40 (SD)		0.6 L/kg	3–6		60–100	Yes	
Micafungin	150 mg IV q24h	C			16.4 (SS)	>99	0.39 L/kg	15–17			No	167 (24 hr)
ANTIMYCOBACTERIALS												
Ethambutol	25 mg/kg po	Safe	Tab + food	80	2–6 (SD)	10–30	6 L/kg Vss/F	4		10-50	No	29.6
Isoniazid	300 mg po	C	Tab/syrup no food	100	3–5 (SD)		0.6-1.2 L/kg	0.7–4		Up to 90	Yes	20.1
Pyrazinamide	20–25 mg/kg po	C	Tab ± food	95	30–50 (SD)	5–10		10–16		100	Yes	500
Rifampin	600 mg po	C	Cap no food	70–90	4–32 (SD)	80	0.65 L/kg Vss	2–5	10,000	7–56	Yes	58
Streptomycin	1 gm IV	D			25–50 (SD)	0–10	0.26 L/kg	2.5	10–60	0–30	No; Intrathecal: 5–10 mg	
ANTIPARASITICS												
Albendazole	400 mg po	C	Tab + food		0.5–1.6	70						
Artemether/ Lumefantrine	4 tabs po: 80/480 mg	C	Tab + food		Art: 9 (SS), D-Art: 1 Lum: 5.6-9 (not SS)			Art: 1.6, D-Art: 1.6, Lum: 101				
Atovaquone	750 mg po bid	C	Susp + food	47	24 (SS)	99.9	0.6 L/kg Vss	67		<1	No	801 (750 mg x 1)
Dapsone	100 mg po q24h	C	Tab ± food	100	1.1 (SS)		1.5 L/kg	10–50				
Ivermectin	12 mg po	C	Tab no food		0.05–0.08 (SD)		9.9 L/kg					
Mefloquine	1.25 gm po	C	Tab + food		0.5–1.2 (SD)	98	20 L/kg	13–24 days				
Miltefosine	50 mg po tid	X	Cap + food		31 (SD)	95		7–31 (long) *AAC 52:2855, 2008*				
Nitazoxanide	500 mg po tab	B	Tab/susp + food		9–10 (SD)	99						41.9 Tizoxanide
Proguanil[8]	100 mg	C	Tab + food		No data	75	1600-2000 L V/F					
Pyrimethamine	25 mg po	C	Tab ± food	"High"	0.1–0.3 (SD)	87	3 L/kg	96				
Praziquantel	20 mg per kg po	B	Tab + food	80	0.2–2.0 (SD)		8000 L V/F	0.8–1.5				1.51
Tinidazole	2 gm po	B	Tab + food	48	48 (SD)	12	50 L	13				902

Preg Risk: FDA risk categories: A = no risk, **B** = No risk – human studies, **C** = toxicity in animals - inadequate human studies, **D** = human risk, but benefit may outweigh risk **X** = fetal abnormalities – risk > benefit; **Food Effect (PO dosing): + food** = take with food, **no food** = take without food, **± food** = take with or without food; **Oral % AB** = % absorbed; **Peak Serum Level: SD** = after single dose, **SS** = steady state after multiple doses; **Volume of Distribution (Vd): V/F** = Vd/oral bioavailability, **Vss** = Vd at steady state, **Vss/F** = Vd at steady state/oral bioavailability; **CSF Penetration:** therapeutic efficacy comment based on dose, usual susceptibility or target organism & penetration into CSF. **AUC** = area under drug concentration curve; **24hr** = AUC 0-24.

TABLE 9A (6) *(Footnotes at the end of table)*

DRUG	REFERENCE DOSE/ROUTE	PREG RISK	FOOD EFFECT (PO Prep)[1]	ORAL %AB	PEAK SERUM LEVEL (μg/mL)	PROTEIN BINDING (%)	VOLUME OF DISTRIB (Vd)	AVER SERUM T½, hrs[2]	BILIARY PENETRATION (%)[3]	CSF[4]/ BLOOD (%)	CSF PENETRATION[5]	AUC (μg*hr/mL)
ANTIVIRAL DRUGS—NOT HIV												
Acyclovir	400 mg po bid	B	Tab/cap/susp ± food	10–20	1.21 (SS)	9–33	0.7 L/kg	2.5–3.5				7.4 (24 hr)
Adefovir	10 mg po	C	Tab ± food	59	0.02 (SD)	≤4	0.37 L/kg Vss	7.5				0.22
Entecavir	0.5 mg po q24h	C	Tab/soln no food	100	4.2 ng/mL (SS)	13	>0.6 L/kg V/F	128–149				0.14
Famciclovir	500 mg po	B	Tab ± food	77	3–4 (SD)	<20	1.1 L/kg*	2–3				8.9 Penciclovir
Foscarnet	60 mg/kg IV	C			155 (SD)	4	0.46 L/kg	<1	No			2195 μM*hr
Ganciclovir	5 mg/kg IV	C			8.3 (SD)	1–2	0.7 L/kg Vss	3.5				24.5
Oseltamivir	75 mg po bid	C	Cap/susp ± food	75	0.065/0.35[9] (SS)	3	23-26 L/kg Vss*	1–3				5.4 (24 hr) Carboxylate
Ribavirin	600 mg po	X	Tab/cap/soln + food	64	0.8 (SD)		2825 L V/F	44				25.4
Rimantadine	100 mg po	C	Tab ± food		0.05–0.1 (SD)		17-19 L/kg	25				3.5
Telbivudine	600 mg po q24h	B	Tab/soln ± food		3.7 (SS)	3.3	>0.6 L/kg V/F	40-49				26.1 (24 hr)
Valacyclovir	1000 mg po	B	Tab ± food	55	5.6 (SD)	13–18	0.7 L/kg	3				19.5 Acyclovir
Valganciclovir	900 mg po q24h	C	Tab/soln + food	59	5.6 (SS)	1–2	0.7 L/kg	4				29.1 Ganciclovir

DRUG	REFERENCE DOSE/ROUTE	PREG RISK	FOOD EFFECT (PO Prep)	ORAL %AB	PEAK SERUM LEVEL (μg/mL)	PROTEIN BINDING (%)	VOLUME OF DISTRIB (Vd)	AVER SERUM T½, hrs[2]	INTRA CELLULAR T½, HOURS	CSF[4]/ BLOOD (%)	CSF PENETRATION[5]	AUC (μg*hr/mL)
ANTI-HIV VIRAL DRUGS												
Abacavir	600 mg po q24h	C	Tab/soln ± food	83	4.3 (SS)	50	0.86 L/kg	1.5	12–26	Low	No	12 (24 hr)
Atazanavir	400 mg po q24h	B	Cap + food	Good	2.3 (SS)	86	88.3 L V/F	7		Intermed	?	22.3 (24 hr)
Darunavir	(600 mg+100 mg RTV) bid	B	Tab + food	82	3.5 (SS)	95	2 L/kg	15		Intermed	?	116.8 (24 hr)
Delavirdine	400 mg po tid	C	Tab ± food	85	19 ± 11(SS)	98		5.8				180 μM*hr
Didanosine	400 mg EC[10] po	B	Cap no food	30–40	?	<5	308-363 L	1.4	25–40	Intermed	?	2.6
Efavirenz	600 mg po q24h	D	Cap/tab no food	42	4.1 (SS)	99	252 L V/F	52–76				184 μM*hr (24 hr)
Emtricitabine	200 mg po q24h	B	Cap/soln ± food	93	1.8 (SS)	<4		10	39	Intermed	?	10 (24 hr)
Enfuvirtide	90 mg sc bid	B		84	5 (SS)	92	5.5 L	4				97.4 (24 hr)
Etravirine	200 mg po bid	B	Tab + food		0.3 (SS)	99.9		41				9 (24 hr)

Preg Risk: FDA risk categories: A = no risk, **B** = No risk – human studies, **C** = toxicity in animals - inadequate human studies, **D** = human risk, but benefit may outweigh risk, **X** = fetal abnormalities – risk > benefit; **Food Effect (PO dosing): + food** = take with food, **no food** = take without food, **± food** = take with or without food; **Oral % AB** = % absorbed; **Peak Serum Level: SD** = after single dose, **SS** = steady state after multiple doses; **Volume of Distribution (Vd): V/F** = Vd/oral bioavailability, **Vss** = Vd at steady state, **Vss/F** = Vd at steady state/oral bioavailability; **CSF Penetration:** therapeutic efficacy comment based on dose, usual susceptibility or target organism & penetration into CSF; **AUC** = area under drug concentration curve; **24hr** = AUC 0-24.

TABLE 9A (7) (*Footnotes at the end of table*)

DRUG	REFERENCE DOSE/ROUTE	PREG RISK	FOOD EFFECT (PO Prep)	ORAL %AB	PEAK SERUM LEVEL (μg/mL)	PROTEIN BINDING (%)	VOLUME OF DISTRIB (Vd)	AVER SERUM T½, hrs[2]	INTRA CELLULAR T½, HOURS	CSF[4]/ BLOOD (%)	CSF PENETRA-TION[5]	AUC (μg*hr/mL)
ANTI-HIV VIRAL DRUGS *(continued)*												
Fosamprenavir	(700 mg po+ 100 mg RTV) bid	C	Boosted ped susp + food Adult susp no food Tab ± food	No data	6 (SS)	90		7.7	No data	Intermed	?	79.2 (24 hr)
Indinavir	800 mg po tid	C	Boosted cap + food, Cap alone no food	65	9 (SS)	60		1.2–2		High	Yes	92.1 μM*hr (24 hr)
Lamivudine	300 mg po	C	Tab/soln ± food	86	2.6 (SS)	<36	1.3 L/kg	5–7	18–22	Intermed	?	11
Lopinavir/RTV	400 mg po bid	C	Soln + food	No data	9.6 (SS)	98–99		5–6 (LPV)		Intermed	?	186 LPV
Maraviroc	300 mg po bid	B	Tab ± food	33	0.3–0.9 (SS)	76	194 L	14-18		Intermed	?	3 (24 hr)
Nelfinavir	1250 mg po bid	B	Tab/powd + food	20–80	3–4 (SS)	98	2–7 L/kg V/F	3.5–5		Low	No	53 (24 hr)
Nevirapine	200 mg po	C	Tab/susp ± food	>90	2 (SD)	60	1.2 L/kg Vss	25–30		High	Yes	110 (24 hr)
Raltegravir	400 mg po bid	C	Tab ± food		5.4 (SS)	83	287 L Vss/F	9		Intermed	?	28.6 μM*hr (24 hr)
Ritonavir (RTV)	600 mg po bid	B	Cap/soln + food	65	11.2 (SS)	98–99	0.41 L/kg V/F	3–5		Low	No	
Saquinavir	(1000 + 100 RTV) mg po bid	B	Tab/cap + food	4	0.37 min (SS conc)	97	700 L Vss	1–2		Low	No	29.2 (24 hr)
Stavudine	40 mg bid	C	Cap/soln ± food	86	0.54 (SS)	<5	46L	1	7.5			2.6 (24 hr)
Tenofovir	300 mg po	B	Tab ± food	25	0.3 (SD)	<1–7	1.3 L/kg Vss	17	>60	Low	No	2.3
Tipranavir	(500 + 200 RTV) mg po bid	C	Cap/soln + food		47–57 (SS)	99.9	7.7-10 L	5.5–6		Low	No	1600 μM*hr (24 hr)
Zidovudine	300 mg po	C	Tab/cap/syrup ± food	60	1–2	<38	1.6 L/kg	0.5–3	11	High	Yes	2.1

[1] Food decreases rate and/or extent of absorption. For adult oral preps; not applicable for peds suspensions.
[2] Assumes CrCl >80 mL per min.
[3] Peak concentration in bile/peak concentration in serum x 100. If blank, no data.
[4] CSF levels with inflammation
[5] Judgment based on drug dose & organ susceptibility. CSF concentration ideally ≥10 above MIC.
[6] Concern over seizure potential; *see Table 10*
[7] Take all po FQs 2–4 hours before sucralfate or any multivalent cations: Ca^{++}, Fe^{++}, Zn^{++}
[8] Given with atovaquone as Malarone for malaria prophylaxis.
[9] Oseltamivir/oseltamivir carboxylate
[10] EC = enteric coated

Preg Risk: FDA risk categories: A = no risk, **B** = No risk – human studies, **C** = toxicity in animals - inadequate human studies, **D** = human risk, but benefit may outweigh risk, **X** = fetal abnormalities – risk > benefit; **Food Effect (PO dosing): + food** = take with food, **no food** = take without food, **± food** = take with or without food; **Oral % AB** = % absorbed; **Peak Serum Level: SD** = after single dose, **SS** = steady state after multiple doses; **Volume of Distribution (Vd): V/F** = Vd/oral bioavailability, **Vss** = Vd at steady state, **Vss/F** = Vd at steady state/oral bioavailability; **CSF Penetration:** therapeutic efficacy comment based on dose, usual susceptibility or target organism & penetration into CSF; **AUC** = area under drug concentration curve; **24hr** = AUC 0-24.

TABLE 9B – PHARMACODYNAMICS OF ANTIBACTERIALS*

BACTERIAL KILLING/PERSISTENT EFFECT	DRUGS	THERAPY GOAL	PK/PD MEASUREMENT
Concentration-dependent/Prolonged persistent effect	Aminoglycosides; daptomycin; ketolides; quinolones; metro	High peak serum concentration	24-hr AUC[1]/MIC
Time-dependent/No persistent effect	Penicillins; cephalosporins; carbapenems; monobactams	Long duration of exposure	Time above MIC
Time-dependent/Moderate to long persistent effect	Clindamycin; erythro/azithro/clarithro; linezolid; tetracyclines; vancomycin	Enhanced amount of drug	24-hr AUC[1]/MIC

* Adapted from *Craig, WA: IDC No. Amer 17:479, 2003 & Drusano, G.L.: CID 44:79, 2007*

TABLE 9C - CYTOCHROME P450 INTERACTIONS OF ANTIMICROBIALS

Cytochrome P450 isoenzyme terminology:
e.g., 3A4 : **3** = family, **A** = subfamily, **4** = gene; **PGP** = an intestinal drug transporter; **P** = glycoprotein; **UGT** = uridine diphosphate glucuronosyltransferase.

	Cytochrome P450 Interactions		
DRUG	**Substrate**	**Inhibits**	**Induces**
Antibacterials			
Azithromycin (all)	PGP	PGP (weak)	
Chloramphenicol		2C19, 3A4	
Ciprofloxacin (all)		1A2, 3A4 (minor)	
Clarithromycin (all)	3A4	3A4, PGP	
Erythromycin (all)	3A4, PGP	3A4, PGP	
Metronidazole		2C9	
Nafcillin			2C9 (?), 3A4
Quinu-Dalfo		Quinu: 3A4	
Rifampin	PGP		1A2, 2C9, 2C19, 2D6 (Weak), 3A4, PGP
Telithromycin		3A4, PGP	
TMP-SMX	SMX: 2C9 (major), 3A4	SMX: 2C9 TMP: 2C8	
Trimethoprim		2C8	
Antifungals			
Fluconazole (400 mg)	3A4 (minor), PGP	2C9, 2C19, 3A4, UGT	
Itraconazole	3A4, PGP	3A4, PGP	
Posaconazole	PGP, UGT	3A4, PGP	
Voriconazole	2C9, 2C19, 3A4	2C9, 2C19 (major), 3A4	
Antimycobacterials (Also Rifampin, above)			
Dapsone	3A4		
Isoniazid	2E1	2C19, 3A4	

	Cytochrome P450 Interactions		
DRUG	**Substrate**	**Inhibits**	**Induces**
Antiparasitics			
Mefloquine	3A4, PGP	PGP	
Praziquantel	3A4		
Proguanil	2C19 (conversion to cycloguanil)		
Tinidazole		2C9	
Antiretrovirals			
Atazanavir	3A4	1A2, 2C9, 3A4	
Darunavir	3A4	3A4	
Delavirdine	2D6, 3A4	2C9, 2C19, 3A4	
Efavirenz	2B6, 3A4	2B6, 2C9, 2C19	2C19, 3A4
Etravirine	2C9, 2C19, 3A4	2C9, 2C19 (weak)	
Fosamprenavir	3A4	2C19, 3A4	
Indinavir	3A4, PGP	3A4, PGP	
Lopinavir/Ritonavir	3A4	3A4	
Maraviroc	3A4, PGP	2D6	
Nelfinavir	2C9, 2C19, 3A4, PGP	3A4, PGP	3A4
Nevirapine	2B6, 3A4		3A4
Raltegravir	UGT		
Ritonavir	2D6, 3A4, PGP	2B6, 2C9, 2C19, 2D6, 3A4, PGP	3A4, 1A2 (?), 2C9 (?), PGP (?)
Saquinavir	3A4, PGP	3A4, PGP	
Tipranavir	3A4, PGP	1A2, 2C9, 2C19, 2D6	3A4, PGP (weak)

Refs: Hansten PD, Horn JR. The top 100 drug interactions: a guide to patient management. 2010 E. Freeland (WA): H&H Publications; 2010; and package inserts.

TABLE 10A – SELECTED ANTIBACTERIAL AGENTS—ADVERSE REACTIONS—OVERVIEW

Adverse reactions in individual patients represent all-or-none occurrences, even if rare. After selection of an agent, the physician should read the manufacturer's package insert [statements in the product labeling (package insert) must be approved by the FDA].

Numbers = frequency of occurrence (%); + = occurs, incidence not available; –+ = significant adverse reaction; 0 = not reported; R = rare, defined as <1%.

NOTE: Important reactions in bold print. A blank means no data found.

	PENICILLINS, CARBAPENEMS, MONOBACTAMS, AMINOGLYCOSIDES																			
		PENICILLINASE-RESISTANT ANTI-STAPH. PENICILLINS			AMINOPENICILLINS				AP PENS				CARBAPENEMS					AMINOGLYCO-SIDES	MISC.	
ADVERSE REACTIONS	Penicillin G,V	Dicloxacillin	Nafcillin	Oxacillin	Amoxicillin	Amox-Clav	Ampicillin	Amp-Sulb	Piperacillin	Pip-Taz	Ticarcillin	Ticar-Clav	Doripenem	Ertapenem	Imipenem	Meropenem	Aztreonam	Amikacin Gentamicin Kanamycin Netilmicin[NUS] Tobramycin	Linezolid	Telithromycin
Rx stopped due to AE						2-4.4			3.2	3.2			3.4			1.2	<1			
Local, phlebitis	+		++	+				3	4	1	3		4-8	4	3	1	4			
Hypersensitivity	+												R		3	3				
Fever	+	+	+	+	+	+	+	+	+	2	+	+	+	+	+		2	+	+	
Rash	**3**	**4**	**4**	**4**	**5**	**3**	**5**	**2**	**1**	**4**	**3**	**2**	**1-5**	**+**	**+**	**+**	**2**			
Photosensitivity	0	0	0	0	0	0	0	0	0	0	0	0			0		+			
Anaphylaxis	R	0	R	R	0	R	R	+	0	0	+	+	R	+	+	+	+			
Serum sickness	4								–	+	+	+			+		+			
Hematologic																				
+ Coombs	3	0	R	R	+	0	+	0	–	+	0	+		1	2	+	R			
Neutropenia	R	0	+	R	+	+	+	+	6	+	0	+	R	+	+	+	+		1.1	
Eosinophilia	+	+	22	22	2	+	22	22	+	+	+	+		+	+	+	8			
Thrombocytopenia	R	0	R	R	R	R	R	R	+	+	R	R	–		+	+	+		3–10 *(see 10C)*	
↑ PT/PTT	R	0	+	0	+	0	+	0	+	+	+	+			R		R			
GI																				
Nausea/vomiting		+	0	0	2	3	2	+	+	7	+	1	4-12	3	2	4	R		3/1	7/2
Diarrhea		+	0	0	**5**	**9**	**10**	**2**	2	11	3	1	6-11	6	2	5	R		4	10
C. difficile colitis		R	R	R	R	+	R	+	+	+	+	+	R		+		+		+	+
Hepatic, ↑ LFTs	R	R	0	+	R	+	R	6	+	+	0	+	+	6	4	4	2		1.3	
Hepatic failure	0	0	0	0	0	0	0	0	0	0	0	0			0					+
Renal: ↑ BUN, Cr	R	0	0	0	R	0	R	R	+	+	0	0			+	0	0	**5–25[1]**		
CNS																				
Headache	R	0	R	R	0	+	R	R	R	8	R	R	4-16	2	+	3	+		2	2
Confusion	R	0	R	R	0	0	R	R	R	R	R	R			+		+		+	

[1] Varies with criteria used.

TABLE 10A (2)

ADVERSE REACTIONS	PENICILLINS, CARBAPENEMS, MONOBACTAMS, AMINOGLYCOSIDES																			
		PENICILLINASE-RESISTANT ANTI-STAPH. PENICILLINS			AMINOPENICILLINS				AP PENS				CARBAPENEMS					AMINOGLYCOSIDES	MISC.	
	Penicillin G,V	Dicloxacillin	Nafcillin	Oxacillin	Amoxicillin	Amox-Clav	Ampicillin	Amp-Sulb	Piperacillin	Pip-Taz	Ticarcillin	Ticar-Clav	Doripenem	Ertapenem	Imipenem	Meropenem	Aztreonam	Amikacin Gentamicin Kanamycin Netilmicin[NUS] Tobramycin	Linezolid	Telithromycin
CNS *(continued)*																				
Seizures	R	0	0	+	0	R	R	0	0	R	R	+	***See footnote***[2]				+			
Special Senses																				
Ototoxicity	0	0	0	0	0	0	0	0	0	0	0	0			R		0	**3–14**[3]		
Vestibular	0	0	0	0	0	0	0	0	0	0	0	0			0		0	**4–6**[3]		
Cardiac																				
Dysrhythmias	R	0		0	0	0	0	0	0	0	0	0			0		+			
Miscellaneous, Unique *(Table 10C)*	+	+	+	+	+	+	+	+		+				+	+		+		+	++
Drug/drug interactions, common *(Table 22)*	0	0	0	0	0	0	0	0	0	0	0	0	+		0		0	+	+	+

ADVERSE REACTIONS	CEPHALOSPORINS/CEPHAMYCINS																			
	Cefazolin	Cefotetan	Cefoxitin	Cefuroxime	Cefotaxime	Ceftazidime	Ceftizoxime	Ceftriaxone	Cefepime	Ceftaroline	Ceftobiprole	Cefaclor/Cef.ER[4] /Loracarb	Cefadroxil	Cefdinir	Cefixime	Cefpodoxime	Cefprozil	Ceftibuten	Cefditoren pivoxil	Cefuroxime axetil	Cephalexin
Rx stopped due to AE									1.5	2.7	4			3		2.7	2	2	2	2.2	
Local, phlebitis	+	R	R	2	5	1	4	2	1	2	1.9										
Hypersensitivity	5	1				2			+		R	2									
Fever	+	+	+			R	+	R			1.3	+				R	+		R	R	
Rash	+		2	R	2	2	2	2	2	3	2.7	1	+	R	1	1	1	R	R	R	1
Photosensitivity	0	0	0	0	0	R	0	0													

[2] **All β-lactams in high concentration can cause seizures** *(JAC 45:5, 2000)*. In rabbit, IMP 10x more neurotoxic than benzylpenicillin *(JAC 22:687, 1988)*. In clinical trial of IMP for pediatric meningitis, trial stopped due to seizures in 7/25 IMP recipients; hard to interpret as purulent meningitis causes seizures *(PIDJ 10:122, 1991)*. Risk with IMP ↓ with careful attention to dosage *(Epilepsia 42:1590, 2001)*.
Postulated mechanism: Drug binding to $GABA_A$ receptor. IMP binds with greater affinity than MER.
Package insert, percent seizures: ERTA 0.5, IMP 0.4, MER 0.7. However, in 3 clinical trials of MER for bacterial meningitis, no drug-related seizures *(Scand J Inf Dis 31:3, 1999; Drug Safety 22:191, 2000)*. In febrile neutropenic cancer pts, IMP-related seizures reported at 2% *(CID 32:381, 2001; Peds Hem Onc 17:585, 2000)*. Also reported for DORI.

[3] Varies with criteria used.

[4] Cefaclor extended release tablets.

TABLE 10A (3)

ADVERSE REACTIONS	CEPHALOSPORINS/CEPHAMYCINS																				
	Cefazolin	Cefotetan	Cefoxitin	Cefuroxime	Cefotaxime	Ceftazidime	Ceftizoxime	Ceftriaxone	Cefepime	Ceftaroline	Ceftobiprole	Cefaclor/Cef.ER[4] /Loracarb	Cefadroxil	Cefdinir	Cefixime	Cefpodoxime	Cefprozil	Ceftibuten	Cefditoren pivoxil	Cefuroxime axetil	Cephalexin
Hypersensitivity *(continued)*																					
Anaphylaxis	R	+				R					R	R				R				R	
Serum sickness												≤0.5[5]	+								+
Hematologic																					
+ Coombs	3	+	2	R	6	4			14	9.8		R							R	R	+
Neutropenia	+		2	R	+	1	+	2	1		+	+	+	R	R	R	R		R		3
Eosinophilia		+	3	7	1	8	4	6	1		+			R	R	3	2	5	R	1	9
Thrombocytopenia	+					+	+		+		+	2			R	R	+	R			
↑ PT/PTT		++	+		+	+	+	+	+												
GI			2									3		3	13			6			2
Nausea/vomiting		1		R	R	R		R	1	4/2	+	2			7	4	4	2	6/1	3	
Diarrhea		4		R	1	1		3	1	5	9.1/4.8	–4		15	16	7	3	3	1.4	4	
C. difficile colitis	+	+	+	+	+	+	+	–	+	+	<1	+	+	+	+	+	+	+	+	+	+
Hepatic, ↑ LFTs	+	1	3	4	1	6	4	3	+	2	<2	3	+	1	R	4	2	R	R	2	+
Hepatic failure	0	0	0	0	0	0	0	0	0												
Renal: ↑ BUN, Cr	+		3			R		1	–		R	+		R	+	4	R	R	R		+
CNS																					
Headache	0					1		R	2		4.5	3		2		1	R	R	2	R	+
Confusion	0											+					R				+
Seizures	0										R										
Special Senses																					
Ototoxicity	0	0	0		0	0	0	0				0	0	0	0	0	0	0		0	0
Vestibular	0	0	0		0	0	0	0				0	0	0	0	0	0	0		0	0
Cardiac																					
Dysrhythmias	0	0	0		0	0	0	0				0	0	0	0	0	0	0		0	0
Miscellaneous, Unique *(Table 10C)*								+			+	+							+		
Drug/drug interactions, common *(Table 22)*	0	0	0	0	0	0	0	0				0	0		0	0	0	0		0	0

[5] Serum sickness requires biotransformation of parent drug plus inherited defect in metabolism of reactive intermediates (*Ped Pharm & Therap 125:805, 1994*).

TABLE 10A (4)

ADVERSE REACTIONS	MACROLIDES			QUINOLONES						OTHER AGENTS													
	Azithromycin, Reg. & ER[6]	Clarithromycin, Reg. & ER[6]	Erythromycin	Ciprofloxacin/Cipro XR	Gatifloxacin[NUS]	Gemifloxacin	Levofloxacin	Moxifloxacin	Ofloxacin	Chloramphenicol	Clindamycin	Colistimethate (Colistin)	Daptomycin	Metronidazole	Quinupristin-dalfopristin	Rifampin	Telavancin	Tetracycline/Doxy/Mino	Tigecycline	TMP-SMX	Vancomycin
Rx stopped due to AE	1	3		3.5	2.9	2.2	4.3	3.8	4				2.8						5		
Local, phlebitis					5		0.1–1				+		6		++			+	2		13
Hypersensitivity																1		R		++	**8**
Fever				R	R		R			+	+	+	2			+		+	7	+	1
Rash	R		+	3	R	1–22[7]	2	R	2	+	+	+	4	+	R		4	+	2.4	+	3
Photosensitivity	R			R	R	R	+	R	R		4							+	+	+	0
Anaphylaxis			+	R		R	+		R												R
Serum sickness							+				+										
Hematologic				R														R			
Neutropenia	R	1		R	R				1	+	+			+				+		+	2
Eosinophilia				R			+		1		+							+		+	+
Thrombocytopenia	R	R		R			0.1–1			+	+			R				+		+	+
↑ PT/PTT		1																	4		0
GI			++																	3	
Nausea/vomiting	3	3[8]	**25**	**5**	**8/<3**	**2.7**	**7/2**	**7/2**	**7**		+	+	6.3	**12**		+	27/14		30/20	+	+
Diarrhea	5	3–6	**8**	2	4	3.6	5	5	4	+	**7**		5	+		+	7		13	3	
C. difficile colitis		+	+	**R**	**R**	**R**	**R**	**R**	**R**		++		+			R		+			+
Hepatic, ↑ LFTs	R	R	+	2	R	1.5	0.1–1		2		+				2	+		+	4		0
Hepatic failure	0	0					+									+		+			0
Renal																					
↑ BUN, Cr	+	4		1					R		0		R			+		+	2	+	5
CNS														++							
Dizziness, light headedness				R	3	0.8	**3**	**2**	**3**								3.1		3.5		
Headache	R	2		1	4	1.2	6	2		+	+		5	+				+		+	
Confusion			+	+			0.1–1	R	2	+				+		+				+	
Seizures			+	+			0.1–1		R					+							

[6] Regular and extended-release formulations.
[7] **Highest frequency:** females <40 years of age after 14 days of rx; with 5 days or less of Gemi, incidence of rash <1.5%.
[8] Less GI upset/abnormal taste with ER formulation.

TABLE 10A (5)

ADVERSE REACTIONS	MACROLIDES			QUINOLONES						OTHER AGENTS											
	Azithromycin, Reg. & ER[6]	Clarithromycin, Reg. & ER[6]	Erythromycin	Ciprofloxacin/Cipro XR	Gatifloxacin[NUS]	Gemifloxacin	Levofloxacin	Moxifloxacin	Ofloxacin	Chloramphenicol	Clindamycin	Colistimethate (Colistin)	Daptomycin	Metronidazole	Quinupristin-dalfopristin	Rifampin	Telavancin	Tetracycline/Doxy/Mino	Tigecycline	TMP-SMX	Vancomycin
Special senses																					
Ototoxicity	+		+	0					0												R
Vestibular																		21[9]			
Cardiac																					
Dysrhythmias			+	F	+[10]	+[10]	R	+[10]	+[10]		R										0
Miscellaneous, Unique *(Table 10C)*	+		+	+	+	+	–	+	+	+	+	+	+	+	+	+	+	+	+	+	+
Drug/drug interactions, common *(Table 22)*	+	+	+	+	+	+	–	+	+						++			+	+	+	

TABLE 10B – ANTIMICROBIAL AGENTS ASSOCIATED WITH PHOTOSENSITIVITY

The following drugs are known to cause photosensitivity in some individuals. There is no intent to indicate relative frequency or severity of reactions.
Source: 2007 Red Book, Thomson Healthcare, Inc. Listed in alphabetical order:

Azithromycin, benznidazole, ciprofloxacin, dapsone, doxycycline, erythromycin ethylsuccinate, flucytosine, ganciclovir, gatifloxacin, gemifloxacin, griseofulvin, interferons, lomefloxacin, ofloxacin, pyrazinamide, saquinavir, sulfonamides, tetracyclines, tigecycline, tretinoins, voriconazole

[9] Minocycline has 21% vestibular toxicity.

[10] Fluoroquinolones as class are associated **with QT_c prolongation**. Ref.: *CID 34:861, 2002*.

TABLE 10C –ANTIBIOTIC DOSAGE* AND SIDE-EFFECTS

CLASS, AGENT, GENERIC NAME (TRADE NAME)	USUAL ADULT DOSAGE*	ADVERSE REACTIONS, COMMENTS (*See Table 10A for Summary*)
NATURAL PENICILLINS		**Allergic reactions a major issue.** 10% of all hospital admissions give history of pen allergy; but only 10% have allergic reaction if given penicillin. Why? Possible reasons: inaccurate history, waning immunity with age, aberrant response during viral illness, if given Bicillin C-R IM (procaine Pen + benzathine Pen) could be reaction to procaine. **Most serious reaction is immediate IgE-mediated anaphylaxis;** incidence only 0.05% but 5-10% fatal. Other IgE-mediated reactions: urticaria, angioedema, laryngeal edema, bronchospasm. Morbilliform rash after 72 hrs is not IgE-mediated and not serious. **Serious late allergic reactions:** Coombs-positive hemolytic anemia, neutropenia, thrombocytopenia, serum sickness, interstitial nephritis, hepatitis, eosinophilia, drug fever. **Cross-allergy to cephalosporins and carbapenems** roughly 10%. **For pen desensitization, see *Table 7*.** For skin testing, suggest referral to allergist. High **CSF** concentrations cause seizures. Reduce dosage with renal impairment, *see Table 17*. Allergy refs: *AJM 121:572, 2008; NEJM 354:601, 2006.*
Benzathine penicillin G (Bicillin L-A)	**600,000–1.2 million units IM q2–4 wks**	
Penicillin G	**Low: 600,000–1.2 million units IM per day High: ≥20 million units IV q24h(=12 gm) div q4h**	
Penicillin V (250 & 500 mg caps)	**0.25–0.5 gm po bid, tid, qid before meals & at bedtime**	
PENICILLINASE-RESISTANT PENICILLINS		
Dicloxacillin (Dynapen) (250 & 500 mg caps)	**0.125–0.5 gm po q6h before meals**	Blood levels ~2 times greater than cloxacillin. Acute hemorrhagic cystitis reported. Acute abdominal pain with GI bleeding without antibiotic-associated colitis also reported.
Flucloxacillin[NUS] (Floxapen, Lutropin, Staphcil)	**0.25–0.5 gm po q6h 1–2 gm IV q4h**	Cholestatic hepatitis [women predominate, age >65, rx mean 2 weeks, onset 3 weeks from starting rx (*Ln 339:679, 1992*)]. 16 deaths since 1980; **recommendation: use only in severe infection** (*Ln 344:676, 1994*).
Nafcillin (Unipen, Nafcil)	**1–2 gm IV/IM q4h.**	Extravasation can result in tissue necrosis. With dosages of 200–300 mg per kg per day hypokalemia may occur. **Reversible neutropenia (over 10% with ≥21-day rx, occasionally WBC <1000 per mm³).**
Oxacillin (Prostaphlin)	**1–2 gm IV/IM q4h.**	**Hepatic dysfunction with ≥12 gm per day**. LFTs usually ↑ 2–24 days after start of rx, reversible. In children, more rash and liver toxicity with oxacillin as compared to nafcillin (*CID 34:50, 2002*).
AMINOPENICILLINS		
Amoxicillin (Amoxil, Polymox)	**250 mg–1 gm po tid**	IV available in UK & Europe. IV amoxicillin rapidly converted to ampicillin. Rash with infectious mono– *see Ampicillin*.
Amoxicillin extended release (Moxatag)	**One 775 mg tab po once daily**	Allergic reactions, C. difficile associated diarrhea, false positive test for urine glucose with clinitest.
Amoxicillin-clavulanate (Augmentin) **AM-CL extra-strength peds suspension (ES-600)** **AM-CL-ER—extended release adult tabs**	*See Comment for adult products* **Peds Extra-Strength susp.: 600/42.9 per 5 mL. Dose: 90/6.4 mg/kg div bid.** For adult formulations, *see Comments* IV amox-clav available in Europe	With bid regimen, less clavulanate & less diarrhea. Clavulanate assoc. with rare reversible cholestatic hepatitis. In pts with immediate allergic reaction to AM-CL, ⅓ due to Clav component (*J Allergy Clin Immunol 125:502, 2010*). Positive blood tests for 1,3-beta D-glucan with IV AM-CL (*NEJM 354:2834, 2006*). **Comparison adult Augmentin product dosage regimens:** Augmentin 500/125 1 tab po tid Augmentin 875/125 1 tab po bid Augmentin-XR 1000/62.5 2 tabs po bid
Ampicillin (Principen) (250 & 500 mg caps)	**0.25–0.5 gm po q6h. 50–200 mg/kg IV/day.**	A maculopapular rash occurs (not urticarial), **not true penicillin allergy**, in 65–100% pts with infectious mono, 90% with chronic lymphocytic leukemia, and 15–20% in pts taking allopurinol.
Ampicillin-sulbactam (Unasyn)	**1.5–3 gm IV q6h.**	Supplied in vials: ampicillin 1 gm, sulbactam 0.5 gm or amp 2 gm, sulbactam 1 gm. AM-SB is not active vs pseudomonas. Total daily dose sulbactam ≤4 gm. Frequent resistance of Enterobacteriaceae.
EXTENDED SPECTRUM PENICILLINS. NOTE: Platelet dysfunction may occur with any of the antipseudomonal penicillins, esp. in renal failure patients.		
Piperacillin (Pipracil) (Hard to find PIP alone; usually PIP-TZ)	**3–4 gm IV q4–6h (max 24 gm/day). For urinary tract infection: 2 gm IV q6h. See *Comment***	1.85 mEq Na^+ per gm. *See PIP-TZ comment on extended infusion.* For P. aeruginosa infections: 3 gm IV q4h.

* NOTE: all dosage recommendations are for adults (unless otherwise indicated) & assume normal renal function.
(See page 2 for abbreviations)

TABLE 10C (2)

CLASS, AGENT, GENERIC NAME (TRADE NAME)	USUAL ADULT DOSAGE*	ADVERSE REACTIONS, COMMENTS *(See Table 10A for Summary)*
ANTIPSEUDOMONAL PENICILLINS		
Piperacillin-tazobactam (PIP-TZ) (Zosyn)	**Formulations:** PIP/TZ: **2/0.25 gm (2.25 gm)** PIP/TZ: **3/0.375 gm (3.375 gm)** PIP/TZ: **4/0.5 gm (4.5 gm)** Standard Dose (no P. aeruginosa): **3.375 gm IV q6h or 4.5 gm IV q8h** Standard Dose for P. aeruginosa: **3.375 gm IV q4h or 4.5 gm IV q6h** *See Comment for more doses.*	Continuous Infusion (CI) or Extended Infusion (EI) Regimens (based on PK/PD data, invitro, animal & clinical studies) • Critically Ill ICU pt: 4/0.5 gm loading dose, then 8/1 gm IV by CI (CrCl > 50 mL/min)*(Int J Antimicrob Agents 35:156, 2010)*. • Patient Not Critically Ill (dose based on CrCl level (mL/min)): CrCl > 40: 3.375 gm IV q8h (4 hr-EI) CrCl 20-40 3.375 gm q12h (EI) CrCl < 20: Dose unclear *(AAC 54:460, 2010)*. • Cystic fibrosis + P. aeruginosa infection: 350-450 mg/kg/day div q4-6h • P. aeruginosa pneumonia: Combine PIP-TZ with CIP or Tobra. Misc: Assoc false-pos galactomannan test for aspergillus, thrombocytopenia *(Mayo CLin Proceed 74:290, 1999)*. 5 mg Na+/gm of PIP-TZ.
Temocillin[NUS]	**1-2 gm IV q12h.**	Semi-synthetic penicillin highly resistant to wide range of beta-lactamases; used to treat beta-lactamase producing aerobic gram-negative bacilli resistant to extended-spectrum cephalosporins. Contact: *eumedica.com*
Ticarcillin disodium (Ticar)	**3 gm IV q4–6h.**	Coagulation abnormalities common with large doses, interferes with platelet function, ↑ bleeding times; may be clinically significant in pts with renal failure. (4.5 mEq Na+ per gm)
Ticarcillin-clavulanate (Timentin)	**3.1 gm IV q4–6h.**	Supplied in vials: ticarcil in 3 gm, clavulanate 0.1 gm per vial. 4.5–5 mEq Na+ per gm. Diarrhea due to clavulanate. Rare reversible cholestatic hepatitis secondary to clavulanate *(ArIM 156:1327, 1996)*.
CARBAPENEMS. NOTE: In pts with pen allergy, 11% had allergic reaction after imipenem or meropenem *(CID 38:1102, 2004)*; 9% in a 2nd study *(JAC 54:1155, 2004)*; and 0% in 2 other studies *(NEJM 354:2835, 2006; AnIM 146:266, 2007)*.		
Doripenem (Doribax) Ref: *CID 49:291, 2009.*	Intra-abdominal & complicated UTI: **500 mg IV q8h (1-hr infusion)**. Hospital-acquired pneumonia[NAI]: **500 mg IV q8h (4-hr infusion)**	Most common adverse reactions (≥5%): Headache, nausea, diarrhea, rash & phlebitis. Seizure reported in post-marketing surveillance. Can lower serum valproic acid levels. Adjust dose if renal impairment. Somewhat more stable in solution than **IMP** or **MER** *(JAC 65:1023, 2010; CID 49:291, 2009)*.
Ertapenem (Invanz)	**1 gm IV/IM q24h.**	**Lidocaine** diluent for IM use; ask about lidocaine allergy. Standard dosage may be inadequate in obesity (BMI ≥40). Reports of DRESS (drug rash eosinophilia systemic symptoms) Syndrome. Visual hallucinations reported *(NZ Med J 122:76, 2009)*.
Imipenem + cilastatin (Primaxin) Ref: *JAC 58:916, 2006*	**0.5 gm IV q6h**; for P. aeruginosa: 1 gm q6–8h *(see Comment)*	For infection due to P. aeruginosa, increase dosage to 3 or 4 gm per day div. q8h or q6h. Continuous infusion of carbapenems may be more efficacious & safer *(AAC 49:1881, 2005)*. Seizure comment, *see footnote², Table 10A, page 88*. Cilastatin decreases risk of toxicity to proximal tubules of kidney.
Meropenem (Merrem)	**0.5–1 gm IV q8h. Up to 2 gm IV q8h for meningitis.**	For seizure incidence comment, *see Table 10A, page 88*. Comments: Does not require a dehydropeptidase inhibitor (cilastatin). Activity vs aerobic gm-neg. slightly ↑ over IMP, activity vs staph & strep slightly ↓; anaerobes: B. ovatus, B. distasonis more resistant to meropenem.
MONOBACTAMS		
Aztreonam (Azactam)	**1 gm q8h–2 gm IV q6h.**	Can be used in pts with allergy to penicillins/cephalosporins. Animal data and a letter raise concern about cross-reactivity with ceftazidime *(Rev Inf Dis 7:613, 1985)*; side-chains of aztreonam and ceftazidime are identical.
Aztreonam for Inhalation (Cayston)	**75 mg inhaled tid x 28 days.** Use bronchodilator before each inhalation.	Improves respiratory symptoms in CF pts colonized with P. aeruginosa. Alternative to inhaled Tobra. AEs: bronchospasm, cough, wheezing. So far, no emergence of other resistant pathogens. Ref: *Chest 135:1223, 2009.*
CEPHALOSPORINS (1st parenteral, then oral drugs). NOTE: Prospective data demonstrate correlation between use of cephalosporins (esp. 3rd generation) and ↑ risk of C. difficile toxin-induced diarrhea. May also ↑ risk of colonization with vancomycin-resistant enterococci. **For cross-allergenicity, see *Oral, on page 95*.**		
1st Generation, Parenteral		
Cefazolin (Ancef, Kefzol)	**1-1.5 gm IV/IM q8h (max. 12 gm/day)**	Do not give into lateral ventricles—seizures! No activity vs. community-associated MRSA.

(See page 2 for abbreviations)

* NOTE: all dosage recommendations are for adults (unless otherwise indicated) & assume normal renal function.

TABLE 10C (3)

CLASS, AGENT, GENERIC NAME (TRADE NAME)	USUAL ADULT DOSAGE*	ADVERSE REACTIONS, COMMENTS *(See Table 10A for Summary)*
CEPHALOSPORINS (1st parenteral, then oral drugs) *(continued)*		
2nd Generation, Parenteral		
Cefotetan (Cefotan)	**1–3 gm IV/IM q12h. (max. dose not >6 gm q24h).**	Increasing resistance of B. fragilis, Prevotella bivia, Prevotella disiens (most common in pelvic infections); do not use for intra-abdominal infections. Methylthiotetrazole (MTT) side chain can inhibit vitamin K activation. Avoid alcohol-disulfiram reaction.
Cefoxitin (Mefoxin)	**1 gm q8h–2 gm IV/IM q6-8h.**	Increasing resistance to B. fragilis.
Cefuroxime (Kefurox, Ceftin, Zinacef)	**0.75–1.5 gm IV/IM q8h.**	*See Cefuroxime axetil for oral preparation.*
3rd Generation, Parenteral—Use correlates with incidence of C. difficile toxin diarrhea; perhaps due to cephalosporin resistance of C. difficile *(CID 38:646, 2004)*.		
Cefoperazone-sulbactamNUS (Sulperazon)	**Usual dose (Cefperazone comp) 1–2 gm IV q12h;** if larger doses, do not exceed 4 gm/day of sulbactam.	Investigational in U.S. In SE Asia & elsewhere, used to treat intra-abdominal, biliary, & gyn. infections. Other uses due to broad spectrum of activity. Possible clotting problem due to side-chain.
Cefotaxime (Claforan)	**1 gm q8–12h to 2 gm IV q4h.**	Maximum daily dose: 12 gm; can give as 4 gm IV q8h.
Ceftazidime (Fortaz, Tazicef)	**1–2 gm IV/IM q8–12h.**	Excessive use may result in ↑ incidence of C. difficile-assoc. diarrhea and/or selection of vancomycin-resistant E. faecium. Ceftaz is susceptible to extended-spectrum cephalosporinases *(CID 27:76 & 81, 1998)*.
Ceftizoxime (Cefizox)	From **1-2 gm IV q8-12h** up to **2 gm IV q4h**.	Maximum daily dose: 12 gm; can give as 4 gm IV q8h.
Ceftriaxone (Rocephin)	Commonly used IV dosage in adults: **1-2 gm once daily** Purulent meningitis: **2 gm q12h.** Can give **IM** in 1% lidocaine.	**"Pseudocholelithiasis"** 2° to sludge in gallbladder by ultrasound (50%), symptomatic (9%) *(NEJM 322:1821, 1990)*. More likely with ≥2 gm per day with pt on total parenteral nutrition and not eating *(AnIM 115:712, 1991)*. Clinical significance still unclear but has led to cholecystectomy *(JID 17:356, 1995)* and gallstone pancreatitis *(Ln 17:662, 1998)*. In pilot study: 2 gm once daily by continuous infusion superior to 2 gm bolus once daily *(JAC 59:285, 2007)*. For Ceftriaxone Desensitization, *see Table 7, page 77*.
Other Generation, Parenteral		
Cefepime (Maxipime)	**1–2 gm IV q12h.**	Active vs P. aeruginosa and many strains of Enterobacter, serratia, C. freundii resistant to ceftazidime, cefotaxime, aztreonam *(LnID 7:338, 2007)*. More active vs MSSA than 3rd generation cephalosporins. Neutropenia after 14 days rx *(Scand J Infect Dis 42:156, 2010)*.
CefpiromeNUS (HR 810)	**1–2 gm IV q12h**	Similar to cefepime; ↑ activity vs enterobacteriaceae, P. aeruginosa, Gm + organisms. Anaerobes: less active than cefoxitin, more active than cefotax or ceftaz.
Ceftaroline fosamil (Teflaro)	**600 mg IV q12h (1-hr infusion)**	Avid binding to PBP 2a; active vs. MRSA. Inactivated by Amp C & ESBL enzymes.
Ceftobiprole	**0.5 gm IV q8h for mixed gm- neg & gm-pos infections. 0.5 gm IV q12h for gm-pos infections**	Infuse over 2 hrs for q8h dosing, over 1 hr for q12h dosing. Associated with caramel-like taste disturbance. Ref.: *Clin Microbiol Infections 13(Suppl 2):17 & 25, 2007*. Active vs. MRSA.

(See page 2 for abbreviations)

* NOTE: all dosage recommendations are for adults (unless otherwise indicated) & assume normal renal function.

TABLE 10C (4)

CLASS, AGENT, GENERIC NAME (TRADE NAME)	USUAL ADULT DOSAGE*	ADVERSE REACTIONS, COMMENTS (*See Table 10A for Summary*)
CEPHALOSPORINS (1st parenteral, then oral drugs) *(continued)*		
Oral Cephalosporins		
1st Generation, Oral		**Cross-Allergenicity: Patients with a history of IgE-mediated allergic reactions to a penicillin (e.g., anaphylaxis, angioneurotic edema, immediate urticaria) should not receive a cephalosporin.** If the history is a "measles-like" rash to a penicillin available data suggest a 5–10% risk of rash in such patients; there is no enhanced risk of anaphylaxis. Cephalosporin skin tests, if available, predictive of reaction *(AnIM 141:16, 2004; AJM 121:572, 2008)*. Even if Pen allergy skin test positive overall only 2% of pts given cephalosporin suffer allergic reaction. Watch for side chain cross-allergenicity; Amox has same side chain as Cefadroxil & Cefprozil; Amp has same side chain as Cefaclor, Cephalexin & Cephadrine. Any of the cephalosporins can result in **C. difficile toxin**-mediated diarrhea/enterocolitis. The reported frequency of nausea/vomiting and non-C. difficile toxin diarrhea is summarized in *Table 10A*. There are **few drug-specific adverse effects, e.g.:** **Cefaclor:** Serum sickness-like reaction 0.1–0.5%—arthralgia, rash, erythema multiforme but no adenopathy, proteinuria or demonstrable immune complexes. Appear due to mixture of drug biotransformation and genetic susceptibility *(Ped Pharm & Therap 125:805, 1994)*. **Cefdinir:** Drug-iron complex causes red stools in roughly 1% of pts **Cefditoren pivoxil:** Hydrolysis yields pivalate. Pivalate absorbed (70%) & becomes pivaloylcarnitine which is renally excreted; 39–63% ↓ **in serum carnitine concentrations**. Carnitine involved in fatty acid (FA) metabolism & FA transport into mitochondria. Effect transient & reversible. No clinical events documented to date *(Med Lett 44:5, 2002)*. Also contains caseinate (milk protein); **avoid if milk allergy** (not same as lactose intolerance). Need gastric acid for optimal absorption. **Cefpodoxime**: There are rare reports of acute liver injury, bloody diarrhea, pulmonary infiltrates with eosinophilia. **Cephalexin:** Can cause false-neg. urine dipstick test for leukocytes.
Cefadroxil (Duricef) (500 mg caps, 1 gm tabs)	**0.5–1 gm po q12h.**	
Cephalexin (Keflex) (250 & 500 mg tabs)	**0.25–1 gm po q6h (max 4 gm/day).**	
2nd Generation, Oral		
Cefaclor (Ceclor, Raniclor) (250 & 500 mg caps)	**0.25–0.5 gm po q8h.**	
Cefprozil (Cefzil) (250 & 500 mg tabs)	**0.25–0.5 gm po q12h.**	
Cefuroxime axetil po (Ceftin)	**0.125–0.5 gm po q12h.**	
3rd Generation, Oral		
Cefdinir (Omnicef) (300 mg cap)	**300 mg po q12h or 600 mg q24h.**	
Cefditoren pivoxil (Spectracef)	**400 mg po bid.**	
Cefixime (Suprax) (400 mg tab)	**0.4 gm po q12–24h.**	
Cefpodoxime proxetil (Vantin)	**0.1–0.2 gm po q12h.**	
Ceftibuten (Cedax) (400 mg tab)	**0.4 gm po q24h.**	
AMINOGLYCOSIDES AND RELATED ANTIBIOTICS—*See Table 10D, page 101, and Table 17A, page 189*		
GLYCOPEPTIDES, LIPOGLYCOPEPTIDES		
Teicoplanin[NUS] (Targocid)	**For septic arthritis—maintenance dose 12 mg/kg per day; S. aureus endocarditis—trough serum levels >20 mcg/mL required (12 mg/kg q12h times 3 loading dose, then 12 mg/kg q24h)**	Hypersensitivity: fever (at 3 mg/kg 2.2%, at 24 mg per kg 8.2%), skin reactions 2.4%. Marked ↓ platelets (high dose ≥15 mg per kg per day). Red neck syndrome less common than with vancomycin.
Telavancin (Vibativ) Lipoglycopeptide Ref: *CID 49:1908, 2009*	10 mg/kg IV q24h if CrCl >50 mL/min. Infuse each dose over 1 hr. No data on dosing for obese patient.	**Avoid during pregnancy: teratogenic in animals.** Adverse events in phase 3 trials vs. vanco: dysgeusia 33% vs. 7%; nausea 27% vs. 15%; vomiting 14% vs. 7%; headache 14% vs. 13%; ↑ creatinine (3.1% vs. 1.1%); foamy urine; flushing if infused rapidly. Potential nephrotoxicity and QTc interval prolongation.
Vancomycin (Vancocin) Guidelines Ref: *CID 49:325, 2009.* ***See Comments for po dose.***	**Initial doses based on actual wt, including for obese pts.** Subsequent doses adjusted based on measured trough serum levels. **For critically ill pts, give loading dose of 25-30 mg/kg IV then 15-20 mg/kg IV q8-12h.** Target trough level is 15-20 μg/mL. For individual doses over 1 gm, infuse over 1.5-2 hrs. **Dosing for morbid obesity (BMI ≥40 kg/m²):** If CrCl ≥50 mL/min & pt not critically ill: 30 mg/kg/day divided q8-12h—no dose over 2 gm. Infuse doses of 1 gm or more over 1.5-2 hrs. Check trough levels.	If MIC of vancomycin vs. S. aureus is ≥2 μg/mL, not possible achieve desired AUC/MIC of >400; consider alternative rx with **daptomycin or linezolid.** **PO vanco for C. difficile colitis: 125 mg po q6h.** Commercial po formulation very expensive (generic soon). Can compound po vanco from IV formulation: 5 g, IV vanco powder + 47.5 mL sterile H_2O, 0.2 gm saccharin, 0.05 gm stevia powder, 40 mL glycerin and then enough cherry syrup to yield 100 mL = 50 mg vanco/mL. Oral dose = 2.5 mL q6h po. **Intrathecal dose:** 5-10 mg/day (infants); 10-20 mg/day (children & adults) to target CSF concentration of 10-20 μg/mL. Higher doses of vanco ↑ risk of **nephrotoxicity** *(AAC 52:1330, 2008; see also CID 49:507, 2009)*. Concomitant hypertension or administration of aminoglycoside or loop diuretic are risk factors with continuous infusion *(JAC 62:168, 2008)*. **Red Neck Syndrome:** consequence of rapid infusion with non-specific histamine release. **Other adverse effects:** rash, immune thrombocytopenia *(NEJM 356:904, 2007)*, fever, neutropenia, **IgA bullous dermatitis** *(CID 38:442, 2004)*. **Obesity dosing:** Frequent underdosing *(AJM 121:515, 2008)*. For CrCl calculation for morbidly obese patient see *Table 10D or Am J Health Sys Pharm 66:642, 2009.*

(See page 2 for abbreviations)

* NOTE: all dosage recommendations are for adults (unless otherwise indicated) & assume normal renal function.

TABLE 10C (5)

CLASS, AGENT, GENERIC NAME (TRADE NAME)	USUAL ADULT DOSAGE*	ADVERSE REACTIONS, COMMENTS *(See Table 10A for Summary)*
CHLORAMPHENICOL, CLINDAMYCIN(S), ERYTHROMYCIN GROUP, KETOLIDES, OXAZOLIDINONES, QUINUPRISTIN-DALFOPRISTIN		
Chloramphenicol (Chloromycetin)	**50-100 mg/kg/day po/IV div q6h (max 4 gm/day)**	No oral drug distrib in U.S. Hematologic (↓ RBC ~1/3 pts, aplastic anemia 1:21,600 courses). Gray baby syndrome in premature infants, anaphylactoid reactions, optic atrophy or neuropathy (very rare), digital paresthesias, minor disulfiram-like reactions.
Clindamycin (Cleocin)	**0.15–0.45 gm po q6h. 600–900 mg IV/IM q8h**.	Based on number of exposed pts, these drugs are the most frequent cause of **C. difficile toxin-mediated diarrhea**. In most severe form can cause pseudomembranous colitis/toxic megacolon. Available as caps, IV sol'n, topical (for acne) & intravaginal suppositories & cream.
Lincomycin (Lincocin)	**0.6 gm IV/IM q8h.**	Risk of C. difficile colitis. Rarely used.
Erythromycin Group (Review drug interactions before use)		
Azithromycin (Zithromax) **Azithromycin ER** (ZMax)	**po preps:** Tabs 250 & 600 mg. Peds suspension: 100 & 200 mg per 5 mL. Adult ER suspension: 2 gm. Dose varies with indication, *see Table 1A*, Acute otitis media *(page 10)*, acute exac. chronic bronchitis *(page 34)*, Comm.-acq. pneumonia *(pages 36–37)*, & sinusitis *(page 47)*. **IV:** 0.5 gm per day.	**Motilin:** activates duodenal/jejunal receptors to initiate peristalsis. Erythro (E) and E esters activate motilin receptors and cause uncoordinated peristalsis with resultant anorexia, nausea or vomiting. Less binding and GI distress with azithromycin/clarithromycin. No peristalsis benefit *(JAC 59:347, 2007)*. Systemic erythro in 1st 2 wks of life associated with **infantile hypertrophic pyloric stenosis** *(J Ped 139:380, 2001)*. **Frequent drug-drug interactions:** *see Table 22, page 200*. Major concern is prolonged QT_c interval on EKG. **Prolonged QTc:** Mutations in 6 genes (LQT 1–3) produce abnormal cardiac K^+/Na^+ channels. Variable penetrance: no symptoms, repeated syncope, to sudden death *(NEJM 358:169, 2008)*. **↑ risk if female & QTc >500 msec! Risk amplified by other drugs** [macrolides, antiarrhythmics, & drug-drug interactions ***(see FQs page 97 for list)***]. Can result in torsades de pointes (ventricular tachycardia) and/or cardiac arrest. Refs.: *CID 43:1603, 2006; www.qtdrugs.org & www.torsades.org*. Cholestatic hepatitis in approx. 1:1000 adults (not children) given E estolate. **Transient reversible tinnitus or deafness** with ≥4 gm per day of erythro IV in pts with renal or hepatic impairment. Reversible sensorineural hearing loss with Azithro *(J Otolaryngol 36:257, 2007)*. Dosages of oral erythro preparations expressed as base equivalents. With differences in absorption/biotransformation, variable amounts of erythro esters required to achieve same free erythro serum level, e.g., 400 mg Erythro ethyl succinate = 250 mg Erythro base. **Azithromycin** reported to exacerbate symptoms of myasthenia gravis.
Erythromycin Base and esters (Erythrocin) IV name: E. lactobionate	**0.25 gm q6h–0.5 gm po/IV q6h: 15–20 mg/kg up to 4 gm q24h. Infuse over 30+ min.**	
Clarithromycin (Biaxin) or clarithro extended release (Biaxin XL)	**0.5 gm po q12h.** **Extended release: Two 0.5 gm tabs po per day.**	
Ketolide **Telithromycin** (Ketek) *(Med Lett 46:66, 2004; Drug Safety 31:561, 2008)*	**Two 400 mg tabs po q24h.** 300 mg tabs available.	Drug warnings: acute liver failure & serious liver injury post treatment. *(AnIM 144:415, 447, 2006)*. **Uncommon: blurred vision** 2° slow accommodation; may cause exacerbation of **myasthenia gravis (Black Box Warning)**. Potential QT_c prolongation. Several **drug-drug interactions** *(Table 22, pages 200–201) (NEJM 355:2260, 2006)*.
Linezolid (Zyvox) (600 mg tab)	**PO or IV dose: 600 mg q12h.** Available as 600 mg tabs, oral suspension (100 mg per 5 mL), & IV solution.	**Reversible myelosuppression:** thrombocytopenia, anemia, & neutropenia reported. Most often after >2 wks of therapy. Incidence of thrombocytopenia after 2 wks of rx: 7/20 osteomyelitic pts; 5/7 pts treated with vanco & then linezolid. Refs.: *CID 37:1609, 2003 & 38:1058 & 1065, 2004*. 6-fold increased risk in pts with ESRD *(CID 42:66, 2006)*. **Lactic acidosis; peripheral neuropathy, optic neuropathy:** After 4 or more wks of therapy. Data consistent with time and dose-dependent inhibition of intramitochondrial protein synthesis *(CID 42:1111,2006; AAC 50:2042, 2006; Pharmacotherapy 27:771, 2007)*. **Inhibitor of monoamine oxidase;** risk of severe hypertension if taken with foods rich in tyramine. Avoid concomitant pseudoephedrine, phenylpropanolamine, and caution with SSRIs[1]. **Serotonin syndrome** (fever, agitation, mental status changes, tremors). Risk with concomitant SSRIs: *(CID 42:1578 and 43:180, 2006)*. Other adverse effects: black hairy tongue and acute interstitial nephritis *(IDCP 17:61, 2009)*. **Resistance:** Mutational resistance rare. Outbreaks of Linezolid resistant S. epidermidis and MRSA due to mobil gene that methylates ribosomal target of Linezolid *(CID 50:821, 2010)*.
Quinupristin + dalfopristin (Synercid) *(CID 36:473, 2003)*	**7.5 mg per kg IV q8h via central line**	Venous irritation (5%); none with central venous line. Asymptomatic ↑ in unconjugated bilirubin. **Arthralgia** 2%–50% *(CID 36:476, 2003)*. **Drug-drug interactions:** Cyclosporine, nifedipine, midazolam, many more—*see Table 22*.

[1] **SSRI** = selective serotonin reuptake inhibitors, e.g., fluoxetine (Prozac).

(See page 2 for abbreviations) * NOTE: all dosage recommendations are for adults (unless otherwise indicated) & assume normal renal function.

TABLE 10C (6)

CLASS, AGENT, GENERIC NAME (TRADE NAME)	USUAL ADULT DOSAGE*	ADVERSE REACTIONS, COMMENTS (*See Table 10A for Summary*)
TETRACYCLINES (*Mayo Clin Proc 74:727, 1999*)		
Doxycycline (Vibramycin, Doryx, Monodox, Adoxa, Periostat) (20, 50, 75, 100 mg tab)	**0.1 gm po/IV q12h**	Similar to other tetracyclines. ↑ nausea on empty stomach. Erosive esophagitis, esp. if taken at bedtime; **take with lots of water.** Phototoxicity & photo-onycholysis occur but less than with tetracycline. Deposition in teeth less. Can be used in patients with renal failure. *Comments:* Effective in treatment and prophylaxis for malaria, leptospirosis, typhus fevers.
Minocycline (Minocin, Dynacin) (50, 75, 100 mg cap; 45, 90, 135 mg ext rel tab)	**200 mg po loading dose, then 100 mg po q12h** IV minocycline no longer available.	**Vestibular symptoms** (30–90% in some groups, none in others): vertigo 33%, ataxia 43%, nausea 50%, vomiting 3%, women more frequently than men. Hypersensitivity pneumonitis, reversible, ~34 cases reported (*BMJ 310:1520, 1995*). Can increase **pigmentation** of the skin with long-term use. *Comments:* More effective than other tetracyclines vs staph and in prophylaxis of meningococcal disease. P. acnes: many resistant to other tetracyclines, not to mino. Induced autoimmunity reported in children treated for acne (*J Ped 153:314, 2008*). Active vs Nocardia asteroides, Mycobacterium marinum.
Tetracycline, Oxytetracycline (Sumycin)(250, 500 mg cap) (*CID 36:462, 2003*)	**0.25–0.5 gm po q6h, 0.5–1 gm IV q12h**	GI (oxy 19%, tetra 4), anaphylactoid reaction (rare), deposition in teeth, negative N balance, hepatotoxicity, enamel agenesis, pseudotumor cerebri/encephalopathy. Outdated drug: Fanconi syndrome. *See drug-drug interactions, Table 22.* **Contraindicated in pregnancy, hepatotoxicity in mother, transplacental to fetus.** *Comments:* IV dosage over 2.0 gm per day may be associated with fatal hepatotoxicity. False-neg. urine dipstick for leukocytes.
Tigecycline (Tygacil)	**100 mg IV initially, then 50 mg IV q12h with po food, if possible to decrease risk of nausea.** **If severe liver dis. (Child Pugh C):** 100 mg IV initially, then 25 mg IV q12h	Derivative of tetracycline. High incidence of nausea (25%) & vomiting (20%) but only 1% of pts discontinued therapy due to an adverse event. Details on AEs in *JAC 62 (Suppl 1): i17, 2008.* Pregnancy Category D. Do not use in children under age 18. Like other tetracyclines, may cause photosensitivity, pseudotumor cerebri, pancreatitis, a catabolic state (elevated BUN) and maybe hyperpigmentation (*CID 45:136, 2007*). **Tetracycline, minocycline & tigecycline** associated with acute pancreatitis (*Int J Antimicrob Agents, 34:486, 2009*). Dear Doctor Letter (4/27/09): lower cure rate and higher mortality in pts with VAP treated with tigecycline.
FLUOROQUINOLONES (FQs): All can cause false-positive urine drug screen for opiates (*Pharmacother 26:435, 2006*). Toxicity review: *Drugs Aging 27:193, 2010.*		
Ciprofloxacin (Cipro) and **Ciprofloxacin-extended release** (Cipro XR, Proquin XR) (100, 250, 500, 750 mg tab; 500 mg ext rel tab)	Usual Parenteral Dose: **400 mg IV q12h** For P. aeruginosa: **400 mg IV q8h** Uncomplicated Urethritis/cystitis (Oral) Dose: **250 mg po bid or CIP XR 500 mg po once daily** Other Indications (Oral): **500-750 mg po bid**	FQs are a common precipitant of C. difficile toxin-mediated diarrhea. **Children:** No FQ approved for use under age 16 based on joint cartilage injury in immature animals. Articular SEs in children est. at 2–3% (*LnID 3:537, 2003*). The exception is anthrax. Pathogenesis believed to involve FQ chelation of Mg++ damaging chondrocyte interactions (*AAC 51:1022, 2007; Int J Antimicrob Agents 33:194, 2009*). **CNS toxicity:** Poorly understood. Varies from mild (lightheadedness) to moderate (confusion) to severe (seizures). May be aggravated by NSAIDs. **Gemi skin rash:** Macular rash after 8–10 days of rx. Incidence of rash with ≤5 days of therapy only 1.5%. Frequency highest females, < age 40, treated 14 days (22.6%). In men, < age 40, treated 14 days, frequency 7.7%. Mechanism unclear. Indication to DC therapy. **Hypoglycemia/hyperglycemia:** Due to documented hypo and hyperglycemic reactions (*NEJM 354:1352, 2006; CID 49:402, 2009*, US distribution of Gati in US ceased in 6/2006. Gati ophthalmic solution remains available. **Opiate screen false-positives:** FQs can cause false-positive urine assay for opiates (*JAMA 286:3115, 2001; AnPharmacotherapy 38:1525, 2004*). **Photosensitivity:** *See Table 10B, page 91* **QT_c (corrected QT) interval prolongation:** ↑ QT_c (>500 msec or >60 msec from baseline) is considered possible with any FQ. ↑ QT_c can lead to torsades de pointes and ventricular fibrillation. Risk low with current marketed drugs. Risk ↑ in women, ↓ K^+, ↓ mg^{++}, bradycardia. (Refs.: *CID 43:1603, 2006*). Major problem is ↑ risk with concomitant drugs.
Gatifloxacin (Tequin)[NUS] *See comments*	**200–400 mg IV/po q24h.** (*See comment*) Ophthalmic solution (Zymar)	
Gemifloxacin (Factive) (320 mg tab)	**320 mg po q24h.**	

(See page 2 for abbreviations)

* NOTE: all dosage recommendations are for adults (unless otherwise indicated) & assume normal renal function.

TABLE 10C (7)

CLASS, AGENT, GENERIC NAME (TRADE NAME)	USUAL ADULT DOSAGE*	ADVERSE REACTIONS, COMMENTS *(See Table 10A for Summary)*
FLUOROQUINOLONES (FQs) *(continued)*		
Levofloxacin (Levaquin) (250, 500, 750 mg tab)	**250–750 mg po/IV q24h**.	**Avoid concomitant drugs with potential to prolong QTc:** **Antiarrhythmics:** Amiodarone, Disopyramide, Dofetilide, Flecainide, Ibutilide, Procainamide, Quinidine, quinine, Sotalol **Anti-Infectives:** Azoles (not posa), Clarithro/erythro, FQs (not CIP), Halofantrine, NNRTIs, Protease Inhibitors, Pentamidine, Telavancin, Telithromycin **Anti-Hypertensives:** Bepridil, Isradipine, Nicardipine, Moexipril **CNS Drugs:** Fluoxetine, Haloperidol, Phenothiazines, Pimozide, Quetiapine, Risperidone, Sertraline, Tricyclics, Venlafaxine, Ziprasidone **Misc:** Dolasetron, Droperidol, Fosphenytoin, Indapamide, Methadone, Naratriptan, Salmeterol, Sumatriptan, Tamoxifen, Tizanidine **Updates online: www.qtdrugs.org; www.torsades.org**
Moxifloxacin (Avelox)	400 mg po/IV q24h Ophthalmic solution (Vigamox)	**Tendinopathy:** Over age 60, approx. 2–6% of all Achilles tendon ruptures attributable to use of FQ *(ArIM 163:1801, 2003)*. ↑ risk with concomitant steroid, renal disease or post transplant (heart, lung, kidney) *(CID 36:1404, 2003)*. Overall incidence is low *(Eur J Clin Pharm 63:499, 2007)*. **Ca++, Mg++ chelation:** Dairy products ↓ area under curve of CIP by 1/3 after po dose; no effect on moxi *(Clin Pharm Ther 50:498, 1991; Clin Pharmacokinet 40 (Suppl1) 33:2001)*. **Allergic Reactions:** Rare (1:50,000). IgE-mediated: urticaria, anaphylaxis. May be more common with Moxi. 3 pts with Moxi immediate reactions tolerated CIP *(Am Pharmacother 44:740, 2010)*.
Ofloxacin (Floxin)	200–400 mg po bid. Ophthalmic solution (Ocuflox)	
POLYMYXINS		
Polymyxin B (Poly-Rx) 1 mg = 10,000 units	Standard Dose: 15,000–25,000 units/kg/day IV divided q12h **Intrathecal Rx of Meningitis:** 50,000 units/day into CSF daily x 3-4 days, then qod x 2 or more wks	**Adverse effects: Neurologic:** rare but serious is neuromuscular blockade; other, circumoral paresthesias, extremity numbness, blurred vision, drowsy, irritable, ataxia; **Renal:** reversible acute tubular necrosis.
Colistin (Polymyxin E) *(LnID 6:589, 2006; AAC 50:2274 & 4231, 2006)* In U.S., usual drug for IV use is a salt: **colistimethate sodium (Colymycin -M)**.	Dose in mg/kg of "base" using ideal body weight. IV Dose (except CF): **2.5 mg/kg/day IV in 2-4 div doses** Cystic fibrosis Dose: **3-8 mg/kg/day IV in 3 div doses**	**Intrathecal or Intraventricular Dose:** 10 mg/day x several wks; successful with daily dosing for 3-4 days, then qod dosing. **Cystic fibrosis inhalation Rx:** 50-75 mg in 3-4 mL saline via nebulizer 2-3 x/day **Nephrotoxicity:** Reversible tubular necrosis. After **CMS**, 45% pts had evidence of toxicity, most often mild & reversible *(CID 48:1724, 2009)*. **Neurotoxicity:** Frequent vertigo, facial paresthesia, abnormal vision, confusion, ataxia, rarely neuromuscular blockade → respiratory failure. In cystic fibrosis pts, 29% experienced paresthesia, ataxia or both. **Other:** Maybe hyperpigmentation *(CID 45:136, 2007)*. **Dosage:** PK study suggests need for loading dose & higher maintenance dose in critically ill patients *(AAC 53:3430, 2009)*.

(See page 2 for abbreviations)

* NOTE: all dosage recommendations are for adults (unless otherwise indicated) & assume normal renal function.

TABLE 10C (8)

CLASS, AGENT, GENERIC NAME (TRADE NAME)	USUAL ADULT DOSAGE*	ADVERSE REACTIONS, COMMENTS (*See Table 10A for Summary*)
MISCELLANEOUS AGENTS		
Daptomycin (Cubicin) (Ref on resistance: *CID 45:601, 2007; Review: CID 50:S10, 2010)*	**Skin/soft tissue: 4 mg per kg IV q24h** **Bacteremia/right-sided endocarditis: 6 mg per kg IV q24h** **Morbid obesity:** base dose on total body weight *(J Clin Pharm 45:48, 2005)*	**Potential muscle toxicity:** At 4 mg per kg per day., ↑ CPK in 2.8% dapto pts & 1.8% comparator-treated pts. Risk increases ↑ min conc ≥24.3 mg/L *(CID 50:1568, 2010)*. Suggest weekly CPK; DC dapto if CPK exceeds 10x normal level or ↑ symptoms of myopathy and CPK > 1,000. Manufacturer suggests stopping statins during dapto rx). Selected reagents (HemosIL Recombiplastin, Hemoliance Recombiplastin), can falsely prolong PT & INR *(Blood Coag & Fibrinolysis 19:32, 2008)*. **NOTE:** Dapto well-tolerated in healthy volunteers at doses up to 12 mg/kg q24h x 14d *(AAC 50:3245, 2006)* and in pts given mean dose of 8 mg/kg/day *(CID 49:177, 2009)*. *Resistance of S. aureus reported during dapto therapy, post-vanco therapy & de novo.* Eosinophilic pneumonia/chronic steroid-dep pneumonia reported *(CID 50:737, 2010)*.
Fosfomycin (Monurol) (3 gm packet)	**3 gm with water po times 1 dose.**	Diarrhea in 9% compared to 6% of pts given nitrofurantoin and 2.3% given TMP-SMX. Available outside U.S., IV & PO, for treatment of multi-drug resistant bacteria *(CID 46:1069, 2008)*. For MDR-GNB: 6-12 gm/day IV divided q6-8h.
Fusidic acid[NUS] (Fucidin)	**500 mg po/IV tid (Denmark & Canada)**	Jaundice (17% with IV use; 6% with po) *(CID 42:394, 2006)*.
Methenamine hippurate (Hiprex, Urex)	**1 gm po q6h bid**	Nausea and vomiting, skin rash or dysuria. Overall ~3%. Methenamine requires (pH ≤5) urine to liberate formaldehyde. Useful in suppressive therapy after infecting organisms cleared; do not use for pyelonephritis. *Comment:* Do not force fluids; may dilute formaldehyde. Of no value in pts with chronic Foley. If urine pH >5.0, co-administer ascorbic acid (1–2 gm q4h) to acidify the urine; cranberry juice (1200–4000 mL per day) has been used, results ±.
Methenamine mandelate (Mandelamine)	**1 gm po qid**	
Metronidazole (Flagyl) (250, 375, 500 mg tab/cap) Ref.: *Activity vs. B. fragilis* Still drug of choice *(CID 50 (Suppl 1):S16, 2010)*.	Anaerobic infections: **usually IV, 7.5 mg per kg (~500 mg) q6h (not to exceed 4 gm q24h)**. With long T½, **can use IV at 15 mg per kg q12h.** If life-threatening, use loading dose of **IV 15 mg per kg. Oral dose: 500 mg qid; extended release tabs** available 750 mg	Common AEs: nausea (12%), metallic taste, "furry" tongue. Avoid alcohol during 48 hrs after last dose to avoid disulfiram reaction (N/V, flushing, tachycardia, dyspnea). Neurologic AEs with high dose/long Rx: peripheral, autonomic and optic neuropathy *(J Child Neurol 21:429, 2006)*. Aseptic meningitis, encephalopathy, seizures & reversible cerebellar lesion reported *(NEJM 346:68, 2002)*. Also: topical & vaginal gels. Can use IV sol'n as enema for *C. diff colitis*
Nitazoxanide	***See Table 13B, page 141***	
Nitrofurantoin macrocrystals (Macrobid, Macrodantin, Furadantin) (25, 50, 100 mg caps)	Active UTI: **Furadantin/Macrodantin 50-100 mg po qid x 7 days OR Macrobid 100 mg po bid x 7 days** Dose for long-term UTI suppression: **50–100 mg at bedtime**	Absorption ↑ with meals. Increased activity in acid urine, much reduced at pH 8 or over. Not effective in endstage renal disease. Nausea and vomiting, peripheral neuropathy, pancreatitis. **Pulmonary reactions** (with chronic rx): acute ARDS type, **chronic desquamative interstitial pneumonia with fibrosis**. Intrahepatic cholestasis & **hepatitis** similar to chronic active hepatitis. Hemolytic anemia in G6PD deficiency. Drug rash, eosinophilia, systemic symptoms (DRESS) hypersensitivity syndrome reported *(Neth J Med 67:147, 2009)*. **Contraindicated in renal failure**. Should not be used in infants <1 month of age. Birth defects: increased risk reported *(Arch Ped Adolesc Med 163:978, 2009)*.
Rifampin (Rimactane, Rifadin) (150, 300 mg cap)	**300 mg po bid or 600 mg po once daily**	Causes orange-brown discoloration of sweat, urine, tears, contact lens. Many important drug-drug interactions, see *Table 22*. Immune complex flu-like syndrome: fever, headache, myalgias, arthralgia--especially with intermittent rx. Thrombocytopenia, vasculitis reported *(C Ann Pharmacother 42: 727, 2008)*. Can cause interstitial nephritis.
Rifaximin (Xifaxan) (200, 500 mg tab)	Diarrhea: **200 mg tab po tid** times 3 days. Hepatic encephalopathy: **550 mg tab bid**.	For traveler's diarrhea and hepatic encephalopathy *(Med Lett 52:, 87, 2004; NEJM 362:1071, 2010)*. In general, adverse events equal to or less than placebo.
Sulfonamides [e.g., sulfisoxazole (Gantrisin), sulfamethoxazole (Gantanol), (Truxazole), sulfadiazine]	Dose varies with indications. *See Nocardia & Toxoplasmosis*	**CNS:** fever, headache, dizziness; **Derm:** mild rash to life threatening Stevens-Johnson syndrome, toxic epidermal necrolysis, photosensitivity; **Hem:** agranulocytosis, aplastic anemia; **Cross-allergenicity:** other sulfa drugs, sulfonyl ureas, diuretics, crystalluria (esp sulfadiazine-need ≥ 1500 mL po fluid/day); **Other:** serum sickness, hemolysis if G6PD def, polyarteritis, SLE reported.

(See page 2 for abbreviations)

* NOTE: all dosage recommendations are for adults (unless otherwise indicated) & assume normal renal function.

TABLE 10C (9)

CLASS, AGENT, GENERIC NAME (TRADE NAME)	USUAL ADULT DOSAGE*	ADVERSE REACTIONS, COMMENTS *(See Table 10A for Summary)*
MISCELLANEOUS AGENTS *(continued)*		
Tinidazole (Tindamax)	**Tabs 250, 500 mg.** Dose for giardiasis: 2 gm po times 1 with food.	**Adverse reactions:** metallic taste 3.7%, nausea 3.2%, anorexia/vomiting 1.5%. All higher with multi-day dosing. Avoid alcohol during & for 3 days after last dose; cause disulfiram reaction, flushing, N/V, tachycardia.
Trimethoprim (Trimpex, Proloprim, and others) (100, 200 mg tab)	**100 mg po q12h or 200 mg po q24h**.	**CNS:** drug fever, aseptic meningitis; **Derm:** rash (3-7% at 200 mg/day), phototoxicity, Stevens-Johnson syndrome (rare), toxic epidermal necrolysis (rare); **Renal:** ↑ K+, ↓ Na+, ↑ Cr; **Hem:** neutropenia, thrombocytopenia, methaemoglobinemia.
Trimethoprim (TMP)-Sulfamethoxazole (SMX) (Bactrim, Septra, Sulfatrim, Cotrimoxazole) Single-strength (SS) is 80 TMP/400 SMX, double-strength (DS) 160 TMP/800 SMX	**Standard po rx: 1 DS tab bid. P. carinii:** ***see Table 13, page 135*****. IV rx (base on TMP component): standard 8–10 mg per kg per day divided q6h, q8h, or q12h. For shigellosis: 2.5 mg per kg IV q6h**.	Adverse reactions in 10%: GI: nausea, vomiting, anorexia. Skin: Rash, urticaria, photosensitivity. More serious (1–10%): **Stevens-Johnson syndrome & toxic epidermal necrolysis.** Skin reactions may represent toxic metabolites of SMX rather than allergy *(AnPharmacotherapy 32:381, 1998)*. Daily ascorbic acid 0.5–1.0 gm may promote detoxification *(JAIDS 36:1041, 2004)*. Rare hypoglycemia, esp AIDS pts: *(LnID 6:178, 2006)*. **Sweet's Syndrome** can occur. TMP competes with creatinine for tubular secretion; serum creatinine can ↑; TMP also blocks distal renal tubule secretion of K^+. ↑ serum K^+ in 21% of pts *(AnIM 124:316, 1996)*. Risk of hyperkalemia increased 7x if concomitant ace inhibitor *(Arch Int Med 170:1045, 2010)*. TMP one etiology of **aseptic meningitis** *(CID 19:431, 1994)*. TMP-SMX contains sulfites and may trigger asthma in sulfite-sensitive pts. Frequent drug cause of thrombocytopenia *(AnIM 129:886, 1998)*. No cross allergenicity with other sulfonamide non-antibiotic drugs *(NEJM 349:1628, 2003)*. **For TMP-SMX desensitization**, *see Table 7, page 77*.
Topical Antimicrobial Agents Active vs. S. aureus & Strep. pyogenes		
Bacitracin (Baciquent)	20% bacitracin zinc ointment, apply bid.	Active vs. staph, strep & clostridium. Contact dermatitis incidence 9.2% *(IDC No Amer 18:717, 2004)*.
Fusidic acid[NUS] ointment	**2% ointment, apply tid**	*CID 42:394, 2006*. Available in Canada and Europe *(Leo Laboratories)*.
Mupirocin (Bactroban)	**Skin cream or ointment 2%: Apply tid times 10 days. Nasal ointment 2%: apply bid times 5 days.**	Skin cream: itch, burning, stinging 1–1.5%; Nasal: headache 9%, rhinitis 6%, respiratory congestion 5%. Not active vs. enterococci or gm-neg bacteria. Summary of resistance: *CID 49:935, 2009*.
Polymyxin B—Bacitracin (Polysporin)	5000 units/gm; 400 units/gm. Apply 1-3x/day	Polymyxin active vs. gm-neg bacteria but not Proteus sp., Serratia sp. or gm-pos bacteria. *See Bacitracin comment above*.
Polymyxin B—Bacitracin—Neomycin (Neosporin, triple antibiotic ointment (TAO))	5000 units/gm; 400 units/gm; 3.5 mg/gm. Apply 1-3x/day.	*See Bacitracin and polymyxin B comments above*. Neomycin active vs. gm-neg bacteria and staphylococci; not active vs. streptococci. Contact dermatitis incidence 1%; risk of nephro- & oto-toxicity if absorbed. TAO spectrum broader than mupirocin and active mupirocin-resistant strains *(DMID 54:63, 2006)*.
Retapamulin (Altabax)	1% ointment; apply bid. 5, 10 & 15 gm tubes.	Microbiologic success in 90% S. aureus infections and 97% of S. pyogenes infections *(J Am Acd Derm 55:1003, 2006)*. Package insert says **do not use for MRSA** (not enough pts in clinical trials).

* NOTE: all dosage recommendations are for adults (unless otherwise indicated) & assume normal renal function.

TABLE 10D – AMINOGLYCOSIDE ONCE-DAILY AND MULTIPLE DAILY DOSING REGIMENS

(See *Table 17, page 189,* if estimated creatinine clearance <90 mL per min.)

- General Note: dosages are given as **once daily dose (OD)** and **multiple daily dose (MDD)**.
- For **calculation of dosing weight in non-obese patients** use Ideal Body Weight (IBW):
  - **Female:** 45.5 kg + 2.3 kg per inch over 60 inch height = dosing weight in kg;
  - **Male:** 50 kg + 2.3 kg per inch over 60 inch height = dosing weight in kg.
- **Adjustment for calculation of dosing weight in obese patients** (actual body weight (ABW) is ≥ 30% above IBW): IBW + 0.4 (ABW minus IBW) = adjusted weight (*Pharmacotherapy 27:1081, 2007; CID 25:112, 1997*).
- If CrCl >90 mL/min, use doses in this table. If CrCl <90, *use doses in Table 17, page 189.*
- **For non-obese patients, calculate estimated creatinine clearance (CrCl) as follows:**

$$\frac{(140 \text{ minus age})(\text{IBW in kg})}{72 \times \text{serum creatinine}} = \text{CrCl in mL/min for men. Multiply answer by 0.85 for women (estimated)}$$

- **For morbidly obese patients, calculate estimated creatinine clearance (CrCl) as follows** (*AJM 84:1053, 1988*):

$$\frac{(137 \text{ minus age}) \times ((0.285 \times \text{wt in kg}) + (12.1 \times \text{ht in meters}^2))}{51 \times \text{serum creatinine}} = \text{CrCl (obese male)}$$

$$\frac{(146 \text{ minus age}) \times ((0.287 \times \text{wt in kg}) + (9.74 \times \text{ht in meters}^2))}{60 \times \text{serum creatinine}} = \text{CrCl (obese female)}$$

DRUG	MDD AND OD IV REGIMENS/ TARGETED PEAK (P) AND TROUGH (T) SERUM LEVELS	COMMENTS For more data on once-daily dosing, see *AJM 105:182, 1998, and Table 17, page 188*
Gentamicin (Garamycin), **Tobramycin** (Nebcin)	MDD: 2 mg per kg load, then 1.7 mg per kg q8h P 4–10 mcg/mL, T 1–2 mcg per mL OD: 5.1 (7 if critically ill) mg per kg q24h P 16–24 mcg per mL, T <1 mcg per mL	**All aminoglycosides have potential to cause tubular necrosis and renal failure, deafness due to cochlear toxicity, vertigo due to damage to vestibular organs, and rarely neuromuscular blockade.** Risk minimal with oral or topical application due to small % absorption unless tissues altered by disease. Risk of nephrotoxicity ↑ with concomitant administration of cyclosporine, vancomycin, ampho B, radiocontrast. Risk of nephrotoxicity ↓ by concomitant AP Pen and perhaps by once-daily dosing method (especially if baseline renal function normal). In general, same factors influence risk of ototoxicity. **NOTE: There is no known method to eliminate risk of aminoglycoside nephro/ototoxicity. Proper rx attempts to ↓ the % risk.** The clinical trial data of OD aminoglycosides have been reviewed extensively by meta-analysis (*CID 24:816, 1997*). **Serum levels:** Collect peak serum level (PSL) exactly 1 hr after the start of the infusion of the 3rd dose. In critically ill pts, PSL after the 1st dose as volume of distribution and renal function may change rapidly. Other dosing methods and references: For once-daily 7 mg per kg per day of gentamicin—Hartford Hospital method (may underdose if <7 mg/kg/day dose), *see AAC 39:650, 1995.* One in 500 patients (Europe) have mitochondrial mutation that predicts cochlear toxicity (*NEJM 360:640 & 642, 2009*). Aspirin supplement (3 gm/day) attenuated risk of cochlear injury from gentamicin (*NEJM 354:1856, 2006*).
Kanamycin (Kantrex), **Amikacin** (Amikin), Streptomycin	MDD: 7.5 mg per kg q12h P 15–30 mcg per mL, T 5–10 mcg per mL OD: 15 mg per kg q24h P 56–64 mcg per mL, T <1 mcg per mL	
Netilmicin[NUS]	MDD: 2 mg per kg q8h P 4–10 mcg per mL, T 1–2 mcg per mL OD: 6.5 mg per kg q24h P 22–30 mcg per mL, T <1 mcg per mL	
Isepamicin[NUS]	Only OD: Severe infections 15 mg per kg q24h, less severe 8 mg per kg q24h	
Spectinomycin (Trobicin)[NUS]	2 gm IM times 1–gonococcal infections	
Neomycin—oral	Prophylaxis GI surgery: 1 gm po times 3 with erythro, *see Table 15B, page 177* For hepatic coma: 4–12 gm per day po	
Tobramycin—inhaled (Tobi): *See Cystic fibrosis, Table 1A, page 40.* Adverse effects few: transient voice alteration (13%) and transient tinnitus (3%).		
Paromomycin—oral: *See Entamoeba and Cryptosporidia, Table 13, page 131.*		

TABLE 11A – TREATMENT OF FUNGAL INFECTIONS—ANTIMICROBIAL AGENTS OF CHOICE*

TYPE OF INFECTION/ORGANISM/ SITE OF INFECTION	ANTIMICROBIAL AGENTS OF CHOICE		COMMENTS
	PRIMARY	ALTERNATIVE	
Aspergillosis (A. fumigatus most common, also A. flavus and others) *(See NEJM 360:1870, 2009 for excellent review).*			
Allergic bronchopulmonary aspergillosis (ABPA) Clinical manifestations: wheezing, pulmonary infiltrates, bronchiectasis & fibrosis. Airway colonization assoc. with ↑ blood eosinophils, ↑ serum IgE, ↑ specific serum antibodies.	Acute asthma attacks associated with ABPA: **Corticosteroids**	Rx of ABPA: **Itraconazole**[1] 200 mg po q24h times 16 wks or longer	Itra decreases number of exacerbations requiring corticosteroids with improved immunological markers improved lung function & exercise tolerance *(IDSA Guidelines updated CID 46:327, 2008).*
Allergic fungal sinusitis: relapsing chronic sinusitis; nasal polyps without bony invasion; asthma, eczema or allergic rhinitis; ↑ IgE levels and isolation of Aspergillus sp. or other dematiaceous sp. (Alternaria, Cladosporium, etc.)	**Rx controversial:** systemic corticosteroids + surgical debridement (relapse common).	For failures try **Itra**[1] 200 mg po bid times 12 mo or flucon nasal spray.	Controversial area.
Aspergilloma (fungus ball)	No therapy or surgical resection. Efficacy of antimicrobial agents not proven.		Aspergillus may complicate pulmonary sequestration.
Invasive, pulmonary (IPA) or extrapulmonary: *(See Am J Respir Crit Care Med 173:707, 2006). Good website:doctorfungus.org* Post-transplantation and post-chemotherapy in neutropenic pts (PMN <500 per mm³) but may also present with neutrophil recovery. Most common pneumonia in transplant recipients. Usually a late (≥100 days) complication in allogeneic bone marrow & liver transplantation: High mortality *(CID 44:531, 2007).* **Typical x-ray/CT lung lesions** (halo sign, cavitation, or macronodules) *(CID 44:373, 2007).* Initiation of antifungal Rx based on halo signs on CT associated with better response to Rx & improved outcome. An immunologic test that detects circulating **galactomannan** is available for dx of invasive aspergillosis *(Lancet ID 4:349, 2005).* Galactomannan detection in the blood relatively insensitive; antifungal rx may decrease sensitivity *(CID 40:1762,2005).* One study suggests improved sensitivity when performed on BAL fluid. *(Am J Respir Crit Care Med 177:27, 2008).* **False-pos. tests occur with serum from pts receiving PIP-TZ & AM-CL.** Numerous other causes of false positive galactomannan tests reported. For strengths & weaknesses of the test see *CID 42:1417, 2006.* Posaconazole superior to Flu or Itra with fewer invasive fungal infections and improved survival in patients with hematologic malignancies undergoing induction chemotherapy *(NEJM 356:348, 2007).*	**Primary therapy** *(See CID 46:327, 2008):* **Voriconazole 6 mg/kg IV q12h on day 1; then either (4 mg/kg IV q12h) or (200 mg po q12h for body weight ≥40 kg, but 100 mg po q12h for body weight <40 kg)** **Alternative therapies:** **Liposomal ampho B** (L-AmB) 3-5 mg/kg/day IV; OR **Ampho B lipid complex** (ABLC) 5 mg/kg/d IV; OR **Caspofungin** 70 mg/day then 50 mg/day thereafter; OR **Micafungin**[NAI] 100 mg BID *(JAC 64:840, 2009);* OR **Posaconazole**[NAI] 200 mg qid, then 400 mg bid after stabilization of disease; OR **Itraconazole** capsules 600 mg/day for 3 days, then 400 mg/day (or 2.5 mg/kg of oral solution once daily).		**Voriconazole** more effective than ampho B. Vori, both a substrate and an inhibitor of CYP2C19, CYP2C9, and CYP3A4, has potential for deleterious drug interactions (e.g., with protease inhibitors) and careful review of concomitant medications is mandatory. Measurement of serum concentrations advisable with prolonged therapy or for patients with possible drug-drug interactions. In patients with CrCl <50 ml/min, the drug should be given orally, not IV, since the intravenous vehicle (SBECD-sulfobutylether-B cyclodextrin) may accumulate. **Ampho B: not recommended except as a lipid formulation,** either L-AMB or ABLC. 10 mg/kg and 3 mg/kg doses of L-AMB are equally efficacious with greater toxicity of higher dose *(CID 2007; 44:1289–97).* One comparative trial found much greater toxicity with ABLC than with L-AMB: 34.6% vs 9.4% adverse events and 21.2% vs 2.8% nephrotoxicity *(Cancer 112:1282, 2008).* Vori preferred as primary therapy. **Caspo:** ~50% response rate in IPA. Licensed for salvage therapy. Efavirenz, nelfinavir, nevirapine, phenytoin, rifampin, dexamethasone, and carbamazepine, may reduce caspofungin concentrations. **Micafungin:** Favorable responses to micafungin as a single agent in 6/12 patients in primary therapy group and 9/22 in the salvage therapy group of an open-label, non-comparative trial *(J Infect 53: 337, 2006).* Outcomes no better with combination therapy. Few significant drug-drug interactions. *(Continued on next page)*

[1] **Oral solution preferred to tablets because of ↑ absorption** *(see Table 11B, page 114).*

See page 2 for abbreviations. All dosage recommendations are for adults (unless otherwise indicated) and assume normal renal function

TABLE 11A (2)

TYPE OF INFECTION/ORGANISM/ SITE OF INFECTION	ANTIMICROBIAL AGENTS OF CHOICE		COMMENTS
	PRIMARY	ALTERNATIVE	
Aspergillosis *(continued from previous page)*			
			(Continued from previous page) **Itraconazole: Licensed for treatment of invasive aspergillosis in patients refractory to or intolerant of standard antifungal therapy**. Itraconazole formulated as capsules, oral solution in hydroxypropyl-beta-cyclodextrin (HPCD), and parenteral solution with HPCD as a solubilizer; oral solution and parenteral formulation not licensed for treatment of invasive aspergillosis. 2.5 mg/kg oral solution provides dose equivalent to 400 mg capsules. Parenteral HPCD formulation dosage is 200 mg every 12h IV for 2 days, followed by 200 mg daily thereafter. Oral absorption of capsules enhanced by low gastric pH, erratic in fasting state and with hypochlorhydria; measurements of plasma concentrations recommended during oral therapy of invasive aspergillosis; target troughs concentrations > 0.25 mcg/ml. Itraconazole is a substrate of CYP3A4 and non-competitive inhibitor of CYP3A4 with potential for significant drug-drug interactions. Do not use for azole-non-responders. **Combo therapy:** Uncertain role and not routinely recommended for primary therapy; consider for treatment of refractory disease, although benefit unproven. A typical combo regimen would be an echinocandin in combination with either an azole or a lipid formulation of ampho B.
Blastomycosis *(CID 46: 1801, 2008)* (Blastomyces dermatitidis) Cutaneous, pulmonary or extrapulmonary.	**LAB**, 3 -5 mg/kg per day; OR **Ampho B**, 0.7 -1 mg/kg per day, for 1 -2 weeks, **then itra**[2] 200 mg tid for 3 days followed by itra 200 mg bid for 6 -12 months	**Itra** 200 mg tid for 3 days then once or twice per day for 6 -12 months for mild to moderate disease; OR **Flu** 400-800 mg per day for those intolerant to itra	Serum levels of **itra** should be determined after 2 weeks to ensure adequate drug exposure. Flu less effective than itra; role of vori or posa unclear but active in vitro.
Blastomycosis: CNS disease *(CID 50:797, 2010)*	**LAB** 5 mg/kg per day for 4-6 weeks, followed by **Flu** 800 mg per day	**Itra** 200 mg bid or tid; OR **Vori** 200-400 mg q12h	Flu and vori have excellent CNS penetration, perhaps counterbalance their slightly reduced activity compared to itra. Treat for at least 12 months and until CSF has normalized. Document serum itra levels to assure adequate drug concentrations. Recent study suggests more favorable outcome with Voriconazole *(CID 50:797, 2010)*.

[2] **Oral solution preferred to tablets because of ↑ absorption** *(see Table 11B, page 114)*.

See page 2 for abbreviations. All dosage recommendations are for adults (unless otherwise indicated) and assume normal renal function

TABLE 11A (3)

TYPE OF INFECTION/ORGANISM/ SITE OF INFECTION	ANTIMICROBIAL AGENTS OF CHOICE		COMMENTS
	PRIMARY	ALTERNATIVE	
Candidiasis: Candida is a common cause of nosocomial bloodstream infection. A decrease in *C. albicans* & increase in non-albicans species show ↓ susceptibility among candida species to antifungal agents (esp. fluconazole). These changes have predominantly affected immunocompromised pts in environments where antifungal prophylaxis (esp. fluconazole) is widely used. Oral, esophageal, or vaginal candidiasis is a major manifestation of advanced HIV & represents one of the most common AIDS-defining diagnoses. *See CID 48:503, 2009 for updated IDSA Guidelines.*			
Candidiasis: Bloodstream infection			
Bloodstream: non-neutropenic patient Remove all intravascular catheters if possible; replace catheters at a new site (not over a wire). Higher mortality associated with delay in therapy *(CID 43:25, 2006).*	**Fluconazole** 800 mg (12 mg/kg) loading dose, then 400 mg daily IV or PO; OR **Capsofungin** 70 mg IV loading dose, then 50 mg IV daily (35 mg for moderate hepatic insufficiency); OR **Micafungin** 100 mg IV daily; OR **Anidulafungin** 200 mg IV loading dose then 100 mg IV daily.	**Lipid-based ampho B** 3-5 mg/kg IV daily; OR **Ampho B** 0.7 mg/kg IV daily; OR **Voriconazole** 400 mg (6 mg/kg) twice daily for 2 doses then 200 mg q12h.	**Fluconazole** recommended for patients with mild-to-moderate illness, hemodynamically stable, with no recent azole exposure. Fluconazole not recommended for treatment of documented *C. kruseii*: use an echinocandin or voriconazole or posaconazole (note: echinocandins have better in vitro activity than either vori or posa against *C. glabrata*). Fluconazole recommended for treatment of *Candida parapsilosis* because of reduced susceptibility of this species to echinocandins. Transition from echinocandin to fluconazole for stable patients with *Candida albicans* or other azole-susceptible species. **Echinocandin** for patients with recent azole exposure or with moderately severe or severe illness, hemodynamic instability. An echinocandin should be used for treatment of *Candida glabrata* unless susceptibility to fluconazole or voriconazole has been confirmed. Echinocandin may be preferred empirical therapy in centers with high prevalence of non-albicans candida species. A double-blind randomized trial of anidulafungin (n=127) and fluconazole (n=118) showed a 88% microbiologic response rate (119/135 candida species) with anidulafungin vs a 76% (99/130 candida species) with fluconazole (p=0.02) *(NEJM 356: 2472, 2007).* **Voriconazole** with little advantage over fluconazole (more drug-drug interactions) except for oral step-down therapy of *Candida krusei* or voriconazole-susceptible *Candida glabrata*. Recommended **duration of therapy** is 14 days after last positive blood culture. Duration of systemic therapy should be extended to 4-6 weeks for eye involvement. **Funduscopic examination** within first week of therapy to exclude ophthalmic involvement. Intraocular injections of ampho B may be required for endophthalmitis; echinocandins have poor penetration into the eye. For **septic thrombophlebitis**, catheter removal and incision and drainage and resection of the vein, as needed, are recommended; duration of therapy at least 2 weeks after last positive blood culture.
Bloodstream: neutropenic patient Remove all intravascular catheters if possible; replace catheters at a new site (not over a wire).	**Capsofungin** 70 mg IV loading dose, then 50 mg IV daily, 35 mg for moderate hepatic insufficiency; OR **Micafungin** 100 mg IV daily; OR **Anidulafungin** 200 mg IV loading dose then 100 mg IV daily; OR **Lipid-based ampho B** 3-5 mg/kg IV daily.	**Fluconazole** 800 mg (12 mg/kg) loading dose, then 400 mg daily IV or PO; OR **Voriconazole** 400 mg (6 mg/kg) twice daily for 2 doses then 200 mg (3 mg/kg) q12h.	Fluconazole may be considered for less critically ill patients without recent azole exposure. Duration of therapy in absence of metastatic complications is for 2 weeks after last positive blood culture, resolution of signs, and resolution of neutropenia. Perform funduscopic examination after recovery of white count as signs of ophthalmic involvement may not be seen during neutropenia. *See comments above for recommendations concerning choice of specific agents.*

TABLE 11A (4)

TYPE OF INFECTION/ORGANISM/ SITE OF INFECTION	ANTIMICROBIAL AGENTS OF CHOICE		COMMENTS
	PRIMARY	ALTERNATIVE	
Candidiasis: Bone and joint infections			
Osteomyelitis	**Fluconazole** 400 mg (6 mg/kg) daily IV or PO; OR **Lipid-based ampho B** 3–5 mg/kg daily for several weeks, then oral fluconazole.	An **echinocandin** (as above) or **ampho** B 0.5–1 mg/kg daily for several weeks then oral **fluconazole**.	Treat for a total of 6-12 months. **Surgical debridement** often necessary; **remove hardware** whenever possible.
Septic arthritis	**Fluconazole** 400 mg (6 mg/kg) daily IV or PO; OR **Lipid-based ampho B** 3–5 mg/kg daily for several weeks, then oral fluconazole.	An **echinocandin** or **ampho** B 0.5–1 mg/kg daily for several weeks then oral **fluconazole**.	**Surgical debridement** in all cases; removal of prosthetic joints whenever possible. Treat for at least 6 weeks and indefinitely if retained hardware.
Candidiasis: Cardiovascular infections			
Endocarditis *(See Eur J Clin Microbiol Infect Dis 27:519, 2008)*	**An echinocandin:** **Caspofungin** 50–150 mg/day; OR **Micafungin** 100–150 mg/day; OR **Anidulafungin** 100–200 mg/day; OR **Lipid-based ampho B** 3–5 mg/kg daily **+ 5-FC** 25 mg/kg qid.	**Ampho B** 0.6–1 mg/kg daily **+ 5-FC** 25 mg/kg qid	Consider use of higher doses of echinocandins for endocarditis or other endovascular infections. Can switch to **fluconazole 400-800 mg orally in stable patients** with negative blood cultures and fluconazole susceptible organism. Valve replacement strongly recommended, particularly in those with prosthetic valve endocarditis. Duration of therapy not well defined, but treat for at least 6 weeks after valve replacement and longer in those with complications (e.g., perivalvular or myocardial abscess, extensive disease, delayed resolution of candidemia). Long-term (life-long?) suppression with fluconazole 400-800 mg daily for native valve endocarditis and no valve replacement; life-long suppression for prosthetic valve endocarditis if no valve replacement.
Myocarditis	**Lipid-based ampho B** 3–5 mg/kg daily; OR **Fluconazole** 400–800 mg (6–12 mg/kg) daily IV or PO; OR **An echinocandin** *(see endocarditis)*.		Can switch to **fluconazole 400-800 mg orally in stable patients** with negative blood cultures and fluconazole susceptible organism. Recommended duration of therapy is for several months.
Pericarditis	**Lipid-based ampho B** 3–5 mg/kg daily; OR **Fluconazole** 400–800 mg (6–12 mg/kg) daily IV or PO; OR **An echinocandin** *(see endocarditis)*		**Pericardial window or pericardiectomy** also is recommended. Can switch to **fluconazole 400-800 mg orally in stable patients** with negative blood cultures and fluconazole susceptible organism. Recommended duration of therapy is for several months.

See page 2 for abbreviations. All dosage recommendations are for adults (unless otherwise indicated) and assume normal renal function

TABLE 11A (5)

TYPE OF INFECTION/ORGANISM/ SITE OF INFECTION	ANTIMICROBIAL AGENTS OF CHOICE		COMMENTS
	PRIMARY	ALTERNATIVE	
Candidiasis: Mucosal, esophageal, and oropharyngeal			
Candida esophagitis Primarily encountered in HIV-positive patients	**Fluconazole** 200-400 (3-6 mg/kg) mg daily; OR **An echinocandin (caspofungin** 50 mg IV daily; OR **micafungin** 150 mg IV daily; OR **anidulafungin** 200 mg IV loading dose then 100 mg IV daily); OR **Ampho B** 0.5 mg/kg daily.	An azole (**itraconazole** solution 200 mg daily; or **posaconazole** suspension 400 mg bid for 3 days then 400 mg daily or **voriconazole** 200 mg q12h.	**Duration of therapy** 14-21 days. IV echinocandin or ampho B for patients unable to tolerate oral therapy. For fluconazole refractory disease, itra (80% will respond), posa, vori, an echinocandin, or ampho B. Echinocandins associated with higher relapse rate than fluconazole. ARV therapy recommended. Suppressive therapy with fluconazole 200 mg 3x/wk for recurrent infections. Suppressive therapy may be discontinued once CD4 > 200/mm^3.
Oropharyngeal candidiasis **Non-AIDS patient**	**Clotrimazole troches** 10 mg 5 times daily; OR **Nystatin suspension** or pastilles qid; OR **Fluconazole** 100–200 mg daily.	**Itraconazole** solution 200 mg daily; OR **posaconazole** suspension 400 mg bid for 3 days then 400 mg daily; or **voriconazole** 200 mg q12h; OR an echinocandin (**capsofungin** 70 mg loading dose then 50 mg IV daily; or **micafungin** 100 mg IV daily; or **anidulafungin** 200 mg IV loading dose then 100 mg IV daily); OR **Ampho B** 0.3 mg/kg daily.	**Duration of therapy** 7-14 days. Clotrimazole or nystatin recommended for mild disease; fluconazole preferred for moderate-to-severe disease. Alternative agents reserved for refractory disease.
AIDS patient	**Fluconazole** 100-200 mg daily for 7-14 days.	Same as for non-AIDS patient, above, for 7-14 days.	Antiretroviral therapy (ARV) recommended in HIV-positive patients to prevent recurrent disease. Suppressive therapy not necessary, especially with ARV therapy and CD4 > 200/mm^3, but if required fluconazole 100 mg thrice weekly recommended. Itra, posa, or vori for 28 days for fluconazole-refractory disease. IV echinocardin also an option. Dysphagia or odynophagia predictive of esophageal candidiasis.
Vulvovaginitis **Non-AIDS Patient**	**Topical azole therapy: Butoconazole 2% cream** (5 gm) q24h at bedtime x 3 days or 2% cream SR 5 gm x 1; OR **Clotrimazole 100 mg vaginal tabs** (2 at bedtime x 3 days) or 1% cream (5 gm) at bedtime times 7 days (14 days may ↑ cure rate) or 100 mg vaginal tab x 7 days or 500 mg vaginal tab x 1; OR **Miconazole 200 mg vaginal suppos** (1 at bedtime x 3 days) or 100 mg vaginal suppos. q24h x 7 days or 2% cream (5 gm) at bedtime x 7 days; OR **Terconazole 80 mg vaginal tab** (1 at bedtime x 3 days) or 0.4% cream (5 gm) at bedtime x 7 days or 0.8% cream 5 gm intravaginal q24h x 3 days; or tioconazole 6.5% vag. ointment x 1 dose. **Oral therapy:** **Fluconazole** 150 mg po x 1; OR **Itraconazole** 200 mg po bid x 1 day.		**Recurrent vulvovaginal candidiasis:** fluconazole 150 mg weekly for 6 months.

TABLE 11A (6)

TYPE OF INFECTION/ORGANISM/ SITE OF INFECTION	ANTIMICROBIAL AGENTS OF CHOICE		COMMENTS
	PRIMARY	ALTERNATIVE	
Candidiasis: Mucosal, esophageal, and oropharyngeal/Vulvovaginitis *(continued)*			
AIDS Patient	Topical **azoles** (clotrimazole, buto, mico, tico, or tercon) x3–7d; OR Topical **nystatin** 100,000 units/day as vaginal tablet x14d; OR Oral **flu** 150 mg x1 dose.		For recurrent disease 10-14 days of topical azole or oral flu 150 mg, then flu 150 mg weekly for 6 mo.
Candidiasis: Other infections			
CNS Infection	**Lipid-based ampho B** 3–5 mg/kg daily ± 5-FC 25 mg/kg qid.	**Fluconazole** 400–800 mg (6–12 mg/kg) IV or PO.	Removal of **intraventricular devices** recommended. Flu 400-800 mg as stepdown therapy in the stable patient and in patient intolerant of ampho B. Experience too limited to recommend echinocandins at this time. **Treatment duration** for several weeks until resolution of CSF, radiographic, and clinical abnormalities.
Cutaneous *(including paronychia, Table 1A, page 25)*	Apply topical ampho B, clotrimazole, econazole, miconazole, or nystatin 3-4 x daily for 7–14 days or ketoconazole 400 mg po once daily x 14 days. Ciclopirox olamine 1% cream/lotion; apply topically bid x 7–14 days.		
Disseminated candidiasis	**Fluconazole** 400 mg (6 mg/kg) daily IV or PO; OR **Lipid-based ampho B** 3–5 mg/kg daily OR **An echinocandin** (as for bloodstream infection);	**Ampho B** 0.5–0.7 mg/kg daily.	**Ampho B** recommended for **unstable patients;** flu in stable patients. **Stepdown** to oral flu once patient is stabilized. Other azoles may also be effective. Treatment, usually for several months, should be continued until lesions have resolved and during periods of immunosuppression.
Endophthalmitis • Occurs in 10% of candidemia, thus ophthalmological consult for all pts • Diagnosis: typical white exudates on retinal exam and/or isolation by vitrectomy	**Ampho B**-0.7–1 mg/kg + **Flucytosine** 25 mg/kg qid OR **Fluconazole** 6-12 mg/kg daily.	**Lipid-based ampho** 3-5 mg/kg daily; OR **voriconazole** 6 mg/kg q12h for 2 doses, then 3–4 mg/kg q12h; OR an echinocandin (**capsofungin** 70 mg loading dose then 50 mg IV daily; or **micafungin** 100 mg IV daily; or **anidulafungin** 200 mg IV loading dose then 100 mg IV daily).	**Duration of therapy:** 4-6 weeks or longer, based on resolution determined by repeated examinations. Patients with chorioretinitis only often respond to systemically administered antifungals. Intravitreal amphotericin and/or vitrectomy may be necessary for those with vitritis or endophthalmitis (*Br J Ophthalmol 92;466, 2008; Pharmacotherapy 27:1711, 2007*).
Neonatal candidiasis	**Ampho B** 1 mg/kg daily; OR **Fluconazole** 12 mg/kg daily.	**Lipid-based ampho B** 3-5 mg/kg daily.	**Lumbar puncture** to rule out CNS disease, **dilated retinal examination**, and **intravascular catheter removal** strongly recommended. Lipid-based ampho B used only if there is no renal involvement. Echinocandins considered 3rd line therapy. Duration of therapy is at least 3 weeks.
Peritonitis (Chronic Ambulatory Peritoneal Dialysis) *See Table 19, page 196.*	**Fluconazole** 400 mg po q24h x 2–3 wks; or **caspofungin** 70 mg IV on day 1 followed by 50 mg IV q24h for 14 days; or **micafungin** 100 mg q24h for 14 days.	**Ampho B**, continuous intraperitoneal dosing at 1.5 mg/L of dialysis fluid times 4–6 wk.	Remove cath immediately or if no clinical improvement in 4–7 days.
Candidiasis: Urinary tract infections			
Cystitis **Asymptomatic**	**If possible, remove catheter or stent.** **No therapy indicated except in patients at high risk for dissemination or undergoing a urologic procedure.**		**High risk patients** include neonates and neutropenic patients; these patients should be managed as outlined for treatment of bloodstream infection. For patients undergoing urologic procedures, flu 200 mg (3 mg/kg) daily or ampho B 0.5 mg/kg daily (for flu-resistant organisms) for several days pre- and post-procedure.

See page 2 for abbreviations. All dosage recommendations are for adults (unless otherwise indicated) and assume normal renal function

TABLE 11A (7)

TYPE OF INFECTION/ORGANISM/ SITE OF INFECTION	ANTIMICROBIAL AGENTS OF CHOICE		COMMENTS
	PRIMARY	ALTERNATIVE	
Candidiasis: Urinary tract infections *(continued)*			
Symptomatic	**Fluconazole** 200 mg (3 mg/kg) daily for 14 days.	**Ampho B** 0.5 mg/kg daily (for fluconazole resistant organisms) for 7-10 days.	Concentration of echinocandins in urine are low; case reports of efficacy versus azole resistant organisms *(Can J Infect Dis Med Microbiol 18:149, 2007; CID 44:e46, 2007)*. Persistent candiduria in immunocompromised pt warrants ultrasound or CT of kidneys to rule out fungus ball.
Pyelonephritis	**Fluconazole** 200–400 mg (3–6 mg/kg) once daily orally.	**Ampho B** 0.5 mg/kg daily IV ± 5-FC 25 mg/kg orally qid.	**Treat for 2 weeks**. For suspected disseminated disease treat as if bloodstream infection is present.
Chromoblastomycosis *(Clin Exp Dermatol, 34:849, 2009)*. (Cladophialophora, Phialophora, or Fonsecaea); Cutaneous (usually feet, legs): raised scaly lesions, most common in tropical areas	If lesions small & few, **surgical excision or cryosurgery with liquid nitrogen**. If lesions chronic, extensive, burrowing: **itraconazole**.	**Itraconazole:** 200-400 mg po q24h or 400 mg pulse therapy once daily for 1 week monthly for 6-12 months (or until response)[NAI].	**Terbinafine**[NAI] 500-1000 mg once daily alone or in combination with itraconazole 200-400 mg; or **posaconazole** (800 mg/d) also may be effective.
Coccidioidomycosis (Coccidioides immitis) *(IDSA Guidelines 2005: CID 41:1217, 2005; see also Mayo Clin Proc 83:343, 2008)*			
Primary pulmonary (San Joaquin or Valley Fever): **Pts low risk persistence/complication**	**Antifungal rx not generally recommended.** Treat if fever, wt loss and/or fatigue do not resolve within several wks to 2 mo *(see below)*		Uncomplicated pulmonary in normal host common in endemic areas *(Emerg Infect Dis 12:958, 2006)* Influenza -like illness of 1–2 wk duration.
Primary pulmonary in pts with ↑ risk for complications or dissemination. Rx indicated: • Immunosuppressive disease, post-transplantation, hematological malignancies or therapies (steroids, TNF-α antagonists) • Pregnancy in 3rd trimester. • Diabetes • CF antibody >1:16 • Pulmonary infiltrates • Dissemination (identification of spherules or culture of organism from ulcer, joint effusion, pus from subcutaneous abscess or bone biopsy, etc.)	**Mild to moderate severity:** **Itraconazole** solution 200 mg po or IV bid; OR **Fluconazole** 400 mg po q24h for 3–12 mo **Locally severe or disseminated disease** **Ampho B** 0.6–1 mg/kg per day x 7 days then 0.8 mg/kg every other day or **liposomal ampho B** 3-5 mg/kg/d IV or **ABLC** 5 mg/kg/d IV, until clinical improvement (usually several wks or longer in disseminated disease), followed by **itra** or **flu** for at least 1 year. Some use combination of Ampho B & Flu for progressive severe disease; controlled series lacking. **Consultation with specialist recommended:** surgery may be required. Lifetime suppression in HIV+ patients or until CD4 >250 & infection controlled: flu 200 mg po q24h or itra 200 mg po bid *(Mycosis 46:42, 2003)*.		**Ampho B cure rate 50–70%. Responses to azoles are similar. Itra** may have slight advantage esp. in soft tissue infection. Relapse rates after rx 40%: Relapse rate ↑ if ↑ CF titer ≥1:256. Following CF titers after completion of rx important; rising titers warrant retreatment. **Posaconazole** reported successful in 73% of pts with refractory non-meningeal cocci *(Chest 132:952, 2007)*. Not frontline therapy.
Meningitis: occurs in 1/3 to 1/2 of pts with disseminated coccidioidomycosis			
Adult *(CID 42:103, 2006)*	**Fluconazole** 400–1,000 mg po q24h indefinitely	**Ampho B** IV as for pulmonary *(above)* + 0.1–0.3 mg daily intra-thecal (intraventricular) via reservoir device. **OR itra** 400–800 mg q24h **OR voriconazole** *(see Comment)*	**80% relapse rate, continue flucon indefinitely, Voriconazole** successful in high doses (6 mg/kg IV q12h) followed by oral suppression (200 mg po q12h)
Child	**Fluconazole** (po) (Pediatric dose not established, 6 mg per kg q24h used)		

See page 2 for abbreviations. All dosage recommendations are for adults (unless otherwise indicated) and assume normal renal function

TABLE 11A (8)

TYPE OF INFECTION/ORGANISM/ SITE OF INFECTION	ANTIMICROBIAL AGENTS OF CHOICE		COMMENTS
	PRIMARY	ALTERNATIVE	
Cryptococcosis *(IDSA Guideline: CID 30:710, 2000)*. New Guidelines CID 50:291, 2010. Excellent review: *Brit Med Bull 72:99, 2005*			
Non-meningeal (non-AIDS) Risk 57% in organ transplant & those receiving other forms of immunosuppressive agents *(EID 13:953, 2007)*.	**Fluconazole** 400 mg/day IV or po for 8 wk to 6 mo **For more severe disease:** **Ampho B** 0.5–0.8 mg/kg per day IV till response then change to **fluconazole** 400 mg po q24h for 8–10 wk course	**Itraconazole** 200-400 mg solution q24h for 6-12 mo OR **Ampho B** 0.3 mg/kg per day IV + **flucytosine** 37.5 mg/kg[3] po qid times 6 wk	**Flucon alone 90% effective for meningeal and non-meningeal forms**. Fluconazole as effective as ampho B. Addition of **interferon-γ** (IFN-γ-Ib 50 mcg per M^2 subcut. 3x per wk x 9 wk) to liposomal ampho B assoc. with response in pt failing antifungal rx *(CID 38: 910, 2004)*. Posaconazole 400-800 mg also effective in a small series of patients *(CID 45:562, 2007; Chest 132:952, 2007)*
Meningitis (non-AIDS)	**Ampho B** 0.5–0.8 mg/kg per day IV + **flucytosine** 37.5 mg/kg[3] po q6h until pt afebrile & cultures neg (~6 wk) *(NEJM 301:126, 1979)*, then stop ampho B/flucyt, start **fluconazole** 200 mg po q24h *(AnIM 113:183, 1990)*; OR **Fluconazole** 400 mg po q24h x 8–10 wks (less severely ill pt). Some recommend flu for 2 yr to reduce relapse rate *(CID 28:297, 1999)*. Some recommend AMB plus fluconazole as induction Rx. Studies underway.		If CSF opening pressure >25 cm H_2O, repeat LP to drain fluid to control pressure. Outbreaks of C. gattii meningitis have been reported in the Pacific Northwest *(EID 13:42, 2007)*; severity of disease and prognosis appear to be worse than with C. neoformans; initial therapy with ampho B + flucytosine recommended. C. gattii less susceptible to flucon than C. neoformans *(Clin Microbiol Inf 14:727, 2008)*. Outcomes in both AIDS and non-AIDS cryptococcal meningitis improved with Ampho B + 5-FC induction therapy for 14 days in those with neurological abnormalities or high organism burden *(PLoS ONE 3:e2870, 2008)*.
HIV+/AIDS: Cryptococcemia and/or Meningitis			
Treatment *See Clin Infect Dis 50:291, 2010 (IDSA Guidelines)*. ↓ with ARV but still common presenting OI in newly diagnosed AIDS pts. Cryptococcal infection may be manifested by positive blood culture or positive serum cryptococcal antigen (CRAG: >95% sens). CRAG no help in monitoring response to therapy. With ARV, symptoms of acute meningitis may return: immune reconstitution inflammatory syndrome (IRIS). ↑ CSF pressure **(> 250 mm H_2O)** associated with high mortality: lower with CSF removal. If frequent LPs not possible, ventriculoperitoneal shunts an option *(Surg Neurol 63:529 & 531, 2005)*.	**Ampho B** 0.7 mg/kg IV q24H + **flucytosine**[4] 25 mg/kg po q6h for at least two weeks or longer until CSF is sterilized. *See Comment.* **Then** **Consolidation therapy: Fluconazole** 400-800 mg po q24h to complete a 10-wk course then suppression *(see below)*. Start Antiretroviral Therapy (ARV) if possible.	**Amphotericin B** or **liposomal ampho B plus fluconazole** 400 mg PO or IV daily; **OR Amphotericin B** 0.7 mg/kg **or liposomal ampho B** 4 mg/kg IV q24h alone; **OR Fluconazole** ≥ 800 mg/day (1200 mg preferred) (PO or IV) **plus flucytosine** 25 mg/kg po q6h for 4–6 weeks.	Outcome of treatment: treatment failure associated with dissemination of infection & high serum antigen titer, indicative of high burden of organisms and lack of 5FC use during inductive Rx, abnormal neurological evaluation & underlying hematological malignancy. Mortality rates still high, particularly in those with concomitant pneumonia *(Postgrad Med 121:107, 2009)*. Early Dx essential for improved outcome *(PLOS Medicine 4:e47, 2007)*. Ampho B + 5FC treatment ↓ crypto CFUs more rapidly than ampho + flu or ampho + 5FC + flu. Ampho B 1 mg/kg/d alone much more rapidly fungicidal in vivo than flu 400 mg/d *(CID 45:76&81, 2007)*. Use of lipid-based ampho B associated with lower mortality compared to ampho B deoxycholate in solid organ transplant recipients *(CID 48:1566, 2009)*. Monitor 5-FC levels: peak 70 -80 mg/L, trough 30 -40 mg/L. Higher levels assoc. with bone marrow toxicity. No difference in outcome if given IV or po *(AAC 51:1038, 2007)*. If normal mental status, >20 cells/mm³ CSF, & CSF CRAG <1:1024, flu alone may be reasonable. Failure of flu may rarely be due to resistant organism, especially if burden of organism high at initiation of Rx. Although 200 mg qd = 400 mg qd of flu: median survival 76 & 82 days respectively, authors prefer 400 mg po qd *(BMC Infect Dis 6:118, 2006)*. *(Continued on next page)*

[3] Some experts would reduce to 25 mg per kg q6h
[4] Flucytosine = 5-FC

See page 2 for abbreviations. All dosage recommendations are for adults (unless otherwise indicated) and assume normal renal function

TABLE 11A (9)

TYPE OF INFECTION/ORGANISM/ SITE OF INFECTION	ANTIMICROBIAL AGENTS OF CHOICE		COMMENTS
	PRIMARY	ALTERNATIVE	
Cryptococcosis/ HIV+/AIDS: Cryptococcemia and/or Meningitis *(continued)*			
			(Continued from previous page) Trend toward improved outcomes with fluconazole 400-800 mg combined with ampho B versus ampho B alone in AIDS patients *(CID 48:1775, 2009)*. Role of other azoles uncertain: successful outcomes were observed in 14/29 (48%) subjects with cryptococcal meningitis treated with posaconazole *(JAC 56:745, 2005)*. Voriconazole also may be effective. Survival probably improved with ART but IRIS may complicate its use. There is considerable controversy as to the timing of initiation of ART *(see CID 50:1532, 2010 and CID 51: 984, 985, 986, 987, 2010)*. One study suggests higher mortality with initiation of ART within 72 hrs of diagnosis *(CID 50:1532, 2010)*, but the generalization of this study is an issue. Among others, most authorities continue to recommend ART within 2-6 wks of diagnosis.
Suppression (chronic maintenance therapy) Discontinuation of antifungal rx can be considered among pts who remain asymptomatic, with CD4 >100–200/mm³ for ≥6 months. Some perform a lumbar puncture before discontinuation of maintenance rx. Reappearance of pos. serum CRAG may predict relapse	**Fluconazole** 200 mg/day po [If CD4 count rises to >100/mm³ with effective antiretroviral rx, some authorities recommend dc suppressive rx. *See www.hivatis.org*. Authors would only dc if CSF culture negative.]	**Itraconazole** 200 mg po q12h if flu intolerant or failure. No data on Vori for maintenance.	Itraconazole less effective than fluconazole & not recommended because of higher relapse rate (23% vs 4%). Recurrence rate of 0.4 to 3.9 per 100 patient-years with discontinuation of suppressive therapy in 100 patients on ARV with CD4 >100 cells/mm³.
Dermatophytosis *(See Mycopathologia 166:353, 2008)*			
Onychomycosis (Tinea unguium) *(NEJM 360:2108, 2009)* Ciclopirox olamine 8% lacquer daily for 48 weeks; best suited for superficial and distal infections (overall cure rates of approx 30%).	**Fingernail Rx Options:** **Terbinafine**[5] 250 mg po q24h [children <20 kg: 67.5 mg/day, 20–40 kg: 125 mg/day, >40 kg: 250 mg/day] x 6 wk (79% effective) OR **Itraconazole**[6] 200 mg po q24h x 3 mo.[NAI] OR **Itraconazole** 200 mg po bid x 1 wk/mo x 2 mo OR **Fluconazole** 150–300 mg po q wk x 3–6 mo.[NAI]		**Toenail Rx Options:** **Terbinafine**[5] 250 mg po q24h [children <20 kg: 67.5 mg/day, 20–40 kg: 125 mg/day, >40 kg: 250 mg/day] x 12 wks (76% effective) OR **Itraconazole** 200 mg po q24h x 3 mo (59% effective) OR **Itraconazole** 200 mg bid x 1 wk/mo. x 3–4 mo (63% effective)[NAI] OR **Fluconazole** 150–300 mg po q wk x 6–12 mo (48% effective)[NAI]
Tinea capitis ("ringworm") (Trichophyton tonsurans, Microsporum canis, N. America; other sp. elsewhere) *(PIDJ 18:191, 1999)*	**Terbinafine**[5] 250 mg po q 24h x 2-4 wks (adults); 5 mg/kg/day x 4 wks (children).	**Itraconazole**[6] 5 mg/kg per day x 4 wks[NFDA]. **Fluconazole** 6 mg/kg q wk x 8-12 wk.[NAI] Cap at 150 mg po q wk for adults **Griseofulvin:** adults 500 mg po q24h x 6-8 wks, children 10–20 mg/kg per day until hair regrows.	Durations of therapy are for T. tonsurans; treat for approx. twice as long for M. canis. All agents with similar cure rates (60-100%) in clinical studies. Addition of topical ketoconazole or selenium sulfate shampoo reduces transmissibility *(Int J Dermatol 39:261, 2000)*

[5] **Serious but rare cases of hepatic failure** have been reported in pts receiving terbinafine & should not be used in those with chronic or active liver disease *(see Table 11B, page 116)*.
[6] Use of itraconazole has been associated with myocardial dysfunction and with onset of congestive heart failure.

See page 2 for abbreviations. All dosage recommendations are for adults (unless otherwise indicated) and assume normal renal function

TABLE 11A (10)

TYPE OF INFECTION/ORGANISM/ SITE OF INFECTION	ANTIMICROBIAL AGENTS OF CHOICE		COMMENTS
	PRIMARY	ALTERNATIVE	
Dermatophytosis *(continued)*			
Tinea corporis, cruris, or pedis (Trichophyton rubrum, T. mentagrophytes, Epidermophyton floccosum) "Athlete's foot, jock itch," and ringworm	**Topical rx:** Generally applied 2x/day. Available as creams, ointments, sprays, by prescription & "over the counter." Apply 2x/day for 2–3 wks. Recommend: Lotrimin Ultra or Lamisil AT; contain butenafine & terbinafine—both are fungicidal	**Terbinafine** 250 mg po q24h x 2 wks[NAI] OR **ketoconazole** 200 mg po q24h x 4 wks OR **fluconazole** 150 mg po 1x/wk for 2–4 wks[NAI] **Griseofulvin:** adults 500 mg po q24h times 4–6 wks, children 10–20 mg/kg per day. Duration: 2-4 wks for corporis, 4-8 wks for pedis.	**Keto** po often effective in severe recalcitrant infection. Follow for hepatotoxicity; many drug-drug interactions.
Tinea versicolor (Malassezia furfur or Pityrosporum orbiculare) Rule out erythrasma—*see Table 1A, page 52*	**Ketoconazole** (400 mg po single dose[NAI] or (200 mg q24h x 7 days) or (2% cream 1x q24h x 2 wks)	**Fluconazole** 400 mg po single dose or **Itraconazole** 400 mg po q24h x 3–7 days	**Keto** (po) times 1 dose was 97% effective in 1 study. Another alternative: **Selenium sulfide** (Selsun), 2.5% lotion, apply as lather, leave on 10 min then wash off, 1/day x 7 day or 3–5/wk times 2–4 wks
Fusariosis Third most common cause of invasive mould infections, after *Aspergillus* and *Mucorales* and related molds, in patients with hematologic malignancies *(Mycoses 52:197, 2009)*. Pneumonia, skin infections, bone and joint infections, and disseminated disease occur in severely immunocompromised patients. In contrast to other moulds, blood cultures are frequently positive. *Fusarium solani*, *F. oxysporum*, *F. verticillioides* and *F. moniliforme* account for approx. 90% of isolates (*Clin Micro Rev 20: 695, 2007*) Frequently fatal, outcome depends on decreasing the level of immunosuppression.			
	Lipid-based ampho B 5-10 mg/kg/d; OR **Ampho B** 1-1.5 mg/kg/d.	**Posaconazole** 400 mg po bid with meals (if not taking meals, 200 mg qid); OR **Voriconazole** IV: 6 mg per kg q12h times 1 day, then 4 mg per kg q12h; PO: 400 mg q12h, then 200 mg q12h. *See comments.*	**Surgical debridement** for localized disease. *Fusarium* spp. resistance to most antifungal agents, including echinocandins. *F. solani* and *F. verticillioides* typically are resistant to azoles. *F. oxysporum* and *F. moniliforme* may be susceptible to voriconazole and posaconazole. Role of combination therapy not well defined but case reports of response *(Mycoses 50: 227, 2007)*. Outcome dependent on reduction or discontinuation of immunosuppression. Duration of therapy depends on response; long-term suppressive therapy for patients remaining on immunosuppressive therapy.
Histoplasmosis (Histoplasma capsulatum): *See IDSA Guideline: CID 45:807, 2007.* Best diagnostic test is urinary, serum, or CSF histoplasma antigen: MiraVista Diagnostics (1-866-647-2847)			
Acute pulmonary histoplasmosis	**Mild to moderate disease, symptoms <4 wk:** No rx; If symptoms last over one month: **Itraconazole** 200 mg po tid for 3 days then once or twice daily for 6-12 wk. **Moderately severe or severe: Liposomal ampho B,** 3-5 mg/kg/d or **ABLC** 5 mg/kg/d IV or ampho B 0.7-1.0 mg/kg/d for 1-2 wk, then itra 200 mg tid for 3 days, then bid for 12 wk. **+ methylprednisolone** 0.5-1.0 mg/kg/d for 1-2 wk.		Ampho B for patients at low risk of nephrotoxicity.
Chronic cavitary pulmonary histoplasmosis	**Itra** 200 mg po tid for 3 days then once or twice daily for at least 12 mo (some prefer 18-24 mo).		Document therapeutic itraconazole blood levels at 2 wk. Relapses occur in 9-15% of patients.
Mediastinal lymphadenitis, mediastinal granuloma, pericarditis; and rheumatologic syndromes	**Mild cases:** Antifungal therapy not indicated. Nonsteroidal anti-inflammatory drug for pericarditis or rheumatologic syndromes. If no response to non-steroidals, **Prednisone** 0.5-1.0 mg/kg/d tapered over 1-2 weeks for 1) pericarditis with hemodynamic compromise, 2) lymphadenitis with obstruction or compression syndromes, or 3) severe rheumatologic syndromes. **Itra** 200 mg po once or twice daily for 6-12 wk for moderately severe to severe cases, or if prednisone is administered.		Check itra blood levels to document therapeutic concentrations.

See page 2 for abbreviations. All dosage recommendations are for adults (unless otherwise indicated) and assume normal renal function

TABLE 11A (11)

TYPE OF INFECTION/ORGANISM/ SITE OF INFECTION	ANTIMICROBIAL AGENTS OF CHOICE		COMMENTS
	PRIMARY	ALTERNATIVE	
Histoplasmosis *(continued)*			
Progressive disseminated histoplasmosis	**Mild to moderate disease: itra** 200 mg po tid for 3 days then bid for at least 12 mo **Moderately severe to severe disease: Liposomal ampho B,** 3 mg/kg/d or **ABLC** 5 mg/kg/d for 1-2 weeks then **itra** 200 mg tid for 3 days, then bid for at least 12 mo.		**Ampho B** 0.7-1.0 mg/kg/d may be used for patients at low risk of nephrotoxicity. Confirm therapeutic itra blood levels. Azoles are teratogenic; itra should be avoided in pregnancy; use a lipid ampho formulation. Urinary antigen levels useful for monitoring response to therapy and relapse
CNS histoplasmosis	**Liposomal ampho B,** 5 mg/kg/d, for a total of 175 mg/kg over 4-6 wk, then **itra** 200 mg 2-3x a day for at least 12 mo. Vori likely effective for CNS disease or Itra failures. *(Arch Neurology 65: 666, 2008; J Antimicro Chemo 57:1235, 2006).*		Monitor CNS histo antigen, monitor itra blood levels. PCR may be better for Dx than histo antigen. Absorption of Itra (check levels) and CNS penetration may be an issue; case reports of success with Fluconazole *(Braz J Infect Dis 12:555, 2008)* and Posaconazole *(Drugs 65:1553, 2005)* following Ampho B therapy.
Prophylaxis (immunocompromised patients)	**Itra** 200 mg po daily		Consider primary **prophylaxis in HIV-infected** patients with < 150 CD4 cells/mm³ in high prevalence areas. Secondary prophylaxis (i.e., suppressive therapy) indicated in HIV-infected patients with < 150 CD4 cells/mm³ and other immunocompromised patients in who immunosuppression cannot be reversed
Madura foot *(See Nocardia & Scedosporium)*			
Mucormycosis & other related species—Rhizopus, Rhizomucor, Absidia *(CID 41:521, 2005).* Rhinocerebral, pulmonary invasive. Key to successful rx: early dx with symptoms suggestive of sinusitis (or lateral facial pain or numbness): think mucor with palatal ulcers, &/or black eschars, onset unilateral blindness in immunocompromised or diabetic pt. Rapidly fatal without rx. Dx by culture of tissue or stain: wide ribbon-like, non-septated with variation in diameter & right angle branching *(ClinMicro&Infect 12:7, 2006).*	**Liposomal ampho B** 5-10 mg/kg/day; OR **Ampho B** 1-1.5 mg/kg/day.	**Posaconazole** 400 mg po bid with meals (if not taking meals, 200 mg po qid)[NAI].	**Combination therapy** of ampho B or a lipid-based amphoB plus caspofungin associated with improved cure rates (100% vs 45%) in one small retrospective study (6 combo therapy patients. 31 monotherapy, historical control patients); ampho B lipid complex (ABLC) monotherapy relatively ineffective with 20% success rate vs 69% for other polyenes *(CID 47:364, 2008).* Complete or partial response rates of 60-80% in posaconazole salvage protocols *(JAC 61, Suppl 1, i35, 2008).* Resistant to voriconazole: prolonged use of voriconazole prophylaxis predisposes to zygomycetes infections. Total duration of therapy based on response: continue therapy until 1) resolution of clinical signs and symptoms of infection, 2) resolution or stabilization of radiographic abnormalities; and 3) resolution of underlying immunosuppression. Posaconazole for secondary prophylaxis for those on immunosuppressive therapy *(CID 48:1743, 2009).*
Paracoccidioidomycosis (South American blastomycosis) P. brasiliensis *(Dermatol Clin 26:257, 2008; Expert Rev Anti Infect Ther 6:251, 2008).* Important cause of death from fungal infection in HIV-infected patients in Brazil *(Mem Inst Oswaldo Cruz 104:513, 2009).*	**TMP/SMX** 800/160 mg bid-tid for 30 days, then 400/80 mg/day indefinitely (up to 3-5 years); OR **Itraconazole** (100 or 200 mg orally daily)	**Ketoconazole** 200-400 mg daily for 6-18 months; OR **Ampho B** total dose > 30 mg/kg	Improvement in >90% pts on itra or keto.[NAI] **Ampho B** reserved for severe cases and for those intolerant to other agents. TMP-SMX suppression life-long in HIV+.
Lobomycosis (keloidal blastomycosis)/ P. loboi	**Surgical excision**, **clofazimine** or **itraconazole**.		
Penicilliosis (Penicillium marneffei): Common disseminated fungal infection in AIDS pts in SE Asia (esp. Thailand & Vietnam).	**Ampho B** 0.5–1 mg/kg per day times 2 wks followed by **itraconazole** 400 mg/day for 10 wks followed by 200 mg/day po **indefinitely for HIV-infected pts**.	For less sick patients **Itra** 200 mg po tid x 3 days, then 200 mg po bid x 12 wks, then 200 mg po q24h.[7] (IV if unable to take po)	3rd most common OI in AIDS pts in SE Asia following TBc and cryptococcal meningitis. Prolonged fever, lymphadenopathy, hepatomegaly. Skin nodules are umbilicated (mimic cryptococcal infection or molluscum contagiosum). Preliminary data suggests vori effective: *CID 43:1060, 2006.*

[7] **Oral solution preferred to tablets because of ↑ absorption** *(see Table 11B, page 114).*

See page 2 for abbreviations. All dosage recommendations are for adults (unless otherwise indicated) and assume normal renal function

TABLE 11A (12)

TYPE OF INFECTION/ORGANISM/ SITE OF INFECTION	ANTIMICROBIAL AGENTS OF CHOICE		COMMENTS
	PRIMARY	ALTERNATIVE	
Phaeohyphomycosis, Black molds, Dematiaceous fungi *(See CID 48:1033, 2009)* Sinuses, skin, bone & joint, brain abscess, endocarditis, emerging especially in HSCT pts with disseminated disease. **Scedosporium prolificans**, Bipolaris, Wangiella, Curvularia, Exophiala, Phialemonium, Scytalidium, Alternaria.	**Surgery + itraconazole** 400 mg/day po, duration not defined, probably 6 mo[NAI]	Case report of success with **voriconazole + terbinafine** *(Scand J Infect Dis 39:87, 2007)*; OR **itraconazole + terbinafine** synergistic against S. prolificans. No clinical data & combination could show ↑ toxicity *(see Table 11B, page 114)*.	**Posaconazole** successful in case of brain abscess *(CID 34:1648, 2002)* and refractory infection *(Mycosis: 519, 2006)*. **Notoriously resistant to antifungal rx including amphotericin & azoles.** 44% of patients in compassionate use/salvage therapy study responded to voriconazole *(AAC 52:1743, 2008)*. >80% mortality in immunocompromised hosts.
Scedosporium apiospermum (Pseudallescheria boydii) (not considered a true dematiaceous mold) *(Medicine 81:333, 2002)* Skin, subcut (Madura foot), brain abscess, recurrent meningitis. May appear after near-drowning incidents. Also emerging especially in hematopoietic stem cell transplant (HSCT) pts with disseminated disease	**Voriconazole** 6 mg/kg IV q12h on day 1, then either (4 mg/kg IV q12h) or (200 mg po q12h for body weight ≥40 kg, but 100 mg po q12h for body weight <40 kg) *(AAC 52:1743, 2008)*. 300 mg bid if serum concentrations are subtherapeutic, i.e., < 1 mcg/mL *(CID 46:201, 2008)*.	Surgery + **itraconazole** 200 mg po bid until clinically well.[NAI] (Many species now resistant or refractory to itra); OR **Posa** 400 mg po bid with meals (if not taking meals, 200 mg po qid).	**Resistant to many antifungal drugs including amphotericin**. In vitro voriconazole more active than itra and posaconazole in vitro *(Clin Microbiol Rev 21:157, 2008)*. Case reports of successful rx of disseminated and CNS disease with voriconazole *(AAC 52:1743, 2008)*. Posaconazole active *in vitro* and successful in several case reports
Sporotrichosis *IDSA Guideline: CID 45:1255, 2007.*			
Cutaneous/Lymphocutaneous	**Itraconazole** po 200 mg/day for 2-4 wks after all lesions resolved, usually 3-6 mos.	If no response, **itra** 200 mg po bid or **terbinafine** 500 mg po bid or **SSKI** 5 drops (eye drops) tid & increase to 40-50 drops tid	Fluconazole 400-800 mg daily only if no response to primary or alternative suggestions. Pregnancy or nursing: local hyperthermia *(see below)*.
Osteoarticular	**Itra** 200 mg po bid x 12 mos.	**Liposomal ampho B** 3-5 mg/kg/d IV or **ABLC** 5 mg/kg/d IV or **ampho B deoxycholate** 0.7-1 mg/kg IV daily; if response, change to **itra** 200 mg po bid x total 12 mos.	After 2 wks of therapy, document adequate serum levels of itraconazole.
Pulmonary	If severe, **lipid ampho B** 3-5 mg/kg IV or **standard ampho B** 0.7-1 mg/kg IV once daily until response, then **itra** 200 mg po bid. Total of 12 mos.	Less severe: **itraconazole** 200 mg po bid x 12 mos.	After 2 weeks of therapy document adequate serum levels of itra. Surgical resection plus ampho B for localized pulmonary disease.
Meningeal or Disseminated	**Lipid ampho B** 5 mg/kg IV once daily x 4-6 wks, then—if better—**itra** 200 mg po bid for total of 12 mos.	AIDS/Other immunosuppressed pts: chronic therapy with **itra** 200 mg po once daily.	After 2 weeks, document adequate serum levels of itra.
Pregnancy and children	**Pregnancy:** Cutaneous—local hyperthermia. Severe: **lipid ampho B** 3-5 mg/kg IV once daily. **Avoid itraconazole**.	**Children:** Cutaneous: **Itra** 6-10 mg/kg (max of 400 mg) daily. Alternative is **SSKI** 1 drop tid increasing to max of 1 drop/kg or 40-50 drops tid/day, whichever is lowest.	For children with disseminated sporotrichosis: Standard ampho B 0.7 mg/kg IV once daily & after response, itra 6-10 mg/kg (max 400 mg) once daily.

See page 2 for abbreviations. All dosage recommendations are for adults (unless otherwise indicated, and assume normal renal function

TABLE 11B – ANTIFUNGAL DRUGS: DOSAGE, ADVERSE EFFECTS, COMMENTS

DRUG NAME, GENERIC (TRADE)/USUAL DOSAGE	ADVERSE EFFECTS/COMMENTS
Non-lipid amphotericin B deoxycholate (Fungizone): 0.3–1 mg/kg per day as single infusion **Ampho B predictably not active vs. Scedosporium, Candida lusitaniae & Aspergillus terreus** *(Table 11C, page 117)*	**Admin:** Ampho B is a colloidal suspension that must be prepared in electrolyte-free D5W at 0.1 mg/mL to avoid precipitation. No need to protect suspensions from light. Infusions cause chills/fever, myalgia, anorexia, nausea, rarely hemodynamic collapse/hypotension. Postulated due to proinflammatory cytokines, doesn't appear to be histamine release *(Pharmacol 23:966, 2003)*. Infusion duration usu. 4+ hrs. No difference found in 1 vs 4 hr infus. except chills/fever occurred sooner with 1 hr infus. Febrile reactions ↓ with repeat doses. Rare pulmonary reactions (severe dyspnea & focal infiltrates suggest pulmonary edema) assoc with rapid infus. **Severe rigors respond to meperidine (25–50 mg IV).** Premedication with acetaminophen, diphenhydramine, hydrocortisone (25–50 mg) and heparin (1000 units) had no influence on rigors/fever. If cytokine postulate correct, NSAIDs or high-dose steroids may prove efficacious but their use may risk worsening infection under rx or increased risk of **nephrotoxicity** (i.e., NSAIDs). Clinical side effects ↓ with ↑ age. **Toxicity:** Major concern is nephrotoxicity. Manifest initially by kaliuresis and hypokalemia, then fall in serum bicarbonate (may proceed to renal tubular acidosis), ↓ in renal erythropoietin and anemia, and rising BUN/serum creatinine. Hypomagnesemia may occur. Can reduce risk of renal injury by **(a) pre- & post-infusion hydration with 500 mL saline (if clinical status allows salt load), (b)** avoidance of other nephrotoxins, eg, radiocontrast, aminoglycosides, cis-platinum, **(c)** use of lipid prep of ampho B.
Lipid-based ampho B products[1]: **Amphotericin B lipid complex (ABLC) (Abelcet):** 5 mg/kg per day as single infusion	**Admin:** Consists of ampho B complexed with 2 lipid bilayer ribbons. Compared to standard ampho B, larger volume of distribution, rapid blood clearance and high tissue concentrations (liver, spleen, lung). Dosage: **5 mg/kg once daily;** infuse at 2.5 mg/kg per hr; adult and ped. dose the same. Do NOT use an in-line filter. Do not dilute with saline or mix with other drugs or electrolytes.[2] **Toxicity:** Fever and chills in 14–18%; nausea 9%, vomiting 8%; serum creatinine ↑ in 11%; renal failure 5%; anemia 4%; ↓ K 5%; rash 4%. A fatal case of fat embolism reported following ABLC infusion *(Exp Mol Path 177:246, 2004)*.
Liposomal amphotericin B (LAB, AmBisome): 1–5 mg/kg per day as single infusion.	**Admin:** Consists of vesicular bilayer liposome with ampho B intercalated within the membrane. Dosage: **3–5 mg/kg per day** IV as single dose infused over a period of approx. 120 min. If well tolerated, infusion time can be reduced to 60 min. *(see footnote[2])*. Tolerated well in elderly pts *(J Inf 50:277, 2005)*. **Major toxicity:** Gen less than ampho B. Nephrotoxicity 18.7% vs 33.7% for ampho B, chills 47% vs 75%, nausea 39.7% vs 38.7%, vomiting 31.8% vs 43.9%, rash 24% for both, ↓ Ca 18.4% vs 20.9%, ↓ K 20.4% vs 25.6%, ↓ mg 20.4% vs 25.6%. Acute infusion-related reactions common with liposomal ampho B, 20–40%. 86% occur within 5 min of infusion, incl chest pain, dyspnea, hypoxia or severe abdom, flank or leg pain; 14% dev flushing & urticaria near end of 4 hr infusion. All responded to diphenhydramine (1 mg/kg) & interruption of infusion. Reactions may be due to complement activation by liposome *(CID 36:1213, 2003)*.
Caspofungin (Cancidas) 70 mg IV on day 1 followed by 50 mg IV q24h (reduce to 35 mg IV q24h with moderate hepatic insufficiency)	An echinocandin which inhibits synthesis of β-(1,3)-D-glucan. Fungicidal against candida (MIC <2 mcg/mL) including those resistant to other antifungals & active against aspergillus (MIC 0.4–2.7 mcg/mL). Approved indications for caspo incl: empirical rx for febrile, neutropenic pts; rx of candidemia, candida intraabdominal abscesses, peritonitis, & pleural space infections; esophageal candidiasis; & invasive aspergillosis in pts refractory to or intolerant of other therapies. Serum levels on rec. dosages = peak 12, trough 1.3 (24 hrs) mcg/mL. **Toxicity:** remarkably non-toxic. Most common adverse effect: pruritus at infusion site & headache, fever, chills, vomiting, & diarrhea assoc with infusion. ↑ serum creatinine in 8% on caspo vs 21% short-course ampho B in 422 pts with candidemia *(Ln, Oct. 12, 2005, online)*. Drug metab in liver & dosage ↓ to 35 mg in moderate to severe hepatic failure. Class C for preg (embryotoxic in rats & rabbits). *See Table 22, page 200 for drug-drug interactions, esp. cyclosporine (hepatic toxicity) & tacrolimus (drug level monitoring recommended)*. Reversible thrombocytopenia reported *(Pharmacother 24:1408, 2004)*. **No drug in CSF or urine.**
Micafungin (Mycamine) 50 mg/day for prophylaxis post-bone marrow stem cell trans; 100 mg candidemia, 150 mg candida esophagitis.	The 2nd echinocandin approved by FDA for rx of esophageal candidiasis & prophylaxis against candida infections in HSCT[3] recipients. Active against most strains of candida sp. & aspergillus sp. incl those resist to fluconazole such as C. glabrata & C. krusei. No antagonism seen when combo with other antifungal drugs. No dosage adjust for severe renal failure or moderate hepatic impairment. Watch for drug-drug interactions with sirolimus or nifedipine. Micafungin well tolerated & common adverse events incl nausea 2.8%, vomiting 2.4%, & headache 2.4%. Transient ↑ LFTs, BUN, creatinine reported; rare cases of significant hepatitis & renal insufficiency. *See CID 42:1171, 2006.* **No drug in CSF or urine.**

[1] Published data from patients intolerant of or refractory to conventional ampho B deoxycholate (Amp B d). **None of the lipid ampho B preps has shown superior efficacy compared to ampho B in prospective trials (except liposomal ampho B was more effective vs ampho B in rx of disseminated histoplasmosis at 2 wks). Dosage equivalency has not been established** *(CID 36:1500, 2003)*. Nephrotoxicity ↓ with all lipid ampho B preps.

[2] Comparisons between Abelcet & AmBisome suggest higher infusion-assoc. toxicity (rigors) & febrile episodes with Abelcet (70% vs 36%) but higher frequency of mild hepatic toxicity with AmBisome (59% vs 38%, p=0.05). Mild elevations in serum creatinine were observed in 1/3 of both *(BJ Hemat 103:198, 1998; Focus on Fungal Inf #9, 1999; Bone Marrow Tx 20:39, 1997; CID 26:1383, 1998)*.

[3] HSCT = hematopoietic stem cell transplant.

TABLE 11B (2)

DRUG NAME, GENERIC (TRADE)/USUAL DOSAGE	ADVERSE EFFECTS/COMMENTS
Anidulafungin (Eraxis) For Candidemia: 200 mg IV on day 1 followed by 100 mg/day IV). Rx for EC: 100 mg IV x 1, then 50 mg IV once/d.	An echinocandin with antifungal activity (cidal) against candida sp. & aspergillus sp. including ampho B- & triazole-resistant strains. FDA approved for treatment of esophageal candidiasis (EC), candidemia, and other complicated Candida infections. Effective in clinical trials of esophageal candidiasis & in 1 trial was superior to fluconazole in rx of invasive candidiasis/candidemia in 245 pts (75.6% vs 60.2%). Like other echinocandins, remarkably non-toxic; most common side-effects: nausea, vomiting, ↓ mg, ↓ K & headache in 11–13% of pts. No dose adjustments for renal or hepatic insufficiency. *See CID 43:215, 2006.* **No drug in CSF or urine.**
Fluconazole (Diflucan) 100 mg tabs 150 mg tabs 200 mg tabs 400 mg IV Oral suspension: 50 mg per 5 mL.	IV=oral dose because of excellent bioavailability. **Pharmacology:** absorbed po, water solubility enables IV. For peak serum levels *(see Table 9A, page 82)*. T½ 30hr (range 20–50 hr). 12% protein bound. **CSF levels 50–90% of serum in normals,** ↑ in meningitis. No effect on mammalian steroid metabolism. **Drug-drug interactions common, see *Table* 22.** Side-effects overall 16% [more common in HIV+ pts (21%)]. Nausea 3.7%, headache 1.9%, skin rash 1.8%, abdominal pain 1.7%, vomiting 1.7%, diarrhea 1.5%, ↑ SGOT 20%. Alopecia (scalp, pubic crest) in 12–20% pts on ≥400 mg po q24h after median of 3 mo (reversible in approx. 6mo). Rare: severe hepatotoxicity *(CID 41:301, 2005)*, exfoliative dermatitis. **Note: Candida krusei and Candida glabrata resistant to Flu.**
Flucytosine (Ancobon) 500 mg cap	AEs: Overall 30%. GI 6% (diarrhea, anorexia, nausea, vomiting); hematologic 22% [leukopenia, thrombocytopenia, when serum level >100 mcg/mL (esp. in azotemic pts)]; hepatotoxicity (asymptomatic ↑ SGOT, reversible); skin rash 7%; aplastic anemia (rare—2 or 3 cases). False ↑ in serum creatinine on EKTACHEM analyzer.
Griseofulvin (Fulvicin, Grifulvin, Grisactin) 500 mg, susp 125 mg/mL.	Photosensitivity, urticaria, GI upset, fatigue, leukopenia (rare). Interferes with warfarin drugs. Increases blood and urine porphyrins, should not be used in patients with porphyria. Minor disulfiram-like reactions. Exacerbation of systemic lupus erythematosus.
Imidazoles, topical For vaginal and/or skin use	Not recommended in 1st trimester of pregnancy. Local reactions: 0.5-1.5%: dyspareunia, mild vaginal or vulvar erythema, burning, pruritus, urticaria, rash. Rarely similar symptoms in sexual partner.
Itraconazole (Sporanox) 100 mg cap 10 mg/mL oral solution IV usual dose 200 mg bid x 4 doses followed by 200 mg q24h for a max of 14 days	**Itraconazole tablet & solution forms not interchangeable, solution preferred.** Many authorities recommend measuring drug serum concentration after 2 wk to ensure satisfactory absorption. To obtain highest plasma concentration, tablet is given with food & acidic drinks (e.g., cola) while solution is taken in fasted state; under these conditions, the peak conc. of capsule is approx. 3 mcg/mL & of solution 5.4 mcg/mL. Peak levels reached faster (2.2 vs 5 hrs) with solution. **Peak plasma concentrations after IV injection (200 mg) compared to oral capsule (200 mg): 2.8 mcg/mL (on day 7 of rx) vs 2 mcg/mL (on day 36 of rx).** Protein-binding for both preparations is over 99%, which explains virtual absence of penetration into CSF **(do not use to treat meningitis).** Adverse effects: dose-related nausea 10%, diarrhea 8%, vomiting 6%, & abdominal discomfort 5.7%. Allergic rash 8.6%, ↑ bilirubin 6%, edema 3.5%, & hepatitis 2.7% reported. ↑ doses may produce hypokalemia 8% & ↑ blood pressure 3.2%. Delirium, peripheral neuropathy & tremor reported *(J Neur Neurosurg Psych 81:327, 2010)*. **Reported to produce impairment in cardiac function.** Severe liver failure req transplant in pts receiving pulse rx for onychomycosis: FDA reports 24 cases with 11 deaths out of 50 mill people who received the drug prior to 2001. Other concern, as with fluconazole and ketoconazole, is **drug-drug interactions; see *Table* 22.** Some can be life-threatening.
Ketoconazole (Nizoral) 200 mg tab	Gastric acid required for absorption—cimetidine, omeprazole, antacids block absorption. In achlorhydria, dissolve tablet in 4 mL 0.2N HCl, drink with a straw. Coca-Cola ↑ absorption by 65%. CSF levels "none." **Drug-drug interactions important, see *Table* 22. Some interactions can be life-threatening. Dose- dependent nausea and vomiting.** Liver toxicity of hepatocellular type reported in about 1:10,000 exposed pts—usually after several days to weeks of exposure. At doses of ≥800 mg per day serum testosterone and plasma cortisol levels fall. With high doses, adrenal (Addisonian) crisis reported.
Miconazole (Monistat IV) 200 mg—*not available in U.S.*	IV miconazole indicated in patient critically ill with Scedosporium (Pseudallescheria boydii) infection. Very toxic due to vehicle needed to get drug into solution.
Nystatin (Mycostatin) 30 gm cream 500,000 units oral tab	Topical: virtually no adverse effects. Less effective than imidazoles and triazoles. PO: large doses give occasional GI distress and diarrhea.

See page 2 for abbreviations. All dosage recommendations are for adults (unless otherwise indicated) and assume normal renal function

TABLE 11B (3)

DRUG NAME, GENERIC (TRADE)/USUAL DOSAGE	ADVERSE EFFECTS/COMMENTS
Posaconazole *(Noxafil)* 400 mg po bid with meals (if not taking meals, 200 mg qid). 200 mg po TID (with food) for prophylaxis. 40 mg/mL suspension. **Takes 7-10 days to achieve steady state**. No IV formulation.	An oral triazole with activity against a wide range of fungi refractory to other antifungal rx including: aspergillosis, zygomycosis, fusariosis, Scedosporium (Pseudallescheria), phaeohyphomycosis, histoplasmosis, refractory candidiasis, refractory coccidioidomycosis, refractory cryptococcosis, & refractory chromoblastomycosis. **Should be taken with high fat meal for maximum absorption.** Approved for prophylaxis *(NEJM 356:348, 2007)*. Clinical response in 75% of 176 AIDS pts with azole-refractory oral/esophageal candidiasis. Posaconazole has similar toxicities as other triazoles: nausea 9%, vomiting 6%, abd. pain 5%, headache 5%, diarrhea, ↑ ALT, AST, & rash (3% each). In pts rx for >6 mos., serious side-effects have included adrenal insufficiency, nephrotoxicity, & QTc interval prolongation. Significant drug-drug interactions; inhibits CYP3A4 *(see Table 22)*. *(See Drugs 65:1552, 2005)*
Terbinafine (Lamisil) 250 mg tab	In pts given terbinafine for onychomycosis, rare cases (8) of idiosyncratic & symptomatic hepatic injury & more rarely liver failure leading to death or liver transplant. The drug is **not recommended** for pts with **chronic or active liver disease;** hepatotoxicity may occur in pts with or without pre-existing disease. Pretreatment serum transaminases (ALT & AST) advised & alternate rx used for those with abnormal levels. Pts started on terbinafine should be warned about symptoms suggesting liver dysfunction (persistent nausea, anorexia, fatigue, vomiting, RUQ pain, jaundice, dark urine or pale stools). If symptoms develop, drug should be discontinued & liver function immediately evaluated. In controlled trials, changes in ocular lens and retina reported—clinical significance unknown. Major drug-drug interaction is 100% ↑ in rate of clearance by rifampin. AEs: usually mild, transient and rarely caused discontinuation of rx. % with AE, terbinafine vs placebo: nausea/diarrhea 2.6–5.6 vs 2.9; rash 5.6 vs 2.2; taste abnormality 2.8 vs 0.7. Inhibits CYP2D6 enzymes *(see Table 22)*. An acute generalized exanthematous pustulosis and subacute cutaneous lupus erythematosus reported.
Voriconazole (Vfend) **IV:** Loading dose 6 mg per kg q12h times 1 day, then 4 mg per kg q12h IV for invasive aspergillus & serious mold infections; **3 mg per kg IV q12h** for serious candida infections. **Oral: >40 kg body weight:** 400 mg po q12h, then 200 mg po q12h. **<40 kg body weight:** 200 mg po q12h, then 100 mg po q12h **Take oral dose 1 hour before or 1 hour after eating**. Oral suspension (40 mg per mL). Oral suspension dosing: Same as for oral tabs. Reduce to ½ maintenance dose for moderate hepatic insufficiency	A triazole with activity against Aspergillus sp., **including Ampho resistant strains of A. terreus.** Active vs Candida sp. (including krusei), Fusarium sp., & various molds. Steady state serum levels reach 2.5–4 mcg per mL. Up to 20% of patients with subtherapeutic levels with oral administration: check levels for suspected treatment failure, life threatening infections. 300 mg bid oral dose or 8 mg/kg/d IV dose may be required to achieve target steady-state drug concentrations of 1-6 mcg/mL. Toxicity similar to other azoles/triazoles including uncommon serious hepatic toxicity (hepatitis, cholestasis & fulminant hepatic failure. Liver function tests should be monitored during rx & drug dc'd if abnormalities develop. Rash reported in up to 20%, occ. photosensitivity & rare Stevens-Johnson, hallucinations & anaphylactoid infusion reactions with fever and hypertension. 1 case of QT prolongation with ventricular tachycardia in a 15 y/o pt with ALL reported. **Approx. 21% experience a transient visual disturbance** following IV or po ("altered/enhanced visual perception", blurred or colored visual change or photophobia) within 30–60 minutes. Visual changes resolve within 30–60 min. after administration & are attenuated with repeated doses **(do not drive at night for outpatient rx)**. Persistent visual changes occur rarely. Cause unknown. In patients with ClCr <50 mL per min., the drug should be given orally, not IV, since the intravenous vehicle (SBECD-sulfobutylether-B cyclodextrin) may accumulate. Cyclodextrin couses vacuoles in cells of urinary tract in animals *(Eur J Med Res 7:242, 2002)*. Hallucinations, hypoglycemia, electrolyte disturbance & pneumonitis attributed to ↑ drug concentrations. Potential for drug-drug interactions high—*see Table 22*. **NOTE: Not in urine in active form. No activity vs. zygomycetes, e.g., mucor.**

See page 2 for abbreviations. All dosage recommendations are for adults (unless otherwise indicated) and assume normal renal function

Table 11C – AT A GLANCE SUMMARY OF SUGGESTED ANTIFUNGAL DRUGS AGAINST TREATABLE PATHOGENIC FUNGI

Microorganism	Antifungal[1, 2, 3, 4]					
	Fluconazole[5]	Itraconazole	Voriconazole	Posaconazole	Echinocandin[6]	Polyenes
Candida albicans	+++	+++	+++	+++	+++	+++
Candida dubliniensis	+++	+++	+++	+++	+++	+++
Candida glabrata	±	±	+	+	+++	++
Candida tropicalis	+++	+++	+++	+++	+++	+++
Candida parapsilosis[7]	+++	+++	+++	+++	−+ (higher MIC)	+++
Candida krusei	-	+	++	++	+++	++
Candida guilliermondii	+++	+++	+++	+++	−+ (higher MIC)	++
Candida lusitaniae	+	+	++	++	++	-[8]
Cryptococcus neoformans	+++	+	+++	+++	-	+++
Aspergillus fumigatus[9]	-	++	+++	+++	++	++
Aspergillus flavus[9]	-	++	+++	+++	++	++ (higher MIC)
Aspergillus terreus	-	++	+++	+++	++	-
Fusarium sp.	-	±	++	++	-	++ (lipid formulations)
Scedosporium apiospermum (*Pseudoallescheria boydii*)	-	-	−++	+++	-	-
Scedosporium prolificans[10]	-	-	±	±	-	-
Trichosporon spp.	±	+	++	++	-	+
Zygomycetes (e.g., *Absidia*, *Mucor*, *Rhizopus*)	-	-	-	+++	-	+++ (lipid formulations)
Dematiaceous molds[11] (e.g., *Alternaria*, *Bipolaris*, *Curvularia*, *Exophiala*)	-	++	++−	+++	+	+
Dimorphic Fungi						
Blastomyces dermatitidis	+	+−±	++	++	-	+++
Coccidioides immitis/posadasii	+++	++	++	++	-	+++
Histoplasma capsulatum	+	+++	++	++	-	+++
Sporothrix schenckii	-	++	-	+	-	+++

\- = no activity; ± = possibly activity; + = active, 3rd line therapy (least active clinically)
++ = Active, 2nd line therapy (less active clinically); +++ = Active, 1st line therapy (usually active clinically)

[1] Minimum inhibitory concentration values do not always predict clinical outcome.
[2] Echinocandins, voriconazole, posaconazole and polyenes have poor urine penetration.
[3] During severe immune suppression, success requires immune reconstitution.
[4] **Flucytosine** has activity against *Candida* sp., *Cryptococcus* sp., and dematiaceous molds, but is primarily used in combination therapy.
[5] For infections secondary to *Candida* sp., patients with prior triazole therapy have higher likelihood of triazole resistance.
[6] Echinocandin pharmacodynamics, *see JAC 65:1108, 2010.*
[7] Successful treatment of infections from *Candida parapsilosis* requires removal of foreign body or intravascular device.
[8] Treatment failures reported, even for susceptible strains.
[9] Lipid formulations of amphotericin may have greater activity against *A. fumigatus* and *A. flavus* (+++).
[10] *Scedosporium prolificans* is poorly susceptible to single agents and may require combination therapy (e.g., addition of terbinafine).
[11] Infections from zygomycetes, some *Aspergillus* sp., and dematiaceous molds often require surgical debridement.

TABLE 12A – TREATMENT OF MYCOBACTERIAL INFECTIONS*

Tuberculin skin test (TST). Same as PPD *[MMWR 52(RR-2):15, 2003]*.

Criteria for positive TST after 5 tuberculin units (intermediate PPD) read at 48–72 hours:

- ≥5 mm induration: + HIV, immunosuppressed, ≥15 mg prednisone per day, healed TBc on chest x-ray, recent close contact
- ≥10 mm induration: foreign-born, countries with high prevalence; IVD Users; low income; NH residents; chronic illness; silicosis
- ≥15 mm induration: otherwise healthy

Two-stage to detect sluggish positivity: If 1st PPD + but <10 mm, repeat intermediate PPD in 1 wk. Response to 2nd PPD can also happen if pt received BCG in childhood.

BCG vaccine as child: if ≥10 mm induration, & from country with TBc, should be attributed to M. tuberculosis. In areas of low TB prevalence, TST reactions of ≤18 mm more likely from BCG than TB *(CID 40:211, 2005)*. Prior BCG may result in booster effect in 2-stage TST *(ArIM 161:1760, 2001; Clin Micro Inf 10:980, 2005)*.

Routine anergy testing no longer recommended in HIV+ or HIV-negative patients *(JAMA 283:2003, 2000)*.

Interferon Gamma Release Assays (IGRAs): IGRAs detect sensitivities to MTBc by measuring IFN-8 release in response to MTBc antigens. Four such tests have now been approved by the U.S. FDA:

- QuantiFERON-TB (QFT)(approved 2001, but discontinued in 2005)
- QuantiFERON-TB Gold (QFT-G)(approved 2005)
- QuantiFERON-TB Gold In-Tube Test (QFT-GIT)(approved 2007)
- T-Spot (approved 2008)

QFT-G, QFT-GIT & T-Spot each measures different aspects of immune response so test results are not always interchangeable. IGRAs are relatively specific for MTBc and should not cross-react with BCG or most nontuberculous mycobacteria. CDC recommends IGRA over TST for persons unlikely to return for reading TST & for persons who have received BCG. TST is preferred in children age < 5 yrs (but IGRA is acceptable). IGRA or TST may be used without preference for recent contacts of TB with special utility for follow-up testing since IGRAs do not produce "booster effect". May also be used without preference over TBc for occupational exposures. For detailed discussion of IGRAs, see MMWR 59 (RR-5), 2010.

Nucleic acid amplification tests (NAAT) can reliably detect M. tuberculosis in clinical specimens 1 or more weeks earlier than conventional cultures. They are particularly useful in detecting M.Tbc from smear-positive specimens. Sensitivity lower in smear-negative or extrapulmonary specimens *(CID 49:46, 2009; PLoS Medicine 5:e156, 2008)*. CDC currently recommends that NAA testing be performed on at least one respiratory specimen from each patient for whom diagnosis of TB is being considered but has not yet been established, and for whom the test result would alter case management or TB control activities *(MMWR 58:7, 2009)*.

Rapid (24-hr) diagnostic tests for M. tuberculosis: (1) the Amplified Mycobacterium tuberculosis Direct Test amplifies and detects M. tuberculosis ribosomal RNA; (2) the AMPLICOR Mycobacterium tuberculosis Test amplifies and detects M. tuberculosis DNA. Both tests have sensitivities & specificities >95% in sputum samples that are AFB-positive. In negative smears, specificity remains >95% but sensitivity is 40–77% *(AJRCCM 155:1497, 1997; MMWR 58:7, 2009; CID 49:46, 2009)*. Note that MTB may grow out on standard blood agar plates in 1–2 wks *(J Clin Micro 41: 1710,2003)*.

CAUSATIVE AGENT/DISEASE	MODIFYING CIRCUMSTANCES	SUGGESTED REGIMENS	
		INITIAL THERAPY	CONTINUATION PHASE OF THERAPY
I. **Mycobacterium tuberculosis exposure but TST negative** (household members & other close contacts of potentially infectious cases)	Neonate—Rx essential	INH (10 mg/kg/ day for 3 mo)	Repeat tuberculin skin test (TST) in 3 mo. If mother's smear neg & infant's TST neg & chest x-ray (CXR) normal, stop INH. In UK, BCG is then given *(Ln 2:1479, 1990)*, unless mother HIV+. If infant's repeat TST +&/or CXR abnormal (hilar adenopathy &/or infiltrate), INH + RIF (10–20 mg/kg/day) (or SM). Total rx 6 mo. If mother is being rx, separation of infant from mother not indicated.
	Children <5 years of age—Rx indicated	As for neonate for 1st 3 mos	If repeat TST at 3 mo is negative, stop. If repeat TST +, continue INH for total of 9 mo. If INH not given initially, repeat TST at 3 mo, **if + rx** with INH for 9 mos. *(see Category II below)*.
	Older children & adults—	Risk 2–4% 1st yr	No rx

(Continued on next page)

See page 2 for abbreviations, page 127 for footnotes   * Dosages are for adults (unless otherwise indicated) and assume normal renal function   † **DOT** = directly observed therapy

TABLE 12A (2)

CAUSATIVE AGENT/DISEASE	MODIFYING CIRCUMSTANCES	SUGGESTED REGIMENS	
		INITIAL THERAPY	ALTERNATIVE
II. Treatment of latent infection with M. tuberculosis (formerly known as "prophylaxis) *(NEJM 347:1860, 2002; NEJM 350:2060, 2004; JAMA 293:2776, 2005)* **A. INH indicated due to high-risk** Assumes INH susceptibility likely. INH 54–88% effective in preventing active TB for ≥20 yr.	(1) + tuberculin reactor & HIV+ (risk of active disease 10% per yr, AIDS 170 times ↑, HIV+ 113 times ↑). Development of active Tbc in HIV+ pts after INH usually due to reinfection, not INH failure *(CID 34:386, 2002)*. (2) Newly infected persons (TST conversion in past 2 yrs—risk 3.3% 1st yr) (3) Past tuberculosis, not rx with adequate chemotherapy (INH, RIF, or alternatives) (4) + tuberculin reactors with CXR consistent with non-progressive tuberculous disease (risk 0.5–5.0% per yr) (5) + tuberculin reactors with specific predisposing conditions: illicit IV drug use *(MMWR 38:236, 1989)*, silicosis, diabetes mellitus, prolonged adrenocorticoid rx (>15 mg prednisone/day), immunosuppressive rx, hematologic diseases (Hodgkin's, leukemia), endstage renal disease, clinical condition with rapid substantial weight loss or chronic under-nutrition, previous gastrectomy *(CID 45:428, 2007)*. (6) + tuberculin reactors due to start anti-TNF-(alpha) therapy *(CID 46:1738, 2008)*. For management algorithm *see Thorax 60:800, 2005* **NOTE: For HIV, see Sanford Guide to HIV/AIDS Therapy &/or *JID 196:S35, 2007***	**INH** (5 mg/kg/day, max 300 mg/ day for adults; 10 mg/kg/day not to exceed 300 mg/day for children). May use 2x/wk INH with DOT *(MMWR 52:735, 2003)*. Optimal duration 9 mos. (includes children, HIV–, HIV+, old fibrotic lesions on chest x-ray). In some cases, 6 mos. may be given for cost-effectiveness *(AJRCCM 161:S221, 2000)*. Do not use 6 mo. regimen in HIV+ persons <18 yr, or those with fibrotic lesions on chest film *(NEJM 345:189, 2001)*. For current recommendations for monitoring hepatotoxicity on INH, *see MMWR 59:227, 2010*.	If compliance problem: **INH** by DOT[†] 15 mg/kg 2x/wk times 9 mo. 2 mo **RIF + PZA** regimen effective in HIV– and HIV+ *(AJRCCM 161:S221, 2000; JAMA 283:1445, 2000)*. **However, there are descriptions of severe & fatal hepatitis in immunocompetent pts on RIF + PZA** *(MMWR 50:289, 2001)*. Monitoring for cofactors did not seem to allow prediction of fatalities *(CID 42:346, 2006)*. Therefore, regimen is no longer recommended by CDC for LTBI *(MMWR 52:735, 2003; CID 39:488, 2004)*. Not all agree with CDC recommendation and recent study suggests short course therapy is safe with monitoring and more likely to be completed than longer therapy *(CID 43:271, 2006)*. **RIF** 600 mg/day po for 4 mo. (HIV– and HIV+). Meta-analysis suggests 3 mo of INH + RIF may be equiv to "standard" (6–12 mo) INH therapy *(CID 40:670, 2005)*. 3-4 month INH + RIF regimens also as safe and effective as 9 months INH in children *(CID 45:715, 2007)*.
B. TST positive (organisms likely to be INH-susceptible)	Age no longer considered modifying factor *(see Comments)*	**INH** (5 mg per kg per day, max. 300 mg per day for adults; 10 mg per kg per day not to exceed 300 mg per day for children). Results with 6 mos. rx not quite as effective as 12 mos. (65% vs 75% reduction in disease). 9 mos. is current recommendation. *See II.A above for details and alternate rx.*	Reanalysis of earlier studies favors **INH** prophylaxis (if INH related, hepatitis case fatality rate <1% and TB case fatality ≥6.7%, which appears to be the case) *(ArIM 150:2517, 1990)*. Recent data suggest INH prophylaxis has positive risk-benefit ratio in pts ≥35 if monitored for hepatotoxicity *(AnIM 127:1051, 1997)*. Overall risk of hepatotoxicity 0.1–0.15% *(JAMA 281:1014, 1999)*.
	Pregnancy—Any risk factors *(II.A above)*	Treat with **INH** as above. For women at risk for progression of latent to active disease, esp. those who are HIV+ or who have been recently infected, rx should not be delayed even during the first trimester.	Risk of INH hepatitis may be ↑ *(Ln 346:199, 1995)*
	Pregnancy—No risk factors	No initial rx *(see Comment)*	Delay rx until after delivery *(AJRCCM 149:1359, 1994)*
C. TST positive & drug resistance likely (For data on worldwide prevalence of drug resistance, *see NEJM 344:1294, 2001; JID 185:1197, 2002; JID 194:479, 2006; EID 13:380, 2007)*	INH-resistant (or adverse reaction to INH), RIF-sensitive organisms likely	**RIF** 600 mg per day po for 4 mos. (HIV+ or HIV–)	IDSA guideline lists rifabutin in 600 mg per day dose as another alternative; however, current recommended max. dose of rifabutin is 300 mg per day. Estimate RIF alone has protective effect of 56%; 26% of pts reported adverse effects (only 2/157 did not complete 6 mos. rx) *(AJRCCM 155:1735, 1997)*. 4 months therapy with RIF (10 mg/kg/d) produced fewer adverse effects than 9 months of INH *(AIM 149:689, 2008)*.
	INH- and RIF-resistant organisms likely	Efficacy of all regimens unproven. (**PZA** 25–30 mg per kg per day to max. of 2 gm per day + **ETB** 15–25 mg per kg per day po) times 6–12 mos.	[(**PZA** 25 mg per kg per day to max. of 2 gm per day) + (**levo** 500 mg per day or **oflox** 400 mg bid)], all po, times 6–12 mos. — PZA + oflox has been associated with asymptomatic hepatitis *(CID 24:1264, 1997)*.

See page 2 for abbreviations, page 127 for footnotes * Dosages are for adults (unless otherwise indicated) and assume normal renal function [†] **DOT** = directly observed therapy

TABLE 12A (3)

CAUSATIVE AGENT/DISEASE	MODIFYING CIRCUM-STANCES	SUGGESTED REGIMENS: INITIAL THERAPY[8] Regimen: in order of preference	Drugs	Interval/Doses[1] (min. duration)	CONTINUATION PHASE OF THERAPY[7] (in vitro susceptibility known) Regimen	Drugs	Interval/Doses[1,2] (min. duration)	Range of Total Doses (min. duration)
III. Mycobacterium tuberculosis **A. Pulmonary TB** General reference on rx in adults & children: *Ln 362: 887, 2003; MMWR 52(RR-11):1, 2003; CID 40(Suppl.1): S1, 2005.* References on transplant & other immuno-compromised pts: *CID 48:1276, 2009; CID 38:1229, 2004.* In pts with newly diagnosed HIV and TB, Rx for both should be started as soon as possible *(NEJM 362:697, 2010).*	**Rate of INH resistance known to be <4%** (drug-susceptible organisms) *[Modified from MMWR 52 (RR-11):1, 2003]*	**SEE COMMENTS FOR DOSAGE AND DIRECTLY OBSERVED THERAPY (DOT) REGIMENS**						
		1 *(See Figure 1, page 123)*	INH RIF PZA ETB	7 days per wk times 56 doses (8 wk) or 5 days per wk times 40 doses (8 wk)[3]	1a	INH/ RIF[9]	7 days per wk times 126 doses (18 wk) or 5 days per wk times 90 doses (18 wk)[3]	182–130 (26 wk)
					1b	INH/ RIF	2 times per wk times 36 doses (18 wk)	92–76 (26 wk)[4]
					1c[5]	INH/ RFP	1 time per wk times 18 doses (18 wk)	74–58 (26 wk)
Isolation essential! Pts with active TB should be isolated in single rooms, not cohorted *(MMWR 54(RR-17), 2005)*. Older observations on infectivity of susceptible & resistant M. tbc before and after rx *(ARRD 85:5111, 1962)* may not be applicable to MDR M. tbc or to the HIV+ individual. Extended isolation may be appropriate. 10% of immunocompromised pts with susceptible organisms remain culture-pos at day 60 *(CID 51:371, 2010)*.		2 *(See Figure 1, page 123)*	INH RIF PZA ETB	7 days per wk times 14 doses (2 wk), then 2 times per wk times 12 doses (6 wk) or 5 days per wk times 10 doses (2 wk)[3] then 2 times per wk times 12 doses (6 wk)	2a	INH/ RIF	2 times per wk times 36 doses (18 wk)	62–58 (26 wk)[4]
					2b[5]	INH/ RFP	1 time per wk times 18 doses (18 wk)	44–40 (26 wk)
		3 *(See Figure 1, page 123)*	INH RIF PZA ETB	3 times per wk times 24 doses (8 wk)	3a	INH/ RIF	3 times per wk times 54 doses (18 wk)	78 (26 wk)
See footnotes, page 127		4 *(See Figure 1, page 123)*	INH RIF ETB	7 days per wk times 56 doses (8 wk) or 5 days per wk times 40 doses (8 wk)[3]	4a	INH/ RIF[6]	7 days per wk times 217 doses (31 wk) or 5 days per wk times 155 doses (31 wk)[3]	273–195 (39 wk)
USE DOT REGIMENS IF POSSIBLE *(continued on next page)*					4b	INH/ RIF[6]	2 times per wk times 62 doses (31 wk)	118–102 (39 wk)

COMMENTS

Regimen*	Dose in mg per kg (max. q24h dose) INH	RIF	PZA	ETB	SM	RFB
Q24h:						
Child	10–20 (300)	10–20 (600)	15–30 (2000)	15–25	20–40 (1000)	10–20 (300)
Adult	5 (300)	10 (600)	15–30 (2000)	15–25	15 (1000)	5 (300)
2 times per wk (DOT):						
Child	20–40 (900)	10–20 (600)	50–70 (4000)	50	25–30 (1500)	10–20 (300)
Adult	15 (900)	10 (600)	50–70 (4000)	50	25–30 (1500)	5 (300)
3 times per wk (DOT):						
Child	20–40 (900)	10–20 (600)	50–70 (3000)	25–30	25–30 (1500)	NA
Adult	15 (900)	10 (600)	50–70 (3000)	25–30	25–30 (1500)	NA

Second-line anti-TB agents can be dosed as follows to facilitate DOT: Cycloserine 500–750 mg po q24h (5 times per wk)
Ethionamide 500–750 mg po q24h (5 times per wk)
Kanamycin or capreomycin 15 mg per kg IM/IV q24h (3–5 times per wk)
Ciprofloxacin 750 mg po q24h (5 times per wk)
Ofloxacin 600–800 mg po q24h (5 times per wk)
Levofloxacin 750 mg po q24h (5 times per wk)
(CID 21:1245, 1995)

Risk factors for drug-resistant (MDR) TB: Recent immigration from Latin America or Asia or living in area of ↑ resistance (≥4%) or previous rx without RIF; exposure to known MDR TB. Incidence of MDR TB in **U.S. appears** to have stabilized and may be slightly decreasing *(JAMA 278:833, 1997)*. Incidence of primary drug resistance is particularly high (>25%) in parts of China, Thailand, Russia, Estonia & Latvia *(NEJM 344:1294, 2001; NEJM 347:1850, 2002)*.

(continued on next page)

See page 2 for abbreviations, page 127 for footnotes   * Dosages are for adults (unless otherwise indicated) and assume normal renal function   [1] **DOT** = directly observed therapy

TABLE 12A (4)

CAUSATIVE AGENT/DISEASE	MODIFYING CIRCUM-STANCES	SUGGESTED REGIMEN[8]	DURATION OF TREATMENT (mo.)[9]	SPECIFIC COMMENTS[8]	COMMENTS
III. Mycobacterium tuberculosis A. Pulmonary TB *(continued from previous page)* REFERENCES: *CID 22:683, 1996; Clin Micro Rev 19:658, 2006; Med Lett 7:75, 2009*	**INH (± SM) resistance**	**RIF, PZA, ETB** (an **FQ** may strengthen the regimen for pts with extensive disease). Emergence of FQ resistance a concern (*LnID 3:432, 2003; AAC 49:3178, 2005*)	6	*(continued from previous page)* In British Medical Research Council trials, 6-mo. regimens have yielded ≥95% success rates despite resistance to INH if 4 drugs were used in the initial phase & RIF + ETB or SM was used throughout (*ARRD 133: 423, 1986*). Additional studies suggested that results were best if PZA was also used throughout the 6 mos (*ARRD 136:1339, 1987*). FQs were not employed in BMRC studies, but may strengthen the regimen for pts with more extensive disease. INH should be stopped in cases of INH resistance [*see MMWR 52(RR-11):1, 2003 for additional discussion*]. Outcome similar for drug susceptible and INH-monoresistant strains (*CID 48:179, 2009*).	*(continued from previous page)* **For MDR TB, consider rifabutin** (~30% RIF-resistant strains are rifabutin-susceptible). Note that CIP not as effective as PZA + ETB in multi-drug regimen for susceptible TB (*CID 22:287, 1996*). **Moxifloxacin, and levofloxacin have enhanced activity compared with CIP** against M. tuberculosis (*AAC 47:2442, 2003; AAC 47:3117, 2003; JAC 53:441, 2004; AAC 48:780, 2004*). FQ resistance may be seen in pts previously treated with FQ (*CID 37:1448, 2003*). **Linezolid has excellent in vitro activity, including MDR strains** (*AAC 47: 416, 2003*). Several investigational drugs with activity against MDR- and XDR-TB are undergoing clinical trials, including TMC 207, PA-824, OPC-67683 and SQ 109 (*AAC 53:849, 2009; NEJM 360:2397, 2009*). Mortality reviewed: *Ln 349:71, 1997*. Because RIF, PZA & INH all have potential for hepatotoxicity, question arises as to best method (sequential or simultaneous rechallenge) to resume Rx when clinically indicated. Recent study suggests little difference in rate of subsequent toxicity (8-13%) with either method (*CID 50:833, 2010; CID 50:840, 2010*).
Multidrug-Resistant Tuberculosis (MDR TB): Defined as resistant to at least 2 drugs including INH & RIF. Pt clusters with high mortality (*EJCMID 23: 174, 2004; MMWR 55:305, 2006; JID 194:1194, 2006; AIM 149:123, 2008*).	**Resistance to INH & RIF (± SM)**	**FQ, PZA, ETB, IA**, ± alternative agent[7]	18–24	In such cases, extended rx is needed to ↓ the risk of relapse. In cases with extensive disease, the use of an additional agent (alternative agents) may be prudent to ↓ the risk of failure & additional acquired drug resistance. Resectional surgery may be appropriate.	
	Resistance to INH, RIF (± SM), & ETB or PZA	**FQ (ETB** or **PZA** if active), **IA**, & 2 alternative agents[7]	24	Use the first-line agents to which there is susceptibility. Add 2 or more alternative agents in case of extensive disease. Surgery should be considered. Survival ↑ in pts receiving active FQ & surgical intervention (*AJRCCM 169:1103, 2004*).	
Extensively Drug-Resistant TB (XDR-TB): Defined as resistant to INH & RIF plus any FQ and at least 1 of the 3 second-line drugs: capreomycin, kanamycin or amikacin (*MMWR 56:250, 2007; LnID 9:19, 2009; CID 51:379, 2010*).	**Resistance to RIF**	**INH, ETB, FQ** supplemented with **PZA** for the first 2 mo (an IA may be included for the first 2–3 mos. for pts with extensive disease)	12–18	Q24h & 3 times per wk regimens of INH, PZA, & SM given for 9 mos. were effective in a BMRC trial (*ARRD 115:727, 1977*). However, extended use of an IA may not be feasible. It is not known if ETB would be as effective as SM in these regimens. An all-oral regimen times 12–18 mos. should be effective. But for more extensive disease &/or to shorten duration (e.g., to 12 mos.), an IA may be added in the initial 2 mos. of rx. Linezolid effective (watch for toxicity) in selected cases of MDR-TB and XDR-TB (*JAC 64:1119, 2009; CID 50:49, 2010*).	
See footnotes, page 127 Reviews of therapy for MDR TB: *JAC 54:593, 2004; Med Lett 7:75, 2009. For XDR-TB see MMWR 56:250, 2007 ; NEJM 359:563, 2008*	**XDR-TB**	*See Comments*	18-24	Therapy requires administration of ≥4–6 drugs to which infecting organism is susceptible, including multiple second-line drugs (*MMWR 56:250, 2007*). Increased mortality seen primarily in HIV+ patients. Cure with outpatient therapy likely in non-HIV+ patients when regimens of 4 or 5 or more drugs to which organism is susceptible are employed (*NEJM 359:563, 2008; CID 47:496, 2008*). Successful sputum culture conversion correlates to initial susceptibility to FQs and kanamycin (*CID 46:42, 2008*). Addition of "later generation" FQ (*Levo, Moxi or Sparfloxacin*) beneficial on meta-analysis of XDR-TB (*CID 51:6, 2010*).	

TABLE 12A (5)

CAUSATIVE AGENT/DISEASE; MODIFYING CIRCUMSTANCES	SUGGESTED REGIMENS: INITIAL THERAPY	SUGGESTED REGIMENS: CONTINUATION PHASE OF THERAPY (in vitro susceptibility known)	COMMENTS
III. Mycobacterium tuberculosis *(continued)*			
B. Extrapulmonary TB	**INH** + **RIF** (or **RFB**) + **PZA** q24h times 2 months Authors add **pyridoxine** 25–50 mg po q24h to regimens that include INH.	**INH** + **RIF** (or **RFB**)	6 mo regimens probably effective, Most experience with 9–12 mo regimens. Am Acad Ped (1994) recommends 6 mo rx for isolated cervical adenitis, renal and 12 mo for meningitis, miliary, bone/joint. DOT useful here as well as for pulmonary tuberculosis. IDSA recommends 6 mo for lymph node, pleural, pericarditis, disseminated disease, genitourinary & peritoneal TBc; 6–9 mo for bone & joint; 9-12 mo for CNS (including meningeal) TBc. Corticosteroids "strongly rec" only for pericarditis & meningeal TBc *[MMWR 52(RR-11):1, 2003]*.
C. Tuberculous meningitis Excellent summary of clinical aspects and therapy (including steroids): *CMR 21:243, 2008*	**INH** + **RIF** + **ETB** + **PZA**	May omit ETB when susceptibility to **INH** and **RIF** established. *See Table 9, page 83*, for CSF drug penetration. Initial reg of INH + RIF + SM + PZA also effective, even in patients with INH resistant organisms *(JID 192:79, 2005)*.	3 drugs often rec for initial rx; we prefer 4. May sub ethionamide for ETB. Infection with MDR TB ↑ mortality & morbidity *(CID 38:851, 2004; JID 192:79, 2005)*. Dexamethasone (for 1st mo) has been shown to ↓ complications *(Pediatrics 99:226, 1997)* & ↑ survival in pts >14 yr old *(NEJM 351:1741, 2004)*. PCR of CSF markedly ↑ diagnostic sensitivity and provides rapid dx *(Neurol 45:2228, 1995; ArNeurol 53:771, 1996)* but considerable variability in sensitivity depending on method used *(LnID 3:633, 2003)*. ↓survival in HIV pts *(JID 192:2134, 2005)*.
D. Tuberculosis during pregnancy	**INH** + **RIF** + **ETB** for 9 mo	PZA not recommended: teratogenicity data inadequate. Because of potential ototoxicity to fetus throughout gestation (16%), SM should not be used unless other drugs contraindicated. Add pyridoxine 25 mg per day for pregnant women on INH. Breast-feeding should not be discouraged in pts on first-line drugs *[MMWR 52(RR-11):1, 2003]*.	
E. Treatment failure or relapse: Usually due to poor compliance or resistant organisms *(AJM 102:164, 1997)*	Directly observed therapy (DOT)[†]. Check susceptibilities. *(See section III.A, page 120 & above)*	Pts whose sputum has not converted after 5–6 mos.= treatment failures. Failures may be due to non-compliance or resistant organisms. Check susceptibilities of original isolates and obtain susceptibility on current isolates. Non-compliance common, therefore institute DOT. If isolates show resistance, modify regimen to include at least 2 effective agents, preferably ones which pt has not received. Surgery may be necessary. In HIV+ patients, reinfection is a possible explanation for "failure." NB, patients with MDR-TB usually convert sputum within 12 weeks of successful therapy *(AnIM 144:650, 2006)*.	
F. HIV infection or AIDS—pulmonary or extrapulmonary (NOTE: 60–70% of HIV+ pts with TB have extrapulmonary disease)	**INH** + **RIF** (or **RFB**) + **PZA** q24h times 2 months. (Authors add **pyridoxine** 25–50 mg po q24h to regimens that include INH)	**INH** + **RIF** (or **RFB**) q24h times 4 months (total 6 mos.). May treat up to 9 mos. in pts with delayed response.	1. Because of possibility of developing resistance to RIF in pts with low CD4 cell counts who receive wkly or biwkly (2x/wk) doses of RFB, it is recom. that such pts receive q24h (or min 3x/wk) doses of RFB for initiation & continuation phase of rx *(MMWR 51:214, 2002)*. 2. Clinical & microbiologic response same as in HIV-neg patient although there is considerable variability in outcomes among currently available studies *(CID 32:623, 2001)*. 3. Post-treatment suppression not necessary for drug-susceptible strains. 4. Rate of INH resistance known to be <4% (for ↑ rates of resistance, *see Section III.A*). 5. More info: *see MMWR 47(RR-20):1, 1998; CID 28:139, 1999; MMWR 52(RR-11):1, 2003.* 6. May use partially intermittent therapy: 1 dose per day for 2 weeks followed by 2–3 doses per wk for 24 wk *[MMWR 47(RR-20), 1998]*. 7. Adjunctive prednisolone of NO benefit in HIV+ patients with CD4 counts >200 *(JID 191:856, 2005)* or in patients with TBc pleurisy *(JID 190:869, 2004)*.
Concomitant protease inhibitor (PI) therapy *(Modified from MMWR 49:185, 2000; AJRCCM 162:7, 2001)*	**Initial & cont. therapy: INH** 300 mg + **RFB** *(see below for dose)* + **PZA** 25 mg per kg + **ETB** 15 mg per kg q24h times 2 mos.; then **INH** + **RFB** times 4 mos. (up to 7 mos.)	**Alternative regimen: INH** + **SM** + **PZA** + **ETB** times 2 mo; then **INH** + **SM** + **PZA** 2–3 x per wk for 7 mo. May be used with any PI regimen. May be prolonged up to 12 mo in pts with delayed response.	**Comments:** Rifamycins induce cytochrome CYP450 enzymes (RIF > RFP > RFB) & reduce serum levels of concomitantly administered PIs. Conversely, PIs (ritonavir > amprenavir >indinavir = nelfinavir > saquinavir) inhibit CYP450 & cause ↑ serum levels of RFP & RFB. If dose of RFB is not reduced, toxicity ↑. RFB/PI combinations are therapeutically effective *(CID 30:779, 2000)*. RFB has no effect on nelfinavir levels at dose of 1250 mg bid *(Can JID 10:21B, 1999)*. **Although RFB is preferred, RIF can be used for rx of active TB in pts on regimens containing efavirenz or ritonavir. RIF should not be administered to pts on ritonavir + saquinavir because drug-induced hepatitis with marked transaminase elevations has been seen in healthy volunteers receiving this regimen (www.fda.gov).** Monitor plasma levels of RFB when given with Lopinavir/Ritonavir *(CID 49:1305, 2009)*. Therapy for TB seems to increase Stavudine toxicity *(CID 48:1617, 2009)*. ART regimens containing Efavirenz less compromised by concomitant RIF than Nevirapine *(CID 48:1752, 2009)*.
	PI Regimen	**RFB Dose**	
	Nelfinavir 1250 mg q12h or indinavir 1000 mg q8h or amprenavir 1200 mg q12h.	150 mg q24h or 300 mg intermittently	
	Saquinavir standard dose	300 mg q24h or intermittently	
	Ritonavir standard dose	150 mg 2x weekly	
	Lopinavir/ritonavir—standard dose	150 mg 2x per wk	

See page 2 for abbreviations, page 127 for footnotes   * Dosages are for adults (unless otherwise indicated) and assume normal renal function   [†] **DOT** = directly observed therapy

TABLE 12A (6)

FIGURE 1 *[Modified from MMWR 52(RR-11):1, 2003]*

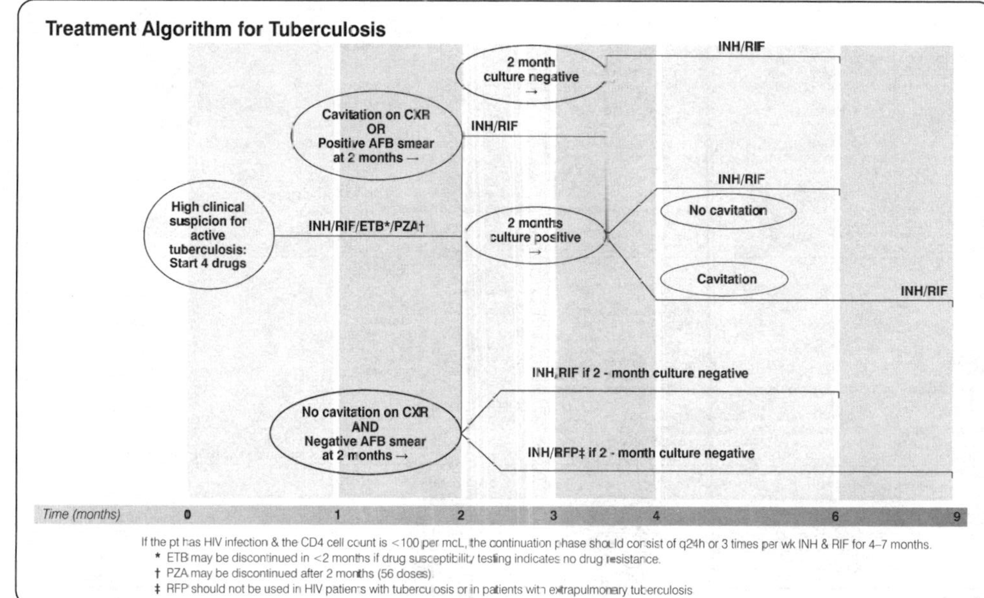

If the pt has HIV infection & the CD4 cell count is <100 per mcL, the continuation phase should consist of q24h or 3 times per wk INH & RIF for 4–7 months.

* ETB may be discontinued in <2 months if drug susceptibility testing indicates no drug resistance.

† PZA may be discontinued after 2 months (56 doses).

‡ RFP should not be used in HIV patients with tuberculosis or in patients with extrapulmonary tuberculosis

See page 2 for abbreviations.

TABLE 12A (7)

CAUSATIVE AGENT/DISEASE	MODIFYING CIRCUMSTANCES	SUGGESTED REGIMENS PRIMARY/ALTERNATIVE		COMMENTS
IV. Other Mycobacterial Disease ("Atypical") *(See ATS Consensus: AJRCCM 175:367, 2007; IDC No. Amer 16:187, 2002; CMR 15:716, 2002; CID 42:1756, 2006)*				
A. M. bovis		**INH + RIF + ETB**		The M. tuberculosis complex includes M. bovis. All isolates resistant to PZA. 9–12 months of rx used by some authorities. Isolation not required. Increased prevalence of extrapulmonary disease in U.S. born Hispanic populations *(CID 47:168, 2008; EID 14:909, 2008)*.
B. Bacillus Calmette-Guerin (BCG) (derived from M. bovis)	Only fever (>38.5°C) for 12–24 hrs	**INH** 300 mg q24h times 3 months		Intravesical BCG effective in superficial bladder tumors and carcinoma in situ. Adverse effects: fever 2.9%, granulomatosis, pneumonitis, hepatitis 0.7%, sepsis 0.4% *(J Urol 147:596, 1992)*. With sepsis, consider initial adjunctive prednisolone. Also susceptible to RFB, cipro, oflox, streptomycin, amikacin, capreomycin *(AAC 53:316, 2009)*. BCG may cause regional adenitis or pulmonary disease in HIV-infected children *(CID 37:1226, 2003)*. **Resistant to PZA.**
	Systemic illness or sepsis	**INH** 300 mg + **RIF** 600 mg + **ETB** 1200 mg po q24h times 6 mos.		
C. M. avium-intracellulare complex (MAC, MAI, or Battey bacillus) *Clin Chest Med 23:633, 2002; ATS/IDSA Consensus Statement: AJRCCM 175:367, 2007; alternative ref: CID 42:1756, 2006.* Anti-tumor necrosis factor-α increases risk of infection with MAI and other non-tuberculous mycobacteria *(EID 15:1556, 2009)*.	**Immunocompetent patients**			See AJRCCM 175:367, 2007 for details of dosing and duration of therapy. Intermittent (tiw) therapy not recommended for patients with cavitary disease, patients who have been previously treated or patients with moderate of severe disease. The primary microbiologic goal of therapy is 12 months of negative sputum cultures on therapy.
	Nodular/Bronchiectatic disease	[**Clarithro** 1000 mg tiw or **azithro** 500-600 mg tiw] + **ETB** 25 mg/kg tiw + **RIF** 600 mg tiw		**"Classic" pulmonary MAC:** Men 50–75, smokers, COPD. May be associated with hot tub use *(Clin Chest Med 23:675, 2002)*.
	Cavitary disease	[**Clarithro** 500-1000 mg/day (lower dose for wt <50 kg) or **azithro** 250-300 mg/day] +**ETB** 15 mg/kg/day + **RIF** 450-600 mg/day ± **streptomycin** or **amikacin**		**"New" pulmonary MAC:** Women 30–70, scoliosis, mitral valve prolapse, (bronchiectasis), pectus excavatum ("Lady Windermere syndrome"). May also be associated with interferon gamma deficiency *(AJM 113:756, 2002)*. For cervicofacial lymphadenitis (localized) in immunocompetent children, surgical excision is as effective as chemotherapy *(CID 44:1057, 2007)*.
	Advanced (severe) or previously treated disease	[**Clarithro** 500-1000 mg/day (lower dose for wt <50 kg) or **azithro** 250-300 mg/day] +**ETB** 15 mg/kg/day ± **streptomycin** or **amikacin**		Moxifloxacin and gatifloxacin, active in vitro & in vivo *(AAC 51:4071, 2007)*.
	Immunocompromised pts: Primary prophylaxis—Pt's CD4 count <50–100 per mm³ Discontinue when CD4 count >100 per mm³ in response to ART *(NEJM 342:1085, 2000; CID 34: 662, 2002)* Guideline: *AnIM 137:435, 2002*	**Azithro** 1200 mg po weekly OR **Clarithro** 500 mg po bid	**RFB** 300 mg po q24h OR **Azithro** 1200 mg po weekly + **RIF** 300 mg po q24h	RFB reduces MAC infection rate by 55% (no survival benefit); clarithro by 68% (30% survival benefit); azithro by 59% (68% survival benefit) *(CID 26:611, 1998)*. Azithro + RFB more effective than either alone but not as well tolerated *(NEJM 335:392, 1996)*. **Many drug-drug interactions,** *see Table 22, pages 202, 205*. Drug-resistant MAI disease seen in 29–58% of pts in whom disease develops while taking clarithro prophylaxis & in 11% of those on azithro but has not been observed with RFB prophylaxis *(J Inf 38:6, 1999)*. Clarithro resistance more likely in pts with extremely low CD4 counts at initiation *(CID 27:807, 1998)*. Need to be sure no active M. tbc; RFB used for prophylaxis may promote selection of rifamycin-resistant M. tbc *(NEJM 335:384 & 428, 1996)*.
	Treatment Either presumptive dx or after + culture of blood, bone marrow, or usually, sterile body fluids, eg liver	(**Clarithro** 500 mg* po bid + **ETB** 15 mg/kg/day + **RFB** 300 mg po q24h *** Higher doses of clari (1000 mg bid) may be associated with ↑ mortality** *(CID 29:125, 1999)*	**Azithro** 500 mg po/day + **ETB** 15 mg/kg/day +/- **RFB** 300-450 mg po/day	Median time to neg. blood culture: clarithro + ETB 4.4 wks vs azithro + ETB >16 wks. At 16 wks, clearance of bacteremia seen in 37.5% of azithro- & 85.7% of clarithro-treated pts *(CID 27:1278, 1998)*. More recent study suggests similar clearance rates for azithro (46%) vs clarithro (56%) at 24 wks when combined with ETB *(CID 31:1245, 2000)*. Azithro 250 mg po q24h not effective, but azithro 600 mg po q24h as effective as 1200 mg q24h & yields fewer adverse effects *(AAC 43: 2869, 1999)*. *(continued on next page)*

     * Dosages are for adults (unless otherwise indicated) and assume normal renal function   [†] **DOT** = directly observed therapy

TABLE 12A (3)

CAUSATIVE AGENT/DISEASE	MODIFYING CIRCUMSTANCES	SUGGESTED REGIMENS PRIMARY	SUGGESTED REGIMENS ALTERNATIVE	COMMENTS
IV. Other Mycobacterial Disease ("Atypical") *(continued)*				
C. M. avium-intracellulare complex *(continued)*				*(continued from previous page)* Addition of RFB to clarithro + ETB ↓ emergence of resistance to clari, ↓ relapse rate & improves survival *(CID 37:1234, 2003)*. Data on clofazimine difficult to assess. Earlier study suggested adding CLO of no value *(CID 25:621, 1997)*. More recent study suggests it may be as effective as RFB in 3 drug regimens containing clari & ETB *(CID 29:125, 1999)* although it may not be as effective as RFB at preventing clari resistance *(CID 28:136, 1999)*. Thus, pending more data, we still do not recommend CLO for MAI in HIV+ pts. Drug toxicity: With clarithro, 23% pts had to stop drug 2° to dose-limiting adverse reaction *(AnIM 121: 905, 1994)*. Combination of clarithro, ETB and RFB led to uveitis and pseudojaundice *(NEJM 330:438, 1994)*; result is reduction in max. dose of RFB to 300 mg. Treatment failure rate is high. Reasons: drug toxicity, development of drug resistance, & inadequate serum levels. Serum levels of clarithro ↓ in pts also given RIF or RFB *(JID 171:747, 1995)*. If pt not responding to initial regimen after 2–4 weeks, add one or more drugs. Several anecdotal reports of pts not responding to usual primary regimen who gained weight and became afebrile with dexamethasone 2–4 mg per day po *(AAC 38:2215, 1994; CID 26:682, 1998)*.
	Chronic post-treatment suppression—secondary prophylaxis	**Always necessary.** [**Clarithro** or azithro] + **ETB** 15 mg/ kg/day *(dosage above)*	**Clarithro** or **azithro** or **RFB** *(dosage above)*	Recurrences almost universal without chronic suppression. However, in patients on ART with robust CD4 cell response, it is possible to discontinue chronic suppression *(JID 178:1446, 1998; NEJM 340:1301, 1999)*.
D. Mycobacterium celatum	Treatment; optimal regimen not defined	May be susceptible to **clarithro**, **FQ** *(Clin Micro Inf 3:582, 1997)*. Suggest rx "like MAI" but often resistant to RIF *(J Inf 38:157, 1999)*. Most reported cases received 3 or 4 drugs, usually clarithro + ETB + CIP ± RFB *(EID 9:399, 2003)*.		Isolated from pulmonary lesions and blood in AIDS patients *(CID 24:144, 1997)*. Easily confused with M. xenopi (and MAC). Susceptibilities similar to MAC, but highly resistant to RIF *(CID 24:140, 1997)*.
E. Mycobacterium chelonae ssp. abscessus **Mycobacterium chelonae ssp. chelonae**	Treatment; Surgical excision may facilitate clarithro rx in subcutaneous abscess and is important adjunct to rx *(CID 24:1147, 1997)*	**Clarithro** 500 mg po bid times 6 mos. *(AnIM 119:482, 1993; CID 24:1147, 1997; EJCMID 19: 43, 2000)*. Azithro may also be effective. For serious disseminated infections add amikacin + IMP or cefoxitin for 1st 2–6 wks *(Clin Micro Rev 15:716, 2002; AJRCCM 175:367, 2007)* or add Moxi or Levo *(CID 49:1365, 2009)*.		M. abscessus susceptible to AMK (70%), clarithro (95%), cefoxitin (70%), CLO, cefmetazole, RFB, FQ, IMP, azithro, cipro, doxy, mino, tigecycline *(CID 42:1756, 2006; JIC 15:46, 2009)*. Single isolates of M. abscessus often not associated with disease. Clarithro-resistant strains now described *(J Clin Micro 39: 2745, 2001)*. M. chelonae susceptible to AMK (80%), clarithro, azithro, tobramycin (100%), IMP (60%), moxifloxacin *(AAC 46:3283, 2002)*, cipro, mino, doxy, linezolid (94%) *(CID 42:1756, 2006)*. Resistant to cefoxitin, FQ *(CID 24:1147, 1997; AJRCCM 156:S1, 1997)*. Tigecycline highly active in vitro *(AAC 52:4184, 2008; CID 49:1358, 2009)*.
F. Mycobacterium fortuitum	Treatment; optimal regimen not defined. Surgical excision of infected areas.	**AMK** + **cefoxitin** + **probenecid** 2–6 wk, then po **TMP- SMX**, or **doxy** 2–6 mo. Usually responds to 6–12 mo of oral rx with 2 drugs to which it is susceptible *(AAC 46: 3283, 2002; Clin Micro Rev 15: 716, 2002)*. Nail salon-acquired infections respond to 4–6 mo of minocycline, doxy, or CIP *(CID 38:38, 2004)*.		**Resistant to all standard anti-TBc drugs.** Sensitive in vitro to doxycycline, minocycline, cefoxitin, IMP, AMK, TMP-SMX, CIP, oflox, azithro, clarithro, linezolid, tigecycline *(Clin Micro Rev 15:716, 2002)*, but some strains resistant to azithromycin, rifabutin *(JAC 39:567, 1997; AAC 52:4184, 2008)*. For M. fortuitum pulmonary disease treat with at least 2 agents active in vitro until sputum cultures negative for 12 months *(AJRCCM 175:367, 2007)*.

See page 2 for abbreviations, page 127 for footnotes * Dosages are for adults (unless otherwise indicated) and assume normal renal function [†] **DOT** = directly observed therapy

TABLE 12A (9)

CAUSATIVE AGENT/DISEASE; MODIFYING CIRCUMSTANCES	SUGGESTED REGIMENS		COMMENTS
	PRIMARY	ALTERNATIVE	
IV. Other Mycobacterial Disease ("Atypical") *(continued)*			
G. Mycobacterium haemophilum	Regimen(s) not defined. In animal model, **clarithro** + **rifabutin** effective *(AAC 39:2316, 1995)*. Combination of **CIP** + **RFB** + **clarithro** reported effective but clinical experience limited *(Clin Micro Rev 9:435, 1996)*. Surgical debridement may be necessary *(CID 26:505, 1998)*.		Clinical: Ulcerating skin lesions, synovitis, osteomyelitis, cervicofacial lymphadenitis in children *(CID 41:1569, 2005)*. Lab: Requires supplemented media to isolate. Sensitive in vitro to: CIP, cycloserine, rifabutin. Over ½ resistant to: INH, RIF, ETB, PZA *(AnIM 120:118, 1994)*. For localized cervicofacial lymphadenitis in immunocompetent children, surgical excision as effective as chemotherapy *(CID 44:1057, 2007)*.
H. Mycobacterium genavense	Regimens used include ≥2 drugs: **ETB**, **RIF**, **RFB**, **CLO**, **clarithro**. In animal model, **clarithro** & **RFB** (& to lesser extent amikacin & **ETB**) shown effective in reducing bacterial counts; CIP not effective *(JAC 42:483, 1998)*.		Clinical: CD4 <50. Symptoms of fever, weight loss, diarrhea. Lab: Growth in BACTEC vials slow (mean 42 days). Subcultures grow only on Middlebrook 7H11 agar containing 2 mcg per mL mycobactin J—growth still insufficient for in vitro sensitivity testing *(Ln 340:76, 1992; AnIM 117:586, 1992)*. Survival ↑ from 81 to 263 days in pts rx for at least 1 month with ≥2 drugs *(ArIM 155:400, 1995)*.
I. Mycobacterium gordonae	Regimen(s) not defined, but consider **RIF** + **ETB** + **KM** or **CIP** *(J Inf 38:157, 1999)* or **linezolid** *(AJRCCM 175:367, 2007)*		In vitro: sensitive to ETB, RIF, AMK, CIP, clarithro, linezolid *(AAC 47:1736, 2003)*. Resistant to INH *(CID 14:1229, 1992)*. Surgical excision.
J. Mycobacterium kansasii	Q24h po: **INH** (300 mg) + **RIF** (600 mg) + **ETB** (25 mg per kg times 2 mos., then 15 mg per kg). Rx for 18 mos. (until culture-neg. sputum times 12 mos; 15 mos. if HIV+ pt.) *(See Comment)*	If RIF-resistant, po q24h: [**INH** (900 mg) + **pyridoxine** (50 mg) + ETB (25 mg per kg)] + **sulfamethoxazole** (1 gm tid). Rx until pt culture-neg. times 12–15 mos. *(See Comment)*. **Clari** + **ETB** + **RIF** also effective in small study *(CID 37:1178, 2003)*.	**All isolates are resistant to PZA.** Rifapentine, azithro, ETB effective alone or in combination in athymic mice *(JAC 42:417, 2001)*. Highly susceptible to linezolid in vitro *(AAC 47:1736, 2003)* and to clarithro and moxifloxacin *(JAC 55:950, 2005)*. If HIV+ pt taking protease inhibitor, substitute either clarithro (500 mg bid) or RFB (150 mg per day) for RIF *(AJRCCM 156:S1, 1997)*. Because of variable susceptibility to INH, some substitute clarithro 500–750 mg q24h for INH. Resistance to clarithro reported *(DMID 31:369, 1998)*, but most strains susceptible to clarithro as well as moxifloxacin *(JAC 55:950, 2005)* & levofloxacin *(AAC 48:4562, 2004)*. Prognosis related to level of immunosuppression *(CID 37:584, 2003)*.
K. Mycobacterium marinum	(**Clarithro** 500 mg bid) or (**minocycline** 100–200 mg q24h) or (**doxycycline** 100–200 mg q24h), or (**TMP-SMX** 160/800 mg po bid), or (**RIF** + **ETB**) for 3 mos. *(AJRCCM 156:S1, 1997; Eur J Clin Microbiol ID 25:609, 2006)*. Surgical excision.		Resistant to INH & PZA *(AJRCCM 156:S1, 1997)*. Also susceptible in vitro to linezolid *(AAC 47:1736, 2003)*. CIP, moxifloxacin also show moderate in vitro activity *(AAC 46:1114, 2002)*.
L. Mycobacterium scrofulaceum	Surgical excision. Chemotherapy seldom indicated. Although regimens not defined, **clarithro** + **CLO** with or **without ETB**. **INH**, **RIF**, **strep** + **cycloserine** have also been used.		In vitro resistant to INH, RIF, ETB, PZA, AMK, CIP *(CID 20: 549, 1995)*. Susceptible to clarithro, strep, erythromycin.
M. Mycobacterium simiae	Regimen(s) not defined. Start 4 drugs as for disseminated MAI.		Most isolates resistant to all 1st-line anti-tbc drugs. Isolates often not clinically significant *(CID 26: 625, 1998)*.
N. Mycobacterium ulcerans (Buruli ulcer)	[**RIF** + **AMK** (7.5 mg per kg IM bid)] or [**ETB** + **TMP-SMX** (160/800 mg po tid)] for 4–6 weeks. Surgical excision most important. WHO recommends **RIF** + **SM** for 8 weeks but overall value of drug therapy not clear *(Lancet Infection 6:288, 2006; Lancet 367:1849, 2006; AAC 51:645, 2007)*. **RIF** + **SM** resulted in 47% cure rate *(AAC 51:4029, 2007)*. **RIF**+ **cipro** recommended as alternatives by WHO *(CMN 31:119, 2009)*.		Susceptible in vitro to RIF, strep, CLO, clarithro, CIP, oflox, amikacin, moxi, linezolid *(AAC 42:2070, 1998; JAC 45: 231, 2000; AAC 46:3193, 2002; AAC 50:1921, 2006)*. Monotherapy with RIF selects resistant mutants in mice *(AAC 47:1228, 2003)*. RIF + moxi; RIF + clarithro; moxi + clarithro similar to RIF + SM in mice *(AAC 51:3737, 2007)*. Treatment generally disappointing—*see review, Ln 354:1013, 1999*. RIF + dapsone only slightly better (82% improved) than placebo (75%) in small study *(Intl J Inf Dis 6:60, 2002)*.
O. Mycobacterium xenopi	Regimen(s) not defined *(CID 24:226 & 233, 1997)*. Some recommend a **macrolide** + (**RIF** or **rifabutin**) + **ETB** ± **SM** *(AJRCCM 156:S1, 1997)* or **RIF** + **INH** ± **ETB** *(Resp Med 97:439, 2003)* but recent study suggests no need to treat in most pts with HIV *(CID 37:1250, 2003)*.		In vitro: sensitive to clarithro *(AAC 36:2841, 1992)* and rifabutin *(JAC 39:567, 1997)* and many standard antimycobacterial drugs. Clarithro-containing regimens more effective than RIF/INH/ETB regimens in mice *(AAC 45:3229, 2001)*. FQs, linezolid also active in vitro.
Mycobacterium leprae (leprosy) Classification: *CID 44:1096, 2007*. Clinical mgmt of leprosy reactions: *IDCP 18:235, 2010*.	There are 2 sets of therapeutic recommendations here: one from USA (National Hansen's Disease Programs [NHDP], Baton Rouge, LA) and one from WHO. Both are based on expert recommendations and neither has been subjected to controlled clinical trial *(P. Joyce & D. Scollard, Conns Current Therapy 2004; J Am Acad Dermatol 51:417, 2004)*.		

See page 2 for abbreviations, page 127 for footnotes * Dosages are for adults (unless otherwise indicated) and assume normal renal function † **DOT** = directly observed therapy

TABLE 12A (10)

Type of Disease	NHDP Regimen	WHO Regimen	COMMENTS
Paucibacillary Forms: (Intermediate, Tuberculoid, Borderline tuberculoid)	(**Dapsone** 100 mg/day + **RIF** 600 mg po/day) for 12 months	(**Dapsone** 100 mg/day (unsupervised) + **RIF** 600 mg 1x/mo (supervised)) for 6 mo	Side effects overall 0.4%
Single lesion paucibacillary	Treat as paucibacillary leprosy for 12 months.	Single dose ROM therapy: (RIF 600 mg + Oflox 400 mg + Mino 100 mg) *(Ln 353:655, 1999)*.	
Multibacillary forms: Borderline Borderline-lepromatous Lepromatous ***See Comment for erythema nodosum leprosum*** Rev.: *Lancet 363:1209, 2004*	(**Dapsone** 100 mg/day + **CLO** 50 mg/day + **RIF** 600 mg/day) for 24 mo **Alternative regimen:** (**Dapsone** 100 mg/day + **RIF** 600 mg/day + **Minocycline** 100 mg/day) for 24 mo if CLO is refused or unavailable.	(**Dapsone** 100 mg/day + **CLO** 50 mg/day (both unsupervised) + **RIF** 600 mg + **CLO** 300 mg once monthly (supervised)). Continue regimen for 12 months.	Side-effects overall 5.1%. For erythema nodosum leprosum: prednisone 60–80 mg/day or thalidomide 100–400 mg/day *(BMJ 44: 775, 1988; AJM 108:487, 2000)*. Thalidomide available in US at 1-800-4-CELGENE. Altho thalidomide effective, WHO no longer rec because of potential toxicity *(JID 193:1743, 2006)* however the majority of leprosy experts feel thalidomide remains drug of choice for ENL under strict supervision. **CLO (Clofazimine)** available from NHDP under ND protocol: contact at 1-800-642-2477. **Ethionamide** (250 mg q24h) or **prothionamide** (375 mg q24h) may be subbed for CLO. Oflox 400 mg po q24h, bactericidal and effective clinically with 4 log ↓ in organisms in small trials *(AAC 38:662, 1994; AAC 38:61, 1994)*. Clarithro also rapidly bactericidal *(AAC 38:515, 1994; Ln 345:4, 1995)*. Regimens incorporating clarithro, minocycline, RIF, moxifloxacin and/or oflox also show promise *(AAC 44:2919, 2000; AAC 50:1558, 2006)*. High relapse rate in pts treated with q24h RIF + oflox for 4 wk *(AAC 41:1953, 1997)*. Resistance to dapsone, RIF & oflox reported *(Ln 349:103, 1997)*. Dapsone monotherapy has been abandoned due to emergence of resistance, but older patients previously treated with dapsone monotherapy may remain on lifelong maintenance therapy. Dapsone (or acedapsone[NUS]) effective for prophylaxis in one study *(J Inf 41:137, 2000)*. Moxifloxacin highly active in vitro and produces rapid clinical response *(AAC 52:3113, 2008)*.

FOOTNOTES:

1 When DOT is used, drugs may be given 5 days/wk & necessary number of doses adjusted accordingly. Although no studies compare 5 with 7 q24h doses, extensive experience indicates this would be an effective practice.
2 Patients with cavitation on initial chest x-ray & positive cultures at completion of 2 mo of rx should receive a 7 mo (31 wk; either 217 doses [q24h] or 62 doses [2x/wk] continuation phase.
3 5 day/wk admin is always given by DOT.
4 Not recommended for HIV-infected pts with CD4 cell counts <100 cells/mcL.
5 Options 1c & 2b should be used only in HIV-neg. pts who have neg. sputum smears at the time of completion of 2 mo rx & do not have cavitation on initial chest x-ray. For pts started on this regimen & found to have a + culture from 2 mo specimen, rx should be extended extra 3 mo.
6 Options 4a & 4b should be considered only when options 1–3 cannot be given.
7 Alternative agents = ethionamide, cycloserine, p-aminosalicylic acid, clarithromycin, AM-CL, linezolid.
8 Modified from *MMWR 52(RR-11):1, 2003. See also IDCP 11:329, 2002.*
9 Continuation regimen with INH/ETB less effective than INH/RIF *(Lancet 364:1244, 2004)*.

See page 2 for abbreviations, page 127 for footnotes   * Dosages are for adults (unless otherwise indicated) and assume normal renal function   [1] **DOT** = directly observed therapy

TABLE 12B – DOSAGE AND ADVERSE EFFECTS OF ANTIMYCOBACTERIAL DRUGS

AGENT (TRADE NAME)[1]	USUAL DOSAGE*	ROUTE/1° DRUG RESISTANCE (RES) US[2, §]	SIDE-EFFECTS, TOXICITY AND PRECAUTIONS	SURVEILLANCE
FIRST LINE DRUGS				
Ethambutol (Myambutol) (100, 400 mg tab)	25 mg/kg/day for 2 mo then 15 mg/ kg/day q24h as 1 dose (<10% protein binding) [Bacteriostatic to both extra-cellular & intracellular organisms]	RES: 0.3% (0–0.7%) po 400 mg tab	**Optic neuritis** with decreased visual acuity, central scotomata, and loss of green and red perception; peripheral neuropathy and headache (~1%), rashes (rare), arthralgia (rare), hyperuricemia (rare). Anaphylactoid reaction (rare). *Comment:* Primarily used to inhibit resistance. Disrupts outer cell membrane in M. avium with ↑ activity to other drugs.	Monthly visual acuity & red/ green with dose >15 mg/kg/ day. ≥10% loss considered significant. Usually reversible if drug discontinued.
Isoniazid (INH) (Nydrazid, Laniazid, Teebaconin) (50, 100, 300 mg tab)	Q24h dose: 5–10 mg/kg/day up to 300 mg/day as 1 dose. 2x/wk dose: 15 mg/kg (900 mg max dose) (< 10% protein binding) [Bactericidal to both extracellular and intracellular organisms] Add pyridoxine in alcoholic, pregnant, or malnourished pts.	RES: 4.1% (2.6–8.5%) po 300 mg tab IM 100 mg/mL in 10 mL (IV route not FDA-approved but has been used, esp. in AIDS)	Overall ~1%. Liver: **Hep** (children 10% mild ↑ SGOT, normalizes with continued rx, age <20 yr rare, 20–34 yr 1.2%, ≥50 yr 2.3%) [also ↑ with q24h alcohol & previous exposure to Hep C (usually asymptomatic—*CID 36:293, 2003*)]. May be fatal. With prodromal sx, dark urine do LFTs; discontinue if SGOT >3–5xnormal. **Peripheral neuropathy** (17% on 6 mg/kg per day, less on 300 mg, incidence ↑ in slow acetylators); **pyridoxine 10 mg q24h will decrease incidence**; other neurologic sequelae, convulsions, optic neuritis, toxic encephalopathy, psychosis, muscle twitching, dizziness, coma (all rare); allergic skin rashes, fever, minor disulfiram-like reaction, flushing after Swiss cheese; blood dyscrasias (rare); + antinuclear (20%). **Drug-drug interactions** common, *see Table 22.*	Pre-rx liver functions. Repeat if symptoms (fatigue, weakness, malaise, anorexia, nausea or vomiting) >3 days (*AJRCCM 152: 1705, 1995*). Some recommend SGOT at 2, 4, 6 mo esp. if age >50 yr. Clinical evaluation every mo.
Pyrazinamide (500 mg tab)	25 mg per kg per day (maximum 2.5 gm per day) q24h as 1 dose [Bactericidal for intracellular organisms]	po 500 mg tab	**Arthralgia; hyperuricemia** (with or without symptoms); hepatitis (not over 2% if recommended dose not exceeded); gastric irritation; photosensitivity (rare).	Pre-rx liver functions. Monthly SGOT, uric acid. Measure serum uric acid if symptomatic gouty attack occurs.
Rifamate®—combination tablet	2 tablets single dose q24h	po (1 hr before meal)	1 tablet contains 150 mg INH, 300 mg RIF	As with individual drugs
Rifampin (Rifadin, Rimactane, Rifocin) (100, 300, 450, 600 mg cap)	10.0 mg per kg per day up to 600 mg per day q24h as 1 dose (60–90% protein binding) [Bactericidal to all populations of organisms]	RES: 0.2% (0–0.3%) po 300 mg cap (IV available, Merrell-Dow)	INH/RIF dc'd in ~3% for toxicity; gastrointestinal irritation, antibiotic-associated colitis, drug fever (1%), pruritus with or without skin rash (1%), anaphylactoid reactions in HIV+ pts, mental confusion, thrombocytopenia (1%), leukopenia (1%), hemolytic anemia, transient **abnormalities in liver function. "Flu syndrome"** (fever, chills, headache, bone pain, shortness of breath) seen if RIF taken irregularly or if q24h dose restarted after an interval of no rx. **Discolors urine, tears, sweat, contact lens an orange-brownish color.** May cause drug-induced lupus erythematosus (*Ln 349: 1521, 1977*).	Pre-rx liver function. Repeat if symptoms. **Multiple significant drug-drug interactions, see *Table 22.***
Rifater®—combination tablet (*See Side-Effects*)	Wt ≥55 kg, 6 tablets single dose q24h	po (1 hr before meal)	1 tablet contains 50 mg INH, 120 mg RIF, 300 mg PZA. Used in 1st 2 months of rx (PZA 25 mg per kg). Purpose is convenience in dosing, ↑ compliance (*AnIM 122: 951, 1995*) but cost 1.58 more. Side-effects = individual drugs.	As with individual drugs, PZA 25 mg per kg
Streptomycin (IV/IM sol'n)	15 mg per kg IM q24h, 0.75–1.0 gm per day initially for 60–90 days, then 1.0 gm 2–3 times per week (15 mg per kg per day) q24h as 1 dose	RES: 3.9% (2.7–7.6%) IM (or IV)	Overall 8%. **Ototoxicity:** vestibular dysfunction (vertigo); paresthesias; dizziness & nausea (all less in pts receiving 2–3 doses per week); tinnitus and high frequency loss (1%); nephrotoxicity (rare); peripheral neuropathy (rare); allergic skin rashes (4–5%); drug fever. Available from X-Gen Pharmaceuticals, 607-732-4411. Ref. re: IV—*CID 19:1150, 1994*. Toxicity similar with qd vs tid dosing (*CID 38:1538, 2004*).	Monthly audiogram. In older pts, serum creatinine or BUN at start of rx and weekly if pt stable

[1] Note: Malabsorption of antimycobacterial drugs may occur in patients with AIDS enteropathy. For review of adverse effects, *see AJRCCM 167:1472, 2003.*

[2] **RES** = % resistance of M. tuberculosis

See page 2 for abbreviations.

* Dosages are for adults (unless otherwise indicated) and assume normal renal function

§ Mean (range) (higher in Hispanics, Asians, and patients <10 years old)

† **DOT** = directly observed therapy

TABLE 12B (2)

AGENT (TRADE NAME)[1]	USUAL DOSAGE*	ROUTE/1° DRUG RESISTANCE (RES) US[2,§]	SIDE-EFFECTS, TOXICITY AND PRECAUTIONS	SURVEILLANCE
SECOND LINE DRUGS (more difficult to use and/or less effective than first line drugs)				
Amikacin (Amikin) (IV soln)	7.5–10.0 mg per kg q24h [Bactericidal for extracellular organisms]	RES: (est. 0.1%) IM/IV 500 mg vial	*See Table 10, pages 87 & 101* Toxicity similar with qd vs tid dosing *(CID 38:1538, 2004)*.	Monthly audiogram. Serum creatinine or BUN weekly if pt stable
Capreomycin sulfate (Capastat sulfate)	1 gm per day (15 mg per kg per day) q24h as 1 dose	RES: 0.1% (0–0.9%) IM/IV	Nephrotoxicity (36%), ototoxicity (auditory 11%), eosinophilia, leukopenia, skin rash, fever, hypokalemia, neuromuscular blockade.	Monthly audiogram, biweekly serum creatinine or BUN
Ciprofloxacin (Cipro) (250, 500, 750 mg tab)	750 mg bid	po 500 mg or 750 mg ER IV 200-400 mg vial	TB not an FDA-approved indication for CIP. Desired CIP serum levels 4–6 mcg per mL, requires median dose 800 mg *(AJRCCM 151:2006, 1995)*. Discontinuation rates 6–7%. CIP well tolerated *(AJRCCM 151:2006, 1995)*. FQ-resistant M. Tb identified in New York *(Ln 345:1148, 1995)*. *See Table 10, pages 90 & 97 for adverse effects.*	None
Clofazimine (Lamprene) (50, 100 mg cap)	50 mg per day (unsupervised) + 300 mg 1 time per month supervised or 100 mg per day	po 50 mg (with meals)	Skin: **pigmentation (pink-brownish black)** 75–100%, dryness 20%, pruritus 5%. GI: abdominal pain 50% (rarely severe leading to exploratory laparoscopy), splenic infarction (VR), bowel obstruction (VR), GI bleeding (VR). Eye: conjunctival irritation, retinal crystal deposits.	None
Cycloserine (Seromycin) (250 mg tab)	750–1000 mg per day (15 mg per kg per day) 2–4 doses per day [Bacteriostatic for both extra-cellular & intracellular organisms]	RES: 0.1% (0–0.3%) po 250 mg cap	Convulsions, **psychoses** (5–10% of those receiving 1.0 gm per day); headache; somnolence; hyperreflexia; increased CSF protein and pressure, **peripheral neuropathy.** 100 mg pyridoxine (or more) q24h should be given concomitantly. Contraindicated in epileptics	None
Dapsone (25, 100 mg tab)	100 mg per day	po 100 mg tab	Blood: ↓ hemoglobin (1–2 gm) & ↑ retics (2–12%), in most pts. Hemolysis in G6PD deficiency. **Methemoglobinemia.** CNS: peripheral neuropathy (rare). GI: nausea, vomiting. Renal: albuminuria, nephrotic syndrome. Erythema nodosum leprosum in pts rx for leprosy (½ pts 1st year).	None
Ethionamide (Trecator-SC) (120, 250 mg tab)	500–1000 mg per day (15–20 mg per kg per day) 1–3 doses per day [Bacteriostatic for extracellular organisms only]	RES: 0.8% (0–1.5%) po 250 mg tab	**Gastrointestinal irritation** (up to 50% on large dose); goiter; peripheral neuropathy (rare); convulsions (rare); changes in affect (rare); difficulty in diabetes control; rashes; hepatitis; purpura; stomatitis; gynecomastia; menstrual irregularity. Give drug with meals or antacids; 50–100 mg pyridoxine per day concomitantly; SGOT monthly. Possibly teratogenic.	
Moxifloxacin (Avelox) (400 mg tab)	400 mg qd	po 400 mg cap IV	Not FDA-approved indication. Concomitant administration of rifampin reduces serum levels of moxi *(CID 45:1001, 2007)*.	None
Ofloxacin (Floxin) (200, 300, 400 mg tab)	400 mg bid	po 400 mg cap IV	Not FDA-approved indication. Overall adverse effects 11%, 4% discontinued due to side-effects. GI: nausea 3%, diarrhea 1%. **CNS:** insomnia 3%, headache 1%, dizziness 1%.	
Para-aminosalicylic acid (PAS, Paser) (Na^+ or K^+ salt) (4 gm cap)	4–6 gm bid (200 mg per kg per day) [Bacteriostatic for extracellular organisms only]	RES: 0.8% (0–1.5%) po 450 mg tab *(see Comment)*	**Gastrointestinal irritation** (10–15%); goitrogenic action (rare); depressed prothrombin activity (rare); G6PD-mediated hemolytic anemia (rare), drug fever, rashes, hepatitis, myalgia, arthralgia. Retards hepatic enzyme induction, may ↓ INH hepatotoxicity. Available from CDC, (404) 639-3670, Jacobus Pharm. Co. (609) 921-7447.	None

See page 2 for abbreviations.

* Dosages are for adults (unless otherwise indicated) and assume normal renal function

§ Mean (range) (higher in Hispanics, Asians, and patients <10 years old)

[1] **DOT** = directly observed therapy

TABLE 12B (3)

AGENT (TRADE NAME)[1]	USUAL DOSAGE*	ROUTE/1° DRUG RESISTANCE (RES) US[2,§]	SIDE-EFFECTS, TOXICITY AND PRECAUTIONS	SURVEILLANCE
SECOND LINE DRUGS *(continued)*				
Rifabutin (Mycobutin) (150 mg cap)	300 mg per day (prophylaxis or treatment)	po 150 mg tab	Polymyalgia, polyarthralgia, leukopenia, granulocytopenia. Anterior uveitis when given with concomitant clarithromycin; avoid 600 mg dose *(NEJM 330:438, 1994)*. Uveitis reported with 300 mg per day *(AnIM 12:510, 1994)*. Reddish urine, orange skin (pseudojaundice).	None
Rifapentine (Priftin) (150 mg tab)	600 mg twice weekly for 1st 2 mos., then 600 mg q week	po 150 mg tab	Similar to other rifabutins. *(See RIF, RFB)*. Hyperuricemia seen in 21%. Causes red-orange discoloration of body fluids. Note ↑ prevalence of RIF resistance in pts on weekly rx *(Ln 353:1843, 1999)*.	None
Thalidomide (Thalomid) (50, 100, 200 mg cap)	100–300 mg po q24h (may use up to 400 mg po q24h for severe erythema nodosum leprosum)	po 50 mg tab	**Contraindicated in pregnancy. Causes severe life-threatening birth defects. Both male and female patients must use barrier contraceptive methods (Pregnancy Category X). Frequently causes drowsiness or somnolence. May cause peripheral neuropathy.** *(AJM 108:487, 2000)* For review, *see Ln 363:1803, 2004*.	Available only through pharmacists participating in System for Thalidomide Education and Prescribing Safety (S.T.E.P.S.)

See page 2 for abbreviations.

* Dosages are for adults (unless otherwise indicated) and assume normal renal function
§ Mean (range) (higher in Hispanics, Asians, and patients <10 years old)

[1] **DOT** = directly observed therapy

TABLE 13A– TREATMENT OF PARASITIC INFECTIONS*

Many of the drugs suggested are not licensed in the US. The following are helpful resources available through the Centers for Disease Control and Prevention (CDC) in Atlanta. Website is www.cdc.gov.
General advice for parasitic diseases other than malaria: (+1) (770) 488-7775 (day), (+1) (770) 488-7100 (after hours).
For CDC Drug Service[1] 8:00 a.m.– 4:30 p.m. EST: (+1) (404) 639-3670; fax: (+1) (404) 639-3717. *See www.cdc.gov/laboratory/drugservice/index.html*
For malaria: Prophylaxis advice (+1) (770) 488-7788; treatment (+1) (770) 488-7788; or after hours (+1) (770) 488-7100 website: www.cdc.gov/malaria
NOTE: All dosage regimens are for adults with normal renal function unless otherwise stated. Many of the suggested regimens are not FDA approved.
For licensed drugs, suggest checking package inserts to verify dosage and side-effects. Occasionally, post-licensure data may alter dosage as compared to package inserts.
For abbreviations of journal titles, *see page 3*. **Reference with peds dosages: *Treat Guide Med Lett 5(Supp 5):1, 2007.*** Sources for Hard-to-Find Antiparasitic Drugs, *see Table 13D, page 144*.

INFECTING ORGANISM	SUGGESTED REGIMENS		COMMENTS
	PRIMARY	ALTERNATIVE	
PROTOZOA—INTESTINAL (non-pathogenic: E. hartmanni, E. dispar, E. coli, Iodamoeba butschlii, Endolimax nana, Chilomastix mesnili)			
Balantidium coli	**Tetracycline** 500 mg po qid x 10 days	**Metronidazole** 750 mg po tid times 5 days	Another alternative: Iodoquinol 650 mg po tid x 20 days.
Blastocystis hominis	Role as pathogen unclear; may serve as marker of exposure to contaminated food/water	**Metronidazole** 1.5 gm po 1x/day x 10 days (placebo-controlled trial in *J Travel Med 10:128, 2003*) or 750 mg po tid x 10 days. **Alternatives: iodoquinol**[2,3] 650 mg po tid x 20 days or **TMP-SMX-DS**, one bid x 7 days	
Cryptosporidium parvum & hominis Treatment is unsatisfactory Ref.: *CID 39:504, 2004*	**Immunocompetent—No HIV: Nitazoxanide** 500 mg po bid x 3 days	**HIV with immunodeficiency:** (1) Effective antiretro-viral therapy best therapy. (2) **Nitazoxanide** is not licensed for immunodeficient pts; no clinical or parasite response compared to placebo	**Nitazoxanide:** Approved in liquid formulation for rx of children & 500 mg tabs for adults who are immunocompetent. Ref.: *CID 40:1173, 2005.* **C. hominis** assoc. with ↑ in post-infection eye & joint pain, recurrent headache, & dizzy spells (*CID 39:504, 2004*).
Cyclospora cayetanensis; cyclosporiasis	Immunocompetent pts: **TMP-SMX-DS** tab 1 po bid x 7–10 days. Other options: *see Comments.*	AIDS pts: **TMP-SMX-DS** tab 1 po qid for up to 3-4 wks. Other options: *see Comments.*	If sulfa-allergic: **CIP** 500 mg po bid x 7 days but results inconsistent.
Dientamoeba fragilis *See AJTMH 82:614, 2010; Clin Micro Infect 14:601, 2008.*	**Iodoquinol** 650 mg po tid x 20 days or **Paromomycin** 25-35 mg/kg/day po in 3 div doses x 7 days. *See footnotes*[2,3] *for drug sources.*	For treatment failures: **Tetracycline** 500 mg po qid x 10 days + **Iodoquinol** 650 mg po tid x 10 days	**Metronidazole** associated with high failure rates.
Entamoeba histolytica; amebiasis. Reviews: *Ln 361:1025, 2003; NEJM 348:1563, 2003.*			
Asymptomatic cyst passer	**Paromomycin** (aminosidine in U.K.) 25-35 mg/kg/day po in 3 divided doses x 7 days OR **iodoquinol** 650 mg po tid x 20 days	**Diloxanide furoate**[NUS] (Furamide) 500 mg po tid x 10 days.	
Patient with diarrhea/dysentery; mild/moderate disease. Oral therapy possible	**Metronidazole** 500–750 mg po tid x 7-10 days or **tinidazole** 2 gm po daily x 3 days, followed by: Either [**paromomycin**[NUS] 25-35 mg/kg/day po divided in 3 doses x 7 days] or [**iodoquinol** 650 mg po tid x 20 days] to clear intestinal cysts. *See comment.*		Colitis can mimic ulcerative colitis; ameboma can mimic adenocarcinoma of colon. **Nitazoxanide** 500 mg po bid x 3 days may be effective (*JID 184:381, 2001 & Tran R Soc Trop Med & Hyg 101:1025, 2007*)
Severe or extraintestinal infection, e.g., hepatic abscess	(**Metronidazole** 750 mg **IV to PO** tid x 10 days or **tinidazole** 2 gm 1x/day x 5 days) followed by **paromomycin**[NUS] 25-35 mg/kg/day po divided in 3 doses x 7 days or **Iodoquinol** 650 mg po tid x 20 days.		**Serology positive (antibody present) with extraintestinal disease.**
Giardia lamblia; giardiasis	(**Tinidazole** 2 gm po x 1) OR (**nitazoxanide** 500 mg po bid x 3 days)	**Metronidazole** 250 mg po tid x 5 days (high frequency of GI side-effects). *See Comment.* Rx if preg: **Paromomycin** 25-35 mg/kg/day po in 3 divided doses x 5-10 days.	**Refractory pts: (metro 750 mg po + quinacrine**[3] **100 mg po)**—both 3x/day x 3 wks (*CID 33:22, 2001*) or furazolidone 100 mg po qid x 7 days. **Nitazoxanide** ref.: *CID 40:1173, 2005.*

[1] **Drugs available from CDC Drug Service: (+1) 404-639-3670 or www.cdc.gov/laboratory/drugservice/index.html: artesunate, Bithionol, dehydroemetine, diethylcarbamazine (DEC), melarsoprol, nifurtimox, sodium stibogluconate (SSG, Pentostoris), suramin.**

[2] Source for Quinacrine, Iodoquinol, Paromomycin, Diloxanide: Gallipot, Inc. (USA) Compounding Pharmacy, +1 651 681 9517 or 800 423 6967; info@gallipot.com

[3] Quinacrine available from Expert Compounding Pharmacy, (800) 247-9767; (+1) (818) 988-7979; www.uniquerx.com.

TABLE 13A (2)

INFECTING ORGANISM	SUGGESTED REGIMENS		COMMENTS
	PRIMARY	ALTERNATIVE	
PROTOZOA—INTESTINAL *(continued)*			
Isospora belli (now Cystoisospora belli); Isosporiasis *(AIDS ref: MMWR 58 (RR-4):1, 2009)*	**TMP-SMX-DS** tab 1 po bid x 7-10 days; if AIDS pt.: TMP-SMX-DS qid for up to 4 wks.	**CIP** 500 mg po bid x 7 days is second-line alternative *(AnIM 132:885, 2000)*. Limited data on CIP for TMP-SMX failure or TMP-SMX allergy.	Chronic suppression in AIDS pts: either **TMP-SMX-DS** 1 tab po 3x/wk OR tab 1 po daily OR (**pyrimethamine** 25 mg/day po + **folinic acid** 10 mg/day po) OR as 2nd-line alternative: **CIP** 500 mg po 3x/wk.
Microsporidiosis	For HIV pts: antiretroviral therapy key		
Ocular: Encephalitozoon hellum or cuniculi, Vittaforma (Nosema) corneae, Nosema ocularum	**Albendazole** 400 mg po bid x 3 wk plus fumagillin eye drops *(see Comment)*.	In HIV+ pts, reports of response of E. hellum to **fumagillin** eyedrops *(see Comment)*. For V. corneae, may need keratoplasty	To obtain fumagillin: 800-292-6773 or www.leiterrx.com. Neutropenia & thrombocytopenia serious adverse events.
Intestinal (diarrhea): Enterocytozoon bieneusi, Encephalitozoon (Septata) intestinalis	**Albendazole** 400 mg po bid x 3 wk; peds dose: 15 mg/kg per day div. into 2 daily doses x 7 days for **E. intestinalis**. Fumagillin equally effective.	Oral **fumagillin 20 mg po tid** reported effective for **E. bieneusi** *(NEJM 346:1963, 2002)—see Comment*	Dx: Most labs use modified trichrome stain. Need electron micrographs for species identification. FA and PCR methods in development. Peds dose ref.: *PIDJ 23:915, 2004*
Disseminated: E. hellum, cuniculi or intestinalis; Pleistophora sp., *others in Comment*	**Albendazole** 400 mg po bid x 3 wk	No established rx for Pleistophora sp.	For Trachipleistophora sp., try itraconazole + albendazole *(NEJM 351:42, 2004)*. Other pathogens: Brachiola vesicularum & algerae *(NEJM 351:42, 2004)*.
PROTOZOA—EXTRAINTESTINAL			
Amebic meningoencephalitis *(Clin Infect Dis 51:e7, 2010 (Bazamuthia))*			
Acanthamoeba sp.— no proven rx Rev.: *FEMS Immunol Med Micro 50:1, 2007*	Success with IV **pentamidine** + **sulfadiazine** + **flucytosine** + (either **fluconazole** or **itraconazole**)*(FEMS Immunol Med Micro 50:1, 2007)*. 2 children responded to po rx: **TMP-SMX** + **rifampin**+ **keto** *(PIDJ 20:623, 2001)*.		For Acanthamoeba keratitis: miltefosine or voriconazole.
Balamuthia mandrillaris	[**Pentamidine** + **Albendazole** + (**Fluconazole** or **Itraconazole**)] or [**Liposomal Ampho B** + **Sulfadiazine** + (**Azithro** or **Clarithro**)]. *See CID 51:e7, 2010.*		Anecdotal response to miltefosine.
Naegleria fowleri. >95% mortality. Ref. *MMWR 57:573, 2008.*	**Ampho B** 1.5 mg/kg per day in 2 div. doses x 3 days; then 1 mg/kg/day x 6 days plus 1.5 mg/day intrathecal x 2 days; then 1 mg/day intrathecal qod x 8 days.		For Naegleria: Ampho B + azithro synergistic in vitro & in mouse model *(AAC 51:23, 2007)*. Ampho B + fluconazole + rifampin may work *(Arch Med Res 36:83, 2005)*.
Sappinia diploidea	**Azithro** + **pentamidine** + **itra** + **flucytosine** *(JAMA 285:2450, 2001)*		
Babesia microti and other Babesia sp.; babesiosis *(CID 43:1089, 2006)*	**For mild/moderate disease:** (**Atovaquone** 750 mg po bid + **Azithro** 600 mg po on day 1, then 500 mg po daily for total of 7-10 days	**For severe babesiosis:** (**Clindamycin** 600 mg po tid) + (**quinine** 650 mg po tid) x 7–10 days For adults, can give **clinda** IV as 1.2 gm bid.	Overwhelming infection in asplenic patients. In immunocompromised patients, treat for 6 or more weeks *(CID 46:370, 2008)*. Consider exchange transfusion if ≥10% parasitemia *(Tranf Med Rev 16:239, 2002)*.
Leishmaniasis *(Suggest consultation – CDC (+1) 770 488 7775; see LnID 7:581, 2007; CID 43:1089, 2006)*			
Cutaneous: Mild Disease (< 4 lesions, none > 5 cm diameter, no lesions in cosmetically sensitive area, non over joints). Otherwise, consider Moderate Disease	**Mild Disease:** Heat therapy **Paromomycin** ointment bid x 20 days (investigational); cryotherapy; intralesional Antimony. Spontaneous resolution in > 50% but may take 6 months *(PLoS Negl Trop Dis 4:e628, 2010)*. Heat therapy, *see www.thermosurgery.com.*	**Moderate Disease:** **Sodium stibogluconate** (Pentostam) or **Meglumine antimoniate** (Glucantime) 20 mg/kg/day IV/IM x 20 days. Dilute in 120 mL of D5W and infuse over 2 hrs. Alternative: **Fluconazole** 200 mg po daily x 6 weeks	Ampho B (lipid & non-lipid) active vs. cutaneous leishmaniasis in some settings. Topical paromomycin[NUS] & other topical treatment only when low potential for mucosal spread. Generic pentavalent antimony varies in quality and safety.

TABLE 13A (3)

INFECTING ORGANISM	SUGGESTED REGIMENS		COMMENTS
	PRIMARY	ALTERNATIVE	
PROTOZOA—EXTRAINTESTINAL *(continued)*			
Mucosal (Espundia). Usually due to L. brasiliensis.	**Pentavalent antimony (Sb)** 20 mg/kg/day IV or IM x 28 days or **liposomal amphotericin B** (regimens vary) with total cumulative dose of 20-60 mg/kg or **amphotericin B** 0.5-1 mg/kg IV daily or qod to total dose of 20-40 mg/kg.	No good alternative; variable efficacy of oral Miltefosine: **Miltefosine**[NUS] 2.5 mg/kg/day (to maximum of 150 mg/day) po x 28 days *(AJTMH 81:387, 2009)*. For sources, *see Table 13D, page 144.*	
Visceral leishmaniasis – Kala-Azar – New World & Old World *L. donovani*: India, Africa *L. infantum*: Mediterranean *L. chagasi*: New World	**Liposomal ampho B** FDA-approved in immunocompetent hosts: 3 mg/kg once daily days 1-5 & days 14, 21. Alternative regimens: 3 mg/kg IV daily on days 1-5 and day 10 or 10 mg/kg on days 1 and 2.	**Standard Ampho B** 1 mg/kg IV daily x 15-20 days or qod x 8 wks (to total of 15-20 mg/kg)	
Malaria (Plasmodia species)—NOTE: CDC Malaria info—prophylaxis/treatment (770) 488-7788. After hours: 770-488-7100. Refs: ***JAMA 297:2251, 2264 & 2285, 2007.*** **Websites: www.cdc.gov/malaria; www.who.int/health-topics/malaria.htm.**			
Prophylaxis—Drugs plus personal protection: screens, nets, 30–35% DEET skin repellent (avoid 95% products in children), permethrin spray on clothing and mosquito nets			
For areas free of chloroquine (CQ)-resistant P. falciparum: Haiti, Dom. Republic, Cen. America west & north of the Panama Canal, & parts of Middle East	**CQ** 500 mg (300 mg base) po per wk starting 1–2 wk before travel, during travel, & 4 wks post-travel **or atovaquone-proguanil (AP)** 1 adult tab per day (1 day prior to, during, & 7 days post-travel). Another option for adults for P. vivax prophylaxis: **primaquine (PQ)** 30 mg base po daily in non-pregnant. G6PD-neg. travelers; >92% effective vs P. vivax *(CID 33:1990, 2001)*. Note: **CQ** may exacerbate psoriasis.	**CQ Peds dose:** 8.3 mg/kg (5 mg/kg of base) po 1x/wk up to 300 mg (base) max. dose **or AP** by weight (peds tabs): 11–20 kg, 1 tab; 21–30 kg, 2 tabs; 31–40 kg, 3 tabs; >40 kg, 1 adult tab per day. **Adults**: **Doxy** or **MQ** as below.	CQ safe during pregnancy. **The areas free of CQ-resistant falciparum malaria continue to shrink:** *See CDC or WHO maps for most current information on CQ resistance.*
For areas with CQ-resistant P. falciparum CDC info on prophylaxis (770) 488-7788 or website: *www.cdc.gov/malaria & LnID 6:139, 2006*	**Atovaquone** 250 mg—**proguanil** 100 mg **(Malarone)** comb. tablet, 1 per day with food 1–2 days prior to, during, & 7 days post-travel. Peds dose in footnote[4]. **Not in pregnancy**	**Doxycycline** 100 mg po daily for adults & children > 8 yrs of age[4]. Take 1-2 days before, during & for 4 wks after travel. **OR** **Mefloquine (MQ)**[4] 250 mg (228 mg base) po once per wk, 1-2 wks before, during, & for 4 wks after travel *(see Comment)*. *Peds dose in footnote[4]*	**Pregnancy: MQ current best option.** Insufficient data with **Malarone**. **Avoid doxycycline and primaquine.** **Primaquine: Can cause hemolytic anemia if G6PD deficiency present.** **MQ not recommended** if cardiac conduction abnormalities, seizures, or psychiatric disorders, e.g., depression, psychosis. MQ outside U.S.: 275 mg tab, contains 250 mg of base. If used, can start 3 wks before travel to assure tolerability.

[4] **Peds prophylaxis dosages** (Ref.: *CID 34:493, 2002*): **Mefloquine** weekly dose by **weight** in kg: <15 = 5 mg/kg; 15–19 = ¼ adult dose; 20–30 = ½ adult dose; 31–45 = ¾ adult dose; >45 = adult dose. **Atovaquone/proguanil** by **weight** in kg, single daily dose using peds tab (62.5 mg atovaquone & 25 mg proguanil): 5-8 kg, 1/2 tab; 8-10 kg, 3/4 tab; 11–20 kg, 1 tab; 21–30 kg, 2 tabs; 31-40 kg, 3 tabs; ≥41 kg, one adult tab. **Doxycycline**, ages >8–12 yrs: 2 mg per kg per day up to 100 mg/day. Continue daily x 4 wks after leaving risk area. Side effects: photosensitivity, nausea, yeast vaginitis

TABLE 13A (4)

INFECTING ORGANISM	SUGGESTED REGIMENS		COMMENTS
	PRIMARY	ALTERNATIVE	

PROTOZOA—EXTRAINTESTINAL/Malaria (Plasmodia species) *(continued)*

Treatment of Malaria. Diagnosis is by microscopy. Alternative: rapid antigen detection test (Binax NOW): detects 96-100% of P. falciparum and 93% of other plasmodia *(CID 49:908, 2009)*. Need microscopy to speciate. Can stay positive for over a month after successful treatment.

Clinical Severity/ Plasmodia sp.	Region Acquired	Suggested Treatment Regimens (Drug)		Comments
		Primary—Adults	Alternative & Peds	
Uncomplicated/ **P. falciparum (or species not identified)** Malaria rapid diagnostic test (Binax NOW) approved: *MMWR 56:686, 2007*	Cen. Amer., west of Panama Canal; Haiti, Dom. Repub., & most of Mid East—**CQ-sensitive**	**CQ** 1 gm salt (600 mg base) po, then 0.5 gm in 6 hrs, then 0.5 gm daily x 2 days. Total: 2500 mg salt	**Peds: CQ** 10 mg/kg of base po; then 5 mg/kg of base at 6, 24, & 48 hrs. Total: 25 mg/kg base	**Peds dose should never exceed adult dose.**
	CQ-resistant or unknown resistance	**Adults:** [(**QS** 650 mg po tid x 3 days (7 days if SE Asia)] + [(**Doxy** 100 mg po bid) or (**tetra** 250 mg po qid) or **clinda** 20 mg/kg/d divided tid) x 7 days] **OR Atovaquone-proguanil** 1 gm–400 mg (4 adult tabs) po 1x/day x 3 days w/ food **OR Artemether-lumefantrine** tabs (20 mg Art/120 mg Lum): 4 tabs po (at time zero & 8 hrs later) then bid x 2 days (total 6 doses); take with food **OR** as an adult alternative, **mefloquine** 750 mg po x 1 dose, then 500 mg po x 1 dose 6-12 hr later.	**Peds:** (**QS** 10 mg/kg po tid x 3 days) + (**clinda** 20 mg/kg per day div. tid) —both x 7 days. **MQ Salt:** 15 mg/kg x 1, then 6-12 hrs later, 10 mg/kg ALL po. **Artemether-lumefantrine** 6 doses over 3 days (see adult regimen) by weight: 5<15 kg: 1 tab/dose 15<25 kg: 2 tab/dose 25<35 kg: 3 tab/dose >35 kg: 4 tab/dose	Can substitute clinda for doxy/tetra: 20 mg/kg per day po div. tid x 7 days. MQ alternative due to neuropsych. reactions. Avoid if malaria acquired in SE Asia due to resistance. **Peds atovaquone-proguanil dose** (all once daily x 3 d) by weight: 5-8 kg: 2 peds tabs; 9-10 kg: 3 peds tabs; 11-20 kg: 1 adult tab; 21-30 kg: 2 adult tabs; 31-40 kg: 3 adult tabs; >40 kg: 4 adult tabs.
Uncomplicated / P. malariae or P. knowlesi *(JID 199: 1107 & 1143, 2009)*.	All regions	**CQ** as above: adults & peds. In South Pacific, beware of P. knowlesi: looks like P. malariae, but behaves like P. falciparum *(CID 46:165, 2007)*.		
Uncomplicated/ P. vivax or P. ovale	All except Papua, New Guinea & Indonesia (CQ-resistant)	**CQ** as above + **PQ** base: 30 mg po once daily x 14 days	**Peds: CQ** as above + **PQ** base 0.5 mg po once daily x 14 days	PQ added to eradicate latent parasites in liver. **Screen for G6PD def. before starting PQ;** if G6PD positive, dose PQ as 45 mg po once weekly x 8 wk. **Note: rare severe reactions.** Avoid PQ in pregnancy.
Uncomplicated/ P. vivax	CQ-resistant: Papua, New Guinea & Indonesia	[**QS** + (**doxy** or **tetra**) + **PQ**] as above or **Artemether-Lumefantrine** (same dose as for P. falciparum)	**MQ** + **PQ** as above. **Peds** (<8 yrs old): **QS** alone x 7 days or **MQ** alone. If latter fail, add **doxy** or **tetra**	Rarely acute. Lung injury and other serious complications: *LnID 8:449, 2008*.
Uncomplicated Malaria/Alternatives for Pregnancy Ref: *LnID 7:118 & 136, 2007*	CQ-sensitive areas	**CQ** as above		Doxy or tetra used if benefits outweigh risks. No controlled studies of AP in pregnancy. Possible association of MQ & ↑ number of stillbirths. If P. vivax or P. ovale, after pregnancy check for G6PD & give PQ 30 mg po daily times 14 days.
	CQ-resistant P. falciparum	**QS** + **clinda** as above	If failing or intolerant, **QS** + **doxy**	
	CQ-resistant P. vivax	**QS** 650 mg po tid x 7 days		

TABLE 13A (5)

INFECTING ORGANISM	SUGGESTED REGIMENS			COMMENTS
	PRIMARY		ALTERNATIVE	
PROTOZOA—EXTRAINTESTINAL/Malaria (Plasmodia species)/Treatment of Malaria *(continued)*				
Clinical Severity/ Plasmodia sp.	**Region Acquired**	**Suggested Treatment Regimens (Drug)**		**Comments**
		Primary—Adults	**Alternative & Peds**	
Severe malaria, i.e., impaired consciousness, severe anemia, renal failure, pulmonary edema, ARDS, DIC, jaundice, acidosis, seizures, parasitemia >5%. One or more of latter. **Almost always P. falciparum.** *Ref: NEJM 358:1829, 2008; Science 320:30, 2008.*	All regions Note: Artesunate is effective but not FDA-approved. Available from CDC Drug Service under specific conditions.	**Quinidine gluconate** in normal saline: 10 mg/kg (salt) IV over 1 hr then 0.02 mg/kg/min by constant infusion OR 24 mg/kg IV over 4 hrs & then 12 mg/kg over 4 hrs q8h. Continue until parasite density <1% & can take po QS. **QS** as above x 7 days (SE Asia) or 3 days elsewhere **PLUS** (**Doxy** 100 mg IV q12h x 7 days) **OR** (**clinda** 10 mg/kg IV load & then 5 mg/kg IV q8h x 7 days)	**Peds**: **Quinidine gluconate IV**—same mg/kg dose as for adults **PLUS** (**Doxy**: if <45 kg, 4 mg per kg IV q12h; if ≥45 kg, dose as for adults) OR **Clinda**, same mg/kg dose as for adults For IV **artesunate**, *see Comment*: artemether po tabs are not indicated for severe malaria.	During quinidine IV: monitor BP, EKG (prolongation of QTc), & blood glucose (hypoglycemia). Consider exchange transfusion if parasitemia >10%. Switch to QS po + (Doxy or Clinda) when patient able to take oral drugs. Steroids not recommended for cerebral malaria. If quinidine not available, or patient intolerant or high level parasitemia, **IV artesunate** available from CDC Malaria Branch (770-488-7788 or 770-488-7100) (Ref: *CID 44:1067 & 1075, 2007*). Dose: 2.4 mg/kg IV at 0, 12, 24 & 48 hrs, followed by one week of doxycycline (use clinda in pregnancy). Alternative: atovaquone-proguanil.
Malaria—self-initiated treatment: Only for people at high risk. Carry a reliable supply of recommended treatment (to avoid counterfeit meds). Use only if malaria diagnosed.	**Atovaquone-proguanil (AP)** 4 adult tabs (1 gm/400 mg) po daily x 3 days		**Peds:** Using adult **AP** tabs for 3 consecutive days: 11–20 kg, 1 tab; 21–30 kg, 2 tabs; 31–40 kg, 3 tabs; >41 kg, 4 tabs.	Do not use for renal insufficiency pts. Do not use if weight <11 kg, pregnant, or breast-feeding.
Pneumocystis carinii pneumonia (PCP). Revised name is **Pneumocystis jiroveci** (yee-row-vek-ee). *Ref: JAMA 301:2578, 2009.*				
Not acutely ill, able to take po meds. PaO_2 >70 mmHg Interest in detection of PCP by serum assay for B-Glucan *(AnIM 147:70, 2007 & Chest 131:1173, 2007).*	(**TMP-SMX-DS**, 2 tabs po q8h x 21 days) OR (**Dapsone** 100 mg po q24h + **trimethoprim** 5 mg/kg po tid x 21 days) NOTE: Concomitant use of corticosteroids usually reserved for sicker pts with PaO_2 <70 *(see below)*		[**Clindamycin** 300–450 mg po q6h + **primaquine** 15 mg base po q24h] x 21 days OR **Atovaquone** suspension 750 mg po bid with food x 21 days	Mutations in gene of the enzyme target (dihydropteroate synthetase) of sulfamethoxazole identified. Unclear whether mutations result in resist to TMP-SMX or dapsone + TMP *(EID 10:1721, 2004)*. Dapsone ref.: *CID 27:191, 1998.* **After 21 days, chronic suppression in AIDS pts *(see below—post-treatment suppression).***
Acutely ill, po rx not possible. PaO_2 <70 mmHg. Still unclear whether antiretroviral therapy (ART) should be started during treatment of PCP *(CID 46: 634, 2008).*	[**Prednisone** (15–30 min. before TMP-SMX): 40 mg po bid times 5 days, then 40 mg q24h times 5 days, then 20 mg po q24h times 11 days] + [**TMP-SMX** (15 mg of TMP component per kg per day) IV div. q6–8h times 21 days] Can substitute IV prednisolone (reduce dose 25%) for po prednisone		**Prednisone** as in primary rx PLUS [(**Clinda** 600 mg IV q8h) + (**primaquine** 30 mg base po q24h)] times 21 days OR **Pentamidine** 4 mg per kg per day IV times 21 days Caspofungin active in animal models: *CID 36:1445, 2003.*	**After 21 days, chronic suppression in AIDS pts (see *post-treatment suppression*).** **PCP can occur in absence of HIV infection & steroids *(CID 25:215 & 219, 1997).*** Wait 4–8 days before declaring treatment failure & switching to clinda + primaquine or pentamidine *(JAIDS 48:63, 2008)*, or adding caspofungin *(Transplant 84:685, 2007).*
Primary prophylaxis and post-treatment suppression	(**TMP-SMX-DS or -SS**, 1 tab po q24h or 1 DS 3x/wk) OR (**dapsone** 100 mg po q24h). DC when CD4 >200 x/3 mo *(NEJM 344:159, 2001).*		(**Pentamidine** 300 mg in 6 mL sterile water by aerosol q4 wks) OR (**dapsone** 200 mg po + **pyrimethamine** 75 mg po + **folinic acid** 25 mg po—**all once a week**) or **atovaquone** 1500 mg po q24h with food.	TMP-SMX-DS regimen provides cross-protection vs toxo and other bacterial infections. Dapsone + pyrimethamine protects vs toxo. Atovaquone suspension 1500 mg once daily as effective as daily dapsone *(NEJM 339:1889, 1998)* or inhaled pentamidine *(JID 180:369, 1999).*

TABLE 13A (6)

INFECTING ORGANISM	SUGGESTED REGIMENS		COMMENTS
	PRIMARY	ALTERNATIVE	
PROTOZOA—EXTRAINTESTINAL/Malaria (Plasmodia species)/Treatment of Malaria *(continued)*			
Toxoplasma gondii (Reference: *Ln 363:1965, 2004*)			
Immunologically normal patients *(For pediatric doses, see reference)*			
Acute illness w/ lymphadenopathy	No specific rx unless severe/persistent symptoms or evidence of vital organ damage		
Acq. via transfusion (lab accident)	Treat as for active chorioretinitis.		
Active chorioretinitis; meningitis; lowered resistance due to steroids or cytotoxic drugs	[**Pyrimethamine** (pyri) 200 mg po once on 1st day, then 50–75 mg q24h] + [**sulfadiazine** *(see footnote[5])* 1–1.5 gm po qid] + [**leucovorin (folinic acid)** 5–20 mg 3x/wk]—***see Comment.*** Treat 1–2 wk beyond resolution of signs/symptoms; continue leucovorin 1 wk after stopping pyri.		For congenital toxo, toxo meningitis in adults, & chorioretinitis, **add prednisone 1 mg/kg/day in 2 div. doses** until CSF protein conc. falls or vision-threatening inflammation subsides. Adjust folinic acid dose by following CBC results.
Acute in pregnant women. Ref: *CID 47:554, 2008.*	**If <18 wks gestation: Spiramycin[NUS]** 1 gm po q8h until delivery if amniotic fluid PCR is negative. **If >18 wks gestation & documented fetal infection by positive amniotic fluid PCR: Pyrimethamine** 50 mg po q12h x 2 days, then 50 mg/day + **sulfadiazine** 75 mg/kg po x 1 dose, then 50 mg/kg q12h (max 4 gm/day) + **folinic acid** 10-20 mg po daily.		Screen patients with IgG/IgM serology at commercial lab. IgG+ /IgM neg = remote past infection; IgG+/IgM+ = seroconversion. Suggest consultation with Palo Alto Medical Foundation Toxoplasma Serology Lab: 650-853-4828 or toxlab@pamf.org
Fetal/congenital	Mgmt complex. Combo rx with pyrimethamine + sulfadiazine + leucovorin—*see Comment*		Details in *Ln 363:1965, 2004*. **Consultation advisable.**
AIDS			
Cerebral toxoplasmosis *Ref: MMWR 58(RR-4) 1, 2009.*	[**Pyrimethamine** (pyri) 200 mg x 1 po, then 75 mg/day po] + (**sulfadiazine** [Wt based dose: 1 gm if <60 kg, 1.5 gm if ≥60 kg] po q6h) + (**folinic acid** 10–25 mg/day po) for minimum of 6 wks after resolution of signs/ symptoms, and then suppressive rx *(see below)* OR **TMP-SMX** 10/50 mg/kg per day po or IV div. q12h x 30 days *(AAC 42:1346, 1998)*	[**Pyri** + **folinic acid** (as in primary regimen)] + 1 of the following: (1) **Clinda** 600 mg po/IV q6h or (2) **TMP=SMX** 5/25 mg/kg/day po or IV bid or (3) **atovaquone** 750 mg po q6h. Treat 4–6 wks after resolution of signs/symptoms, then suppression.	Use alternative regimen for pts with severe sulfa allergy. If multiple ring-enhancing brain lesions (CT or MRI), >85% of pts respond to 7–10 days of empiric rx; if no response, suggest brain biopsy. Pyri penetrates brain even if no inflammation; folinic acid prevents pyrimethamine hematologic toxicity.
Primary prophylaxis, AIDS pts—IgG toxo antibody + CD4 count <100 per mcL	(**TMP-SMX-DS**, 1 tab po q24h or 3x/wk) or (**TMP-SMX-SS**, 1 tab po q24h)	[(**Dapsone** 50 mg po q24h) + (**pyri** 50 mg po q wk) + (**folinic acid** 25 mg po q wk)] OR **atovaquone** 1500 mg po q24h	Prophylaxis for pneumocystis also effective vs toxo. *Ref: MMWR 58(RR-4):1, 2009.* **Another alternative:** (Dapsone 200 mg po + pyrimethamine 75 mg po + folinic acid 25 mg po) once weekly.
Suppression after rx of cerebral toxo	(**Sulfadiazine** 2-4 gm po divided in 2-4 doses/day) + (**pyri** 25–50 mg po q24h) + (**folinic acid** 10–25 mg po q24h). DC if CD4 count >200 x 3 mo	[(**Clinda** 600 mg po q8h) + (**pyri** 25–50 mg po q24h) + (**folinic acid** 10–25 mg po q24h)] OR **atovaquone** 750 mg po q6–12h	(Pyri + sulfa) prevents PCP and toxo; (clinda + pyri) prevents toxo only. Additional drug needed to prevent PCP.
Trichomonas vaginalis	*See Vaginitis, Table 1A, page 24.*		
Trypanosomiasis. Ref.: ***Ln 362:1469, 2003.*** **Note:** Drugs for African trypanosomiasis may be obtained free from WHO. *See Table 13D, page 144.*			
West African sleeping sickness (T. brucei gambiense)			
Early: Blood/lymphatic—CNS OK	**Pentamidine** 4 mg/kg IM daily x 10 days	From CDC drug service: **Suramin** 100 mg IV (test dose), then 1 gm IV on days 1, 3, 7, 14, & 21	
Late: Encephalitis	**Eflornithine** 100 mg/kg q6h IV x 14 days *(CID 41:748, 2005)*. Obtain drug from WHO drug service *(simarrop@who.int or +41 22 791 1345).*	**Melarsoprol** 2.2 mg/kg per day IV x 10 days (melarsoprol/nifurtimox combination superior to melarsoprol alone *(JID 195:311 & 322, 2007)*.	Combination of IV eflornithine, 400 mg/kg/day divided q12h x 7 days, plus nifurtimox, 15 mg/kg/day po, divided q8h x 10 days more efficacious than standard dose eflornithine *(CID 45:1435 & 1443, 2007)*.

[5] Sulfonamides for toxo. Sulfadiazine now commercially available. Sulfisoxazole much less effective.

TABLE 13A (7)

INFECTING ORGANISM	SUGGESTED REGIMENS		COMMENTS
	PRIMARY	ALTERNATIVE	
PROTOZOA—EXTRAINTESTINAL/Trypanosomiasis *(continued)*			
East African sleeping sickness (T. brucei rhodesiense)			
Early: Blood/lymphatic	**Suramin** 100 mg IV (test dose), then 1 gm IV on days 1, 3, 7, 14, & 21	None	
Late: Encephalitis	**Melarsoprol**[6] 2–3.6 mg/kg per day IV x 3 days; repeat after 7 days & for 3rd time 7 days after 2nd course	Prednisone may prevent/attenuate encephalopathy	
T. cruzi—**Chagas disease** or acute American trypanosomiasis Ref.: *Ln 375:1388, 2010; LnID 10:556, 2010.* For chronic disease: *see Comment.*	**Nifurtimox**[6] 8–10 mg/kg per day po div. 4x/day after meals x 90-120 days Ages 11–16 yrs: 12.5–15 mg/kg per day div. qid po x 90 days Children <11yrs: 15–20 mg/kg per day div. qid po x 90 days.	**Benznidazole**[NUS] 5–7 mg/kg per day po div. 2x/day x 30–90 days *(AJTMH 63:111, 2000).* NOTE: Take with meals to alleviate G-I side effects. Contraindicated in pregnancy.	Immunosuppression for heart transplant can reactivate chronic Chagas disease.
NEMATODES—INTESTINAL (Roundworms). Eosinophilia? Think Strongyloides, toxocaria and filariasis: *CID 34:407, 2005; 42:1781 & 1655, 2006-- See Table 13C.*			
Anisakis simplex (**anisakiasis**) Anisakiasis differentiated from Anisakidosis *(CID 51:806, 2010).*	Physical removal: endoscope or surgery IgE antibody test vs *A. simplex* may help diagnosis.	Anecdotal reports of possible treatment benefit from albendazole *(Ln 360:54, 2002; CID 41:1825, 2005)*	Anisakiasis acquired by eating raw fish: herring, salmon, mackerel, cod, squid. Similar illness due to Pseudoterranova species acquired from cod, halibut, red snapper.
Ascaris lumbricoides (**ascariasis**) *Ln 367:1521, 2006*	**Albendazole** 400 mg po daily x 3 days or **mebendazole** 100 mg po daily x 3 days	**Ivermectin** 150–200 mcg/kg po x 1 dose	Review of efficacy of single dose: *JAMA 299:1937, 2008.*
Capillaria philippinensis (**capillariasis**)	**Mebendazole** 200 mg po bid x 20 days	**Albendazole** 400 mg po bid x 10 days	
Enterobius vermicularis (**pinworm**)	**Mebendazole** 100 mg po x 1, repeat in 2 wks	**Pyrantel pamoate** 11 mg/kg base (to max. dose of 1 gm) po x 1 dose; repeat in 2 wks **OR Albendazole** 400 mg po x 1 dose, repeat in 2 wks.	*Side-effects in Table 13B, page 143.*
Gongylonemiasis	Surgical removal or **albendazole** 400 mg/day po x 3 days		Ref: *CID 32:1378, 2001; J Helminth 80:425, 2006.*
Hookworm (Necator americanus and Ancylostoma duodenale)	**Albendazole** 400 mg po daily x 3 days or **mebendazole** 100 mg po bid x 3 days.	**Pyrantel pamoate** 11 mg/kg (to max. dose of 1 gm) po daily x 3 days	NOTE: Ivermectin not effective. Eosinophilia may be absent but eggs in stool *(NEJM 351:799, 2004).*
Strongyloides stercoralis (**strongyloidiasis**)*(See Comment)*	**Ivermectin** 200 mcg/kg per day po x 2 days	**Albendazole** 400 mg po bid x 7 days ; less effective	**For hyperinfections**, repeat at 15 days. For hyperinfection: veterinary ivermectin given subcutaneously or rectally *(CID 49:1411, 2009).*
Trichostrongylus orientalis	**Pyrantel pamoate** 11 mg/kg (max. 1 gm) po x 1	**Albendazole** 400 mg po x 1 dose	**Mebendazole** 100 mg po bid x 3 days
Trichuris trichiura (**whipworm**) *(Ln 367:1521, 2006)*	**Albendazole** 400 mg po 1x/day x 3 days	**Mebendazole** (100 mg po bid x 3 days or 500 mg once) or **Ivermectin** 200 mcg/kg daily po x 3 days	Cure rate of 55% with one 500 mg dose of **Mebendazole** + one dose of **Ivermectin** 200 mcg/kg *(CID 51:1420, 2010).*
NEMATODES—EXTRAINTESTINAL (Roundworms)			
Ancylostoma braziliense & caninum: causes **cutaneous larva migrans** (Dog & cat hookworm)	**Albendazole** 400 mg po bid x 3 days	**Ivermectin** 200 mcg/kg po x 1 dose/day x 1–2 days	Also called "creeping eruption," dog and cat hookworm. Ivermectin cure rate 77% (1 dose) to 97% (2–3 doses) *(CID 31:493, 2000).*
Angiostrongylus cantonensis (Angiostrongyliasis); eosinophilic meningitis	Symptomatic therapy: Analgesics and, only if necessary, serial LPs.	Drug therapy controversial, may consider. **Albendazole** 400 mg po bid x 21 days	Reports of combining steroids with albendazole *(CID 48:322, 2009; LnID 8:621, 2008).*

[6] Available from CDC Drug Service; *Table 13D, page 144.*

TABLE 13A (8)

INFECTING ORGANISM	SUGGESTED REGIMENS		COMMENTS
	PRIMARY	ALTERNATIVE	
NEMATODES—EXTRAINTESTINAL (Roundworms) *(continued)*			
Baylisascariasis (Raccoon ascaris)	No drug proven efficacious. Try po **albendazole**, Peds: 25–50 mg/kg per day; Adults: 400 mg bid. Both x 10 days		Some add steroids *(CID 39:1484, 2004)*.
Dracunculus medinensis: **Guinea worm** *(CMAJ 170:495, 2004)*	Slow extraction of pre-emergent worm	No drugs effective. Oral analgesics, anti-inflammatory drugs, topical antiseptics/antibiotic ointments to alleviate symptoms and facilitate worm removal by gentle manual traction over several days.	
Filariasis. Wolbachia bacteria needed for filarial development. **Rx with doxy 100–200 mg/day x 6-8 wks** ↓ number of wolbachia & number of microfilaria but no effect on adult worms *(BMJ 326:207, 2003)*			
Lymphatic filariasis (**Elephantiasis**): Wuchereria bancrofti or Brugia malayi or B. timori. Ref: *Curr Opin Inf Dis 21:673, 2008.*	**Diethylcarbamazine**[7,8](DEC): Day 1, 50 mg po; Day 2, 50 mg tid; Day 3, 100 mg tid; Days 4-14, 2 mg/kg q8h for total of 72 mg over 14 days *(see comment)* PLUS **doxy** 200 mg/day x 6 wks	Interest in combining albendazole with **DEC**; no trials comparing combination vs. DEC alone. **Doxycycline** 200 mg/day x 6 wks PLUS **DEC** + **albendazole** reduced microfilaremia *(CID 46:1385, 2008).*	**NOTE: DEC can cause irreversible eye damage if concomitant onchocerciasis.** Goal is reducing burden of adult worms. (Albendazole 400 mg po + Ivermectin 200 mg/kg po) or DEC 6 mg/kg po suppresses microfilaria but no effective on adult worms.
Cutaneous			
Loiasis: **Loa loa**, eyeworm disease	**Diethylcarbamazine** (DEC)[7,8]: Day 1, 50 mg; Day 2, 50 mg tid; Day 3, 100 mg tid; Days 4-21, 8-10 mg/kg/day in 3 divided doses	**Albendazole** 200 mg po bid x 21 days	If concomitant oncho & Loa loa, treat oncho first. If over 5,000 microfilaria/mL of blood, DEC can cause encephalopathy. Might start with albendazole x few days ± steroids, then DEC.
Onchocerca volvulus (**onchocerciasis**)—river blindness *(AJTMH 81:702, 2009)*	First give **doxy** 200 mg/day x 6 wks and then **Ivermectin**: Single dose of 150 mcg/kg po; repeat every 6-12 months until asymptomatic.	If **ivermectin** fails, consider **suramin** (from CDC Drug Service)	Oncho & Loa loa may both be present. Check peripheral smear; if Loa loa microfilaria present, treat oncho first with ivermectin before DEC for Loa loa.
Body cavity			
Mansonella perstans (dipetalonemiasis)	In randomized trial, doxy 200 mg po once daily x 6 weeks cleared microfilaria from blood in 67 of 69 patients *(NEJM 361:1448, 2009).*	**Albendazole** in high dose x 3 weeks.	Efficacy of doxy believed to be due to inhibition of endosymbiont wolbachia. Ivermectin has no activity. Ref: *Trans R Soc Trop Med Hyg 100:458, 2006.*
Mansonella streptocerca	**Diethylcarbamazine**[7,8], as above for Wuchereria OR **ivermectin** 150 mcg/kg x 1	Chronic pruritic hypopigmented lesions that may be confused with leprosy. Can be asymptomatic.	
Mansonella ozzardi	**Ivermectin** 200 mcg/kg x 1 dose may be effective	Usually asymptomatic. Articular pain, pruritus, lymphadenopathy reported. May have allergic reaction from dying organisms.	
Dirofilariasis: **Heartworms**			
D. immitis, dog heartworm	No effective drugs; surgical removal only option		Can lodge in pulmonary artery → coin lesion. Eosinophilia rare.
D. tenuis (raccoon), D. ursi (bear), D. repens (dogs, cats)	No effective drugs	Worms migrate to conjunctivae, subcutaneous tissue, scrotum, breasts, extremities	
Gnathostoma spinigerum: eosinophilic myeloencephalitis	**Albendazole** 400 mg po q24h or bid times 21 days	**Ivermectin** 200 μg/kg/day po x 2 days.	
Toxocariasis: *Clin Micro Rev 16:265, 2003*	**Rx directed at relief of symptoms as infection self-limited, e.g., steroids & antihistamines; use of anthelminthics controversial.**		
Visceral larval migrans	**Albendazole** 400 mg po bid x 5 days	**Mebendazole** 100–200 mg po bid times 5 days	Severe lung, heart or CNS disease may warrant steroids. Differential dx of larval migrans syndromes: Toxocara canis & catis, Ancylostoma spp., Gnathostoma spp., Spirometra spp.

[7] Available from CDC Drug Service; *Table 13D, page 144.*

[8] May need antihistamine or corticosteroid for allergic reaction from disintegrating organisms

TABLE 13A (9)

INFECTING ORGANISM	SUGGESTED REGIMENS		COMMENTS
	PRIMARY	ALTERNATIVE	
NEMATODES—EXTRAINTESTINAL (Roundworms)/Toxocariasis *(continued)*			
Ocular larval migrans	First 4 wks of illness: (Oral **prednisone** 30–60 mg po q24h + subtenon **triamcinolone** 40 mg/wk) x 2 wk		No added benefit of antihelminthic drugs. Rx of little effect after 4 wk. Some use steroids *(Clin Micro Rev 16:265, 2003)*.
Trichinella spiralis (**trichinosis**)—muscle infection	**Albendazole** 400 mg po bid x 8–14 days	**Mebendazole** 200–400 mg po tid x 3 days, then 400–500 mg po tid x 10 days	Use albendazole/mebendazole with caution during pregnancy. Eosinophilia, ↑ IgE, ↑ CPK, ESR 0!
	Concomitant **prednisone** 40–60 mg po q24h		
TREMATODES (Flukes)			
Clonorchis sinensis (liver fluke)	**Praziquantel** 25 mg/kg po tid x 2 days or **albendazole** 10 mg/kg per day po x 7 days		Same dose in children
Dicrocoelium dendriticum	**Praziquantel** 25 mg/kg po tid x 1 day		Ingestion of raw or undercooked sheep liver *(CID 44:145, 2007)*.
Fasciola buski (intestinal fluke)	**Praziquantel** 25 mg/kg po tid x 1 day		Same dose in children
Fasciola hepatica (sheep liver fluke)	**Triclabendazole**[NUS] once, may repeat after 24 hrs. (Source: *See Table 13D, page 144*) 10 mg/kg po x 1 dose (Ref.: *Clin Micro Infect 11:859, 2005*)		**Bithionol**[9]. Adults and children: 30–50 mg/kg (max. dose 2 gm/day) every other day times 10–15 doses. In CDC formulary, efficacy unclear.
Heterophyes heterophyes (intestinal fluke); Metagonimus yokogawai (intestinal fluke); Metorchis conjunctus (No Amer liver fluke); Nanophyetus salmincola	**Praziquantel** 25 mg/kg po tid x 1 days		
Opisthorchis viverrini (liver fluke)	**Praziquantel** 25 mg/kg po tid x 2 days		
Paragonimus westermani (lung fluke)	**Praziquantel** 25 mg/kg po tid x 2 days or **bithionol**[9] 30–50 mg/kg po x 1 every other day x 10-15 doses		Same dose in children
Schistosoma haematobium; GU bilharziasis. *(NEJM 346:1212, 2002)*	**Praziquantel** 20 mg/kg po bid x 1 day **(2 doses)**		Same dose in children.
Schistosoma intercalatum	**Praziquantel** 20 mg/kg po bid x 1 day **(2 doses)**		Same dose in children
Schistosoma japonicum; Oriental schisto. *(NEJM 346:1212, 2002)*	**Praziquantel** 20 mg/kg po **tid** x 1 day **(3 doses)**		Same dose in children. Cures 60–90% pts.
Schistosoma mansoni (intestinal bilharziasis) **Possible praziquantel resistance** *(JID 176:304, 1997) (NEJM 346:1212, 2002)*	**Praziquantel** 20 mg/kg po bid x 1 day (2 doses)		Praziquantel: Same dose for children and adults. Cures 60–90% pts. Report of success treating myeloradiculopathy with single po dose of praziquantel, 50 mg/kg, + prednisone for 6 mo *(CID 39:1618, 2004)*.
Schistosoma mekongi	**Praziquantel** 20 mg per kg po **tid** times 1 day **(3 doses)**		Same dose for children
Toxemic schisto; Katayama fever	**Praziquantel** 20 mg per kg po bid or tid x 3-6 days *(LnID 7:213, 2007)*.		Reaction to onset of egg laying 4-6 wks after infection exposure in fresh water.
CESTODES (Tapeworms)			
Echinococcus granulosus (hydatid disease) *(AJTMH 79:301, 2008)*	Meta-analysis supports percutaneous aspiration-injection-reaspiration (**PAIR**) + albendazole for uncomplicated single liver cysts. Before **&** after drainage: **albendazole** ≥60 kg, 400 mg po bid or <60 kg, 15 mg/kg per day div. bid, with meals. Then: Puncture (P) & needle aspirate (A) cyst content. Instill (I) hypertonic saline (15–30%) or absolute alcohol, wait 20–30 min, then re-aspirate (R) with final irrigation. **Continue albendazole x 28 days** Cure in 96% as comp to 90% pts with surgical resection.		
Echinococcus multilocularis (alveolar cyst disease) *(COID 16:437, 2003)*	**Albendazole** efficacy not clearly demonstrated, can try in dosages used for hydatid disease. Wide surgical resection only reliable rx; technique evolving *(AJM 118:195, 2005)*.		

[9] Available from CDC Drug Service; *Table 13D, page 144*.

TABLE 13A (10)

INFECTING ORGANISM	SUGGESTED REGIMENS — PRIMARY	SUGGESTED REGIMENS — ALTERNATIVE	COMMENTS
CESTODES (Tapeworms) *(continued)*			
Intestinal tapeworms			
Diphyllobothrium latum (fish), Dipylidium caninum (dog), Taenia saginata (beef), & Taenia solium (pork)	**Praziquantel** 5–10 mg/kg po x 1 dose for children and adults.		
Hymenolepis diminuta (rats) and H. nana (humans)	**Praziquantel** 25 mg/kg po x 1 dose for children and adults.		
Neurocysticercosis (NCC): Larval form of T. solium Ref.: *AJTMH 72:3, 2005*	**NOTE: Treat T. solium intestinal tapeworms,** if present, with **praziquantel** 5-10 mg/kg po x 1 dose for children & adults.		
Parenchymal NCC "Viable" cysts by CT/MRI Meta-analysis: Treatment assoc with cyst resolution, ↓ seizures, and ↓ seizure recurrence. Ref: *AnIM 145:43, 2006.*	[**Albendazole** ≥60 kg: 400 mg bid with meals or 60 kg: 15 mg/kg per day in 2 div. doses (max. 800 mg/day) + **Dexamethasone** 0.1 mg/kg per day ± Anti-seizure medication] — all x 8 days	(**Praziquantel** 100 mg/kg per day in 3 div. doses po x 1 day, then 50 mg/kg/d in 3 doses plus **Dexamethasone** 0.1 mg/kg per day ± Anti-seizure medication) — all x 29 days. *See Comment*	Albendazole assoc. with 46% ↓ in seizures *(NEJM 350:249, 2004)*. Praziquantel less cysticidal activity. Steroids decrease serum levels of praziquantel. NIH reports methotrexate at ≤20 mg/wk allows a reduction in steroid use *(CID 44:449, 2007)*.
"Degenerating" cysts	**Albendazole + dexamethasone as above**		**Treatment improves prognosis of associated seizures.**
Dead calcified cysts	**No treatment indicated**		
Subarachnoid NCC	(**Albendazole + steroids** as above) + shunting for hydrocephalus. Without shunt, 50% died within 9 yrs *(J Neurosurg 66:686, 1987)*.		
Intraventricular NCC	**Albendazole + dexamethasone + neuroendoscopic removal if obstruction of CSF circulation**		
Sparganosis (Spirometra mansonoides) Larval cysts; source—frogs/snakes	Surgical resection or ethanol injection of subcutaneous masses *(NEJM 330:1887, 1994)*.		

ECTOPARASITES. Ref.: *CID 36:1355, 2003; Ln 363:889, 2004.* **NOTE: Due to potential neurotoxicity and risk of aplastic anemia, lindane not recommended.**

DISEASE	INFECTING ORGANISM	PRIMARY	ALTERNATIVE	COMMENTS
Head lice *Med Lett 51:57, 2009*	Pediculus humanus, var. capitis	**Permethrin** 1% lotion: Apply to shampooed dried hair for 10 min.; repeat in 9-10 days. **OR** **Malathion** 0.5% lotion (Ovide): Apply to dry hair for 8–12 hrs, then shampoo. 2 doses 7-9 days apart.	**Ivermectin** 200 μg/kg po once; 3 doses at 7 day intervals reported effective *(JID 193:474, 2006)*. **Malathion:** Report that 1–2 20-min. applications 98% effective *(Ped Derm 21:670, 2004)*. In alcohol—potentially flammable.	**Permethrin:** success in 78%. Extra combing of no benefit. Resistance increasing. No advantage to 5% permethrin.
Pubic lice (crabs)	Phthirus pubis	**Pubic hair: Permethrin** OR **malathion** as for head lice	**Eyelids: Petroleum jelly** applied qid x 10 days OR **yellow oxide of mercury** 1% qid x 14 days	
Body lice	Pediculus humanus, var. corporis	No drugs for the patient. Organism lives in & deposits eggs in seams of clothing. Discard clothing; if not possible, treat clothing with 1% malathion powder or 0.5% permethrin powder. Success with ivermectin in homeless shelter: 12 mg po on days 0, 7, & 14 *(JID 193:474, 2006)*		
Scabies	Sarcoptes scabiei			
Immunocompetent patients Refs: *LnID 6:769, 2006*		**Permethrin** 5% cream (ELIMITE). Apply entire skin from chin down to and including toes. Leave on 8–14 hrs. Repeat if itching persists for >2-4 wks after treatment or new pustules occur. Safe for children >2 mo old.	**Ivermectin** 200 μg/kg po x 1. As above, second dose if persistent symptoms.	Trim fingernails. Reapply to hands after handwashing. Pruritus may persist times 2 wk after mites gone. **Less effective: Crotamiton** 10% cream, apply x 24 hr, rinse off, then reapply x 24 hr.

TABLE 13A (11)

INFECTING ORGANISM	SUGGESTED REGIMENS		COMMENTS
	PRIMARY	ALTERNATIVE	
ECTOPARASITES/Scabies *(continued)*			
AIDS and HTLV-infected patients (CD4 <150 per mm³), debilitated or developmentally disabled patients (Norwegian scabies—*see Comments*)	For Norwegian scabies: **Permethrin** 5% as above. 2 or more applications a week apart may be needed. After each permethrin dose (days 2-7) apply 6% sulfur in petrolatum.	**Ivermectin** 200 mcg/kg po x 1 reported effective; may need 2 or more doses separated by 14 days.	Norwegian scabies in AIDS pts: Extensive, crusted. Can mimic psoriasis. Not pruritic. Highly contagious—isolate!
Myiasis Due to larvae of flies	Usually cutaneous/subcutaneous nodule with central punctum. Treatment: Occlude punctum to prevent gas exchange with petrolatum, fingernail polish, makeup cream or bacon. When larva migrates, manually remove.		

TABLE 13B – DOSAGE AND SELECTED ADVERSE EFFECTS OF ANTIPARASITIC DRUGS

NOTE: Drugs available from CDC Drug Service indicated by "CDC." Call (+1) (404) 639-3670 (or -2888 (Fax)). *See Table 13D for Sources of hard-to-find antiparasitic drugs.* Doses vary with indication. For convenience, drugs divided by type of parasite; some drugs used for multiple types of parasites, e.g., albendazole.

CLASS, AGENT, GENERIC NAME (TRADE NAME)	USUAL ADULT DOSAGE	ADVERSE REACTIONS/COMMENTS
Antiprotozoan Drugs		
Intestinal Parasites		
Diloxanide furoate[NUS] (Furamide)	500 mg po tid x 10 days	Source: *See Table 13D, page 144.* Flatulence, N/V, diarrhea.
Iodoquinol (Yodoxin)	Adults: 650 mg po tid (or 30-40 mg/kg/day div. tid); children: 40 mg/kg per day div. tid.	Rarely causes nausea, abdominal cramps, rash, acne. Contraindicated if iodine intolerance or hepatic damage.
Metronidazole	Side-effects similar for all. *See metronidazole in Table 10A, page 90, & Table 10C, page 99*	
Nitazoxanide (Alinia)	Adults: 500 mg po q12h. Children 4–11: 200 mg susp. po q12h. Take with food.	Abdominal pain 7.8%, diarrhea 2.1%. Rev.: *CID 40:1173, 2005; Expert Opin Pharmacother 7:953, 2006.* Headaches; rarely yellow schlera (resolves after treatment).
Paromomycin (Humatin) Aminosidine IV in U.K.	Up to 750 mg qid.	Aminoglycoside similar to neomycin; if absorbed due to concomitant inflammatory bowel disease can result in oto/nephrotoxicity. Doses >3 gm daily are associated with nausea, abdominal cramps, diarrhea.
Quinacrine[NUS] (Atabrine, Mepacrine)	100 mg po tid. No longer available in U.S.; 2 pharmacies will prepare as a service: (1) Connecticut (+1) 203-785-6818; (2) California 800-247-9767	Contraindicated for pts with history of psychosis or psoriasis. Yellow staining of skin. Dizziness, headache, vomiting, toxic psychosis (1.5%), hemolytic anemia, leukopenia, thrombocytopenia, urticaria, rash, fever, minor disulfiram-like reactions.
Tinidazole (Tindamax)	250-500 mg tabs, with food. Regimen varies with indication.	Chemical structure similar to metronidazole but better tolerated. Seizures/peripheral neuropathy reported. **Adverse effects:** Metallic taste 4–6%, nausea 3–5%, anorexia 2–3%.
Antiprotozoan Drugs: Non-Intestinal Protozoa		
Extraintestinal Parasites		
Antimony compounds[NUS] Stibogluconate sodium (Pentostam) from CDC or Meglumine antimonate (Glucantime—French trade names	Dilute in 120 mL of D_5W and infuse over 2 hrs. Ideally, monitor EKG.	Fatigue, myalgia, N/V and diarrhea common. ALT/AST ↑s, ↑ amylase and lipase occur. **NOTE: Reversible T wave changes in 30-60%. Risk of QTc prolongation.**
Artemether-Lumefantrine, po	Tablets contain 20 mg Artemether and 120 mg Lumefantrine. Take with food. Can be crushed and mixed with a few teaspoons of water	Can prolong QT_C: avoid in patients with congenital long QT_C, family history of sudden death or long QT_C, or need for drugs known to prolong QT_C *(see list under fluoroquinolones, Table 10C, page 98)*. Artemether induces CYP3A4 and both Artemether & Lumefantrine are metabolized by CYP3A4 *(see drug-drug interactions, Table 22A, page 200)*. Adverse effects experienced by >30% of adults: headache, anorexia, dizziness, arthralgia and myalgia.

TABLE 13B (2)

CLASS, AGENT, GENERIC NAME (TRADE NAME)	USUAL ADULT DOSAGE	ADVERSE REACTIONS/COMMENTS
Antiprotozoan Drugs: Non-Intestinal Protozoa/Extraintestinal Parasites *(continued)*		
Artesunate, IV *Ref: NEJM 358:1829, 2008*	Available from CDC Malaria Branch. 2.4 mg/kg IV at 0, 12, 24, & 48 hrs	More effective than quinine & safer than quinidine. Contact CDC at 770-488-7758 or 770-488-7100 after hours. No dosage adjustment for hepatic or renal insufficiency. No known drug interactions.
Atovaquone (Mepron) Ref.: *AAC 46:1163, 2002*	Suspension: 1 tsp (750 mg) po bid 750 mg/5 mL.	No. pts stopping rx due to side-effects was 9%; rash 22%, GI 20%, headache 16%, insomnia 10%, fever 14%
Atovaquone and proguanil (Malarone) For prophylaxis of P. falciparum; little data on P. vivax	**Prophylaxis:** 1 tab po (250 mg + 100 mg) q24h with food **Treatment:** 4 tabs po (1000 mg + 400 mg) once daily with food x 3 days Adult tab: 250/100 mg; Peds tab 62.5/25 mg. Peds dosage: *prophylaxis footnote 4 page 133; treatment see comment, page 134.*	Adverse effects in rx trials: Adults—abd. pain 17%, N/V 12%, headache 10%, dizziness 5%. Rx stopped in 1%. Asymptomatic mild ↑ in ALT/AST. Children—cough, headache, anorexia, vomiting, abd. pain. *See drug interactions, Table 22.* Safe in G6PD-deficient pts. Can crush tabs for children and give with milk or other liquid nutrients. Renal insufficiency: contraindicated if CrCl <30 mL per min.
Benznidazole[NUS] (Rochagan, Roche, Brazil)	7.5 mg/kg per day po	Photosensitivity in 50% of pts. GI: abdominal pain, nausea/vomiting/anorexia. CNS: disorientation, insomnia, twitching/seizures, paresthesias, polyneuritis. **Contraindicated in pregnancy**
Chloroquine phosphate (Aralen)	Dose varies—*see Malaria Prophylaxis and rx, pages 133-134.*	Minor: anorexia/nausea/vomiting, headache, dizziness, blurred vision, pruritus in dark-skinned pts. Major: protracted rx in rheumatoid arthritis can lead to retinopathy. Can exacerbate psoriasis. Can block response to rabies vaccine. Contraindicated in pts with epilepsy.
Dapsone Ref.: *CID 27:191, 1998*	100 mg po q24h	Usually tolerated by pts with rash after TMP-SMX. Adverse effects: nausea/vomiting, rash, oral lesions *(CID 18:630, 1994)*. Methemoglobinemia (usually asymptomatic); if >10–15%, stop drug. Hemolytic anemia if G6PD deficient. Sulfone syndrome: fever, rash, hemolytic anemia, atypical lymphocytes, and liver injury *(West J Med 156:303, 1992)*.
Eflornithine[NUS] (Ornidyl) (WHO drug service)	Approved in US for trypanosome infections but not marketed. Aventis product.	Diarrhea in ½ pts, vomiting, abdominal pain, anemia/leukopenia in ½ pts, seizures, alopecia, jaundice, ↓ hearing. Contraindicated in pregnancy.
Fumagillin	Eyedrops + po. 20 mg po tid. Leiter's: 800-292-6773.	Adverse events: Neutropenia & thrombocytopenia
Mefloquine (Lariam)	One 250 mg tab/wk for malaria prophylaxis; for rx, 1250 mg x 1 or 750 mg & then 500 mg in 6–8 hrs. In U.S.: 250 mg tab = 228 mg base; outside U.S., 275 mg tab = 250 mg base	Side-effects in roughly 3%. Minor: headache, irritability, insomnia, weakness, diarrhea. Toxic psychosis, seizures can occur. Teratogenic—do not use in pregnancy. Do not use with quinine, quinidine, or halofantrine. Rare: Prolonged QT interval and toxic epidermal necrolysis *(Ln 349:101, 1997)*. Not used for self-rx due to neuropsychiatric side-effects.
Melarsoprol *(CDC)* (Mel B, Arsobal) (Manufactured in France)	See Trypanosomiasis for adult dose. Peds dose: 0.36 mg/kg IV, then gradual ↑ to 3.6 mg/kg q1–5 days for total of 9–10 doses.	Post-rx encephalopathy (10%) with 50% mortality overall, risk of death 2° to rx 4–8%. Prednisolone 1 mg per kg per day po may ↓ encephalopathy. Other: Heart damage, albuminuria, abdominal pain, vomiting, peripheral neuropathy, Herxheimer-like reaction, pruritus.
Miltefosine[NUS] *(Expert Rev Anti Infect Ther 4:177, 2006)*	100–150 mg (approx. 2.25 mg/kg per day) po x 28 days Cutaneous leishmaniasis 2.25 mg/kg po q24h x 6 wk	Source: *See Table 13D, page 144.* **Pregnancy—No**; teratogenic. Side-effects vary: kala-azar pts, vomiting in up to 40%, diarrhea in 17%; "motion sickness", headache & increased creatinine. Daily dose >150 mg can cause severe GI side effects *(Ln 352:1821, 1998)*.
Nifurtimox (Lampit) *(CDC)* (Manufactured in Germany by Bayer)	8–10 mg/kg per day po div. 4 x per day	Side-effects in 40–70% of pts. GI: abdominal pain, nausea/vomiting. CNS: polyneuritis (1/3), disorientation, insomnia, twitching, seizures. Skin rash. Hemolysis with G6PD deficiency.
Pentamidine (NebuPent)	300 mg via aerosol q month. Also used IM.	Hypotension, hypocalcemia, hypoglycemia followed by hyperglycemia, pancreatitis. Neutropenia (15%), thrombocytopenia. Nephrotoxicity. Others: nausea/vomiting, ↑ liver tests, rash.
Primaquine phosphate	26.3 mg (=15 mg base). Adult dose is 30 mg of base po daily.	In G6PD def. pts, can cause hemolytic anemia with hemoglobinuria, esp. African, Asian peoples. Methemoglobinemia. Nausea/abdominal pain if pt. fasting. *(CID 39:1336, 2004)*. **Pregnancy: No.**

TABLE 13B (3)

CLASS, AGENT, GENERIC NAME (TRADE NAME)	USUAL ADULT DOSAGE	ADVERSE REACTIONS/COMMENTS
Antiprotozoan Drugs: Non-Intestinal Protozoa/Extraintestinal Parasites *(continued)*		
Pyrimethamine (Daraprim, Malocide) Also combined with sulfadoxine as **Fansidar** (25–500 mg)	100 mg po, then 25 mg/day. Cost of folinic acid (leucovorin)	Major problem is hematologic: megaloblastic anemia, ↓ WBC, ↓ platelets. Can give 5 mg folinic acid per day to ↓ bone marrow depression and not interfere with antitoxoplasmosis effect. If high-dose pyrimethamine, ↑ folinic acid to 10–50 mg/day. Pyrimethamine + sulfadiazine can cause mental changes due to carnitine deficiency *(AJM 95:112, 1993)*. Other: Rash, vomiting, diarrhea, xerostomia
Quinidine gluconate Cardiotoxicity ref: LnID 7:549, 2007	Loading dose of 10 mg (equiv to 6.2 mg of quinidine base) / kg IV over 1–2 hr, then constant infusion of 0.02 mg of quinidine gluconate / kg per minute. May be available for compassionate use from Lilly.	Adverse reactions of quinidine/quinine similar: (1) IV bolus injection can cause fatal hypotension, (2) hyperinsulinemic hypoglycemia, esp. in pregnancy, (3) ↓ rate of infusion of IV quinidine if QT interval ↑ >25% of baseline, (4) reduce dose 30–50% after day 3 due to ↓ renal clearance and ↓ vol. of distribution.
Quinine sulfate (300 mg salt = 250 mg base). In U.S. only approved product is Qualaquin.	324 mg tabs. No IV prep. in US. Oral rx of chloroquine-resistant falciparum malaria: 624 mg po tid x 3 days, then (tetracycline 250 mg po qid or doxy 100 mg bid) x 7 days	Cinchonism; tinnitus, headache, nausea, abdominal pain, blurred vision. Rarely: blood dyscrasias, drug fever, asthma, hypoglycemia. Transient blindness in <1% of 500 pts *(AnIM 136:339, 2002)*. **Contraindicated if prolonged QTc, myasthenia gravis, optic neuritis.**
Spiramycin (Rovamycin) *(JAC 42:572, 1998)*	1 gm po q8h *(see Comment)*	GI and allergic reactions have occurred. Available at no cost after consultation with Palo Alto Medical Foundation Toxoplasma Serology Lab: 650-853-4828 or from U.S. FDA 301-796-1600.
Sulfadiazine	1–1.5 gm po q6h.	*See Table 10C, page 99, for sulfonamide side-effects*
Sulfadoxine & pyrimethamine combination (Fansidar)	Contains 500 mg sulfadoxine & 25 mg pyrimethamine	Very long mean half-life of both drugs: Sulfadoxine 169 hrs, pyrimethamine 111 hrs allows weekly dosage. Do not use in pregnancy. Fatalities reported due to Stevens-Johnson syndrome and toxic epidermal necrolysis. Renal excretion—use with caution in pts with renal impairment.
DRUGS USED TO TREAT NEMATODES, TREMATODES, AND CESTODES		
Albendazole (Albenza)	Doses vary with indication. Take with food; fatty meal increases absorption.	Teratogenic, Pregnancy Cat. C; give after negative pregnancy test. Abdominal pain, nausea/vomiting, alopecia, ↑ serum transaminase. Rare leukopenia.
Bithionol *(CDC)*	Adults & children: 30–40 mg/kg (to max. of 2 gm/day) po every other day x 10–15 doses	Photosensitivity, skin reactions, urticaria, GI upset.
Diethylcarbamazine *(CDC)*	Used to treat filariasis.	Headache, dizziness, nausea, fever. Host may experience inflammatory reaction to death of adult worms: fever, urticaria, asthma, GI upset (Mazzotti reaction). **Pregnancy—No.**
Ivermectin (Stromectol, Mectizan)	Strongyloidiasis dose: 200 mcg/kg x 2 doses po Onchocerciasis: 150 mcg/kg x 1 po Scabies: 200 mcg/kg po x 1	Mild side-effects: fever, pruritus, rash. In rx of onchocerciasis, can see tender lymphadenopathy, headache, bone/joint pain. Can cause Mazzotti reaction *(see above)*.
Mebendazole (Vermox)	Doses vary with indication.	Rarely causes abdominal pain, nausea, diarrhea. Contraindicated in pregnancy & children <2 yrs old.
Praziquantel (Biltricide)	Doses vary with parasite; *see Table 13A*.	Mild: dizziness/drowsiness, N/V, rash, fever. Only contraindication is ocular cysticercosis. Metab.-induced by anticonvulsants and steroids; can negate effect with cimetidine 400 mg po tid.
Pyrantel pamoate (over-the-counter)	Oral suspension. Dose for all ages: 11 mg/kg (to max. of 1 gm) x 1 dose	Rare GI upset, headache, dizziness, rash
Suramin (Germanin) *(CDC)*	For early trypanosomiasis. Drug powder mixed to 10% solution with 5 mL water and used within 30 min	Does not cross blood-brain barrier; no effect on CNS infection. Side-effects: vomiting, pruritus, urticaria, fever, paresthesias, albuminuria (discontinue drug if casts appear). Do not use if renal/liver disease present. Deaths from vascular collapse reported.

TABLE 13C – PARASITES THAT CAUSE EOSINOPHILIA (EOSINOPHILIA IN TRAVELERS)

Frequent and Intense (>5000 eos/mcL)	Moderate to Marked Early Infections	During Larval Migration; Absent or Mild During Chronic Infections	Other
Strongyloides (absent in compromised hosts); Lymphatic Filariasis; Toxocaria	Ascaris; Hookworm; Clonarchis; Paragonemis	Opisthorchis	Schistosomiasis; Cysticercosis; Trichuris; Angiostrongylus; Non-lymphatic filariasis; Grathasloma; Capillaria; Trichostrongylus

TABLE 13D – SOURCES FOR HARD-TO-FIND ANTIPARASITIC DRUGS

Source	Drugs Available	Contact Information
CDC Drug Service	Artesunate, Diethylcarbamazine (DEC), Melarsoprol, Nifurtimox, Sodium stibogluconate, Suramin	www.cdc.gov/laboratory/drugservice/index.html (+1) 404-639-3670
WHO	Drugs for treatment of African trypanosomiasis	simarrop@who.int; (+41) 794-682-726; (+41) 227-911-345 francoj@who.int; (+41) 796-198-535; (+41) 227-913-313
Compounding Pharmacies, Specialty Labs, Others		
Expert Compounding Pharmacy	Quinacrine, Iodoquinol	www.uniquerx.com 1-800-247-9767; (+1) 818-988-7979
Gallipot Inc. (USA) Compounding Pharmacy	Quinacrine, Iodoquinol, Paromomycin, Diloxanide	www.gallipot.com 1-800-423-6967; (+1) 651-681-9517
Leiter's Pharmacy	Fumagillin	www.leiterrx.com 1-800-292-0773
Paladin Labs	Miltefosine	www.paladin-labs.com
Victoria Apotheke Zurich	Paromomycin, Triclabendazole	www.pharmaworld.com (+41) 43-344-6060
Fast Track Research	Miltefosine (may be free under treatment IND for cutaneous, mucocutaneous leishmaniasis)	jberman@fasttrackresearch.com
Palo Alto Medical Foundation, Toxoplasma Serology Lab	Spiramycin	(+1) 650-853-4828

TABLE 14A – ANTIVIRAL THERAPY (NON-HIV)*

VIRUS/DISEASE	DRUG/DOSAGE	SIDE EFFECTS/COMMENTS
Adenovirus: Cause of RTIs including fatal pneumonia in children & young adults and 60% mortality in transplant pts *(CID 43:331, 2006)*. Frequent cause of cystitis in transplant patients. Adenovirus 14 associated with severe pneumonia in otherwise healthy young adults *(MMWR 56(45):1181, 2007)*. **Findings include:** fever, ↑ liver enzymes, leukopenia, thrombocytopenia, diarrhea, pneumonia, or hemorrhagic cystitis.	In severe cases of pneumonia or post HSCT[1]: **Cidofovir** • 5 mg/kg/wk x 2 wks, then q 2 wks + **probenecid** 1.25 gm/M^2 given 3 hrs before cidofovir and 3 & 9 hrs after each infusion • Or 1 mg/kg IV 3x/wk. For adenovirus hemorrhagic cystitis *(CID 40:199, 2005; Transplantation. 2006; 81:1398)*: Intravesical **cidofovir** (5 mg/kg in 100 mL saline instilled into bladder).	Successful in 3/8 immunosuppressed children *(CID 38:45, 2004)* *& 8 of 10 children with HSCT (CID 41; 1812, 2005)*. ↓ in virus load predicted response to cidofovir. Ribavirin has had mixed activity; appears restricted to group C serotypes. Vidarabine and Ganciclovir have in vitro activity against adenovirus; little to no clinical data.
Coronavirus—SARS-CoV (Severe Acute Respiratory Distress Syn.) A new coronavirus, isolated Spring 2003 *(NEJM 348:1953 & 1967, 2003)* emerged from southern China & spread to Hong Kong and 32 countries. Bats appear to be a primary reservoir for SARS virus *(PNAS 102: 14040, 2005)*.	**Therapy remains predominantly supportive care.** Therapy tried or under evaluation *(see Comments)*: • Ribavirin—ineffective. • Interferon alfa ± steroids—small case series. • Pegylated IFN-α effective in monkeys. • Low dose steroids alone successful in one Beijing hospital. High dose steroids ↑ serious fungal infections. • Inhaled nitric oxide improved oxygenation & improved chest x-ray *(CID 39:1531, 2004)*.	**Transmission by close contact**: effective infection control practices (**mask [changed frequently]**, eye protection, gown, gloves) key to stopping transmission. Other coronaviruses (HCOV-229E, OC43, NL63, etc.) implicated as cause of croup, asthma exacerbations, & other RTIs in children *(CID 40:1721, 2005; JID 191:492, 2005)*. May be associated with Kawasaki disease *(JID 191:489, 2005)*.
Enterovirus—Meningitis: most common cause of aseptic meningitis. Rapid CSF PCR test is accurate; reduces costs and hospital stay for infants *(Peds 120:489, 2007)*	**No rx currently recommended;** however, **pleconaril** (VP 63843) still under investigation.	No clinical benefit demonstrated in double-blind placebo-controlled study in 21 infants with enteroviral aseptic meningitis *(PIDJ 22:335, 2003)*. Large Phase II study underway for enteroviral sepsis syndrome *(www.NIH.gov)*.
Hemorrhagic Fever Virus Infections: For excellent reviews, see *Med Lab Observer, May 2005, p. 16, Lancet Infectious Disease Vol 6 No 4.*		
Congo-Crimean Hemorrhagic Fever (HF) *(CID 39:284, 2004)* Tick-borne; symptoms include N/V, fever, headache, myalgias, & stupor (1/3). Signs: *conjunctival* injection, hepatomegaly, petechiae (1/3). Lab: ↓ platelets, ↓ WBC, ↑ ALT, AST, LDH & CPK (100%).	Oral **ribavirin, 30 mg/kg** as initial loading dose & 15 mg/kg q6h x 4 days & then 7.5 mg/kg/day x 6 days (WHO recommendation) *(see Comment)*. Reviewed *Antiviral Res 78:125, 2008.*	3/3 healthcare workers in Pakistan had complete recovery *(Ln 346:472, 1995)* & 61/69 (89%) with confirmed CCHF rx with ribavirin survived in Iran *(CID 36:1613, 2003)*. Shorter time of hospitalization among ribavirin treated pts (7.7 vs. 10.3 days), but no difference in mortality or transfusion needs in study done in Turkey *(J Infection 52: 207-215, 2006)*
Ebola/Marburg HF (Central Africa) Severe *outbreak* of Ebola in Angola 308 cases with 277 deaths by 5/3/05 *(NEJM 352:2155, 2005; LnID 5:331, 2005)*. Major epidemic of Marburg 1998-2000 in Congo & 2004–5 in Angola *(NEJM 355:866, 2006)*	**No effective antiviral rx** *(J Virol 77: 9733, 2003)*.	Can infect gorillas & chimps that come in contact with other dead animal carcasses *(Science 303.387, 2004)*. Marburg reported in African Fruit Bat, *Rousettus aegyptiacus* *(PLoS ONE 2. e764, 2007)*. Study in Gabon revealed 15% seroprevalence among 4349 healthy volunteers from 220 randomly selected villages. None recalled any illness similar to Ebola. Seroprevalence among children rises until age 15, then plateaus. Seropositive status correlates to location of fruit bats. *PLoS ONE (Feb 9); 5:e9126, 2010*
With pulmonary syndrome: Hantavirus pulmonary syndrome, "sin nombre virus"	**No benefit from ribavirin has been demonstrated** *(CID 39:1307, 2004)*. Early recognition of disease and supportive (usually ICU) care is key to successful outcome.	Acute onset of fever, headache, myalgias, non-productive cough, thrombocytopenia and non-cardiogenic pulmonary edema with respiratory insufficiency following exposure to rodents.
With renal syndrome: Lassa, Venezuelan, Korean, HF, Sabia, Argentinian HF, Bolivian HF, Junin, Machupo	Oral **ribavirin, 30 mg/kg** as initial loading dose & 15 mg/kg q6h x 4 days & then 7.5 mg/kg x 6 days (WHO recommendation) *(see Comment)*.	Toxicity low, hemolysis reported but recovery when treatment stopped. No significant changes in WBC, platelets, hepatic or renal function. *See CID 36:1254, 2003,* for management of contacts.

[1] HSCT = Hematopoietic stem cell transplant

* *See page 2 for abbreviations. NOTE: All dosage recommendations are for adults (unless otherwise indicated) and assume normal renal function.*

TABLE 14A (2)

VIRUS/DISEASE	DRUG/DOSAGE	SIDE EFFECTS/COMMENTS
Hemorrhagic Fever Virus Infections *(continued)*		
Dengue and dengue hemorrhagic fever (DHF) *www.cdc.gov/ncidod/dvbid/dengue/dengue-hcp.htm* Think dengue in traveler to tropics or subtropics (incubation period usually 4-7 days) with fever, bleeding, thrombocytopenia, or hemoconcentration with shock. Dx by viral isolation or serology; serum to CDC (telephone 787-706-2399).	**No data on antiviral rx.** Fluid replacement with careful hemodynamic monitoring critical. Rx of **DHF** with colloids effective: 6% hydroxyethyl starch preferred in 1 study *(NEJM 353:9, 2005)*. Review in *Semin Ped Infect Dis 16: 60-65, 2005.*	Of 77 cases dx at CDC (2001–2004), recent (2-wk) travel to Caribbean island 30%, Asia 17%, Central America 15%, S. America 15% *(MMWR 54:556, June 10, 2005)*. 5 pts with severe **DHF** rx with dengue antibody-neg. gamma globulin 500 mg per kg q24h IV for 3–5 days; rapid ↑ in platelet counts *(CID 36:1623, 2003)*.
West Nile virus *(see AnIM 104:545, 2004)* A flavivirus transmitted by mosquitoes, blood transfusions, transplanted organs *(NEJM 348: 2196, 2003; CID 38:1257, 2004)*, & breast-feeding *(MMWR 51:877, 2002)*. Birds (>200 species) are main host with humans & horses incidental hosts. The US epidemic continues.	**No proven rx to date.** 2 clinical trials in progress: (1) Interferon alfa-N3 *(CID 40:764, 2005). See www.nyhq.org/posting/rahal.html* (2) IVIG from Israel with high titer antibody West Nile *(JID 188:5, 2003; Transpl Inf Dis 4:160, 2003)*. Contact NIH, 301-496-7453; *see www.clinicaltrials.gov/show/NCT00068055.* Reviewed in *Lancet Neurology 6: 171-181, 2007.*	Usually nonspecific febrile disease but 1/150 cases develops meningoencephalitis, aseptic meningitis or polio-like paralysis *(AnIM 104:545, 2004; JCI 113: 1102, 2004)*. Long-term sequelae (neuromuscular weakness & psychiatric) common *(CID 43:723, 2006)*. Dx by ↑ IgM in serum & CSF or CSF PCR (contact State Health Dept./CDC). Blood supply now tested in U.S. ↑ serum lipase in 11/17 cases *(NEJM 352:420, 2005)*.
Yellow fever	**No data on antiviral rx** **Guidelines for use of preventative vaccine: *(MMWR 51: RR17, 2002)***	Reemergence in Africa & S. Amer. due to urbanization of susceptible population -*(Lancet Inf 5:604, 2005)*. Vaccination effective. *(JAMA 276:1157,1996)*. Vaccine safe and effective in HIV patients, especially in those with suppressed VL and higher CD4 counts *(CID 48:659, 2009)*
Chikungunya fever A self limited arborvirus illness spread by Aedes mosquito. High epidemic potential.	**No antiviral therapy.** Mice given purified human polyvalent CHIKV immunoglobulins was therapeutic *(JID 200: 516, 2009)*.	Clinical presentation: high fever, severe myalgias & headache, macular papular rash with occ. thrombocytopenia. Rarely hemorrhagic complications. Dx by increase in IgM antibody.
Hepatitis Viral Infections		
Hepatitis A *(Ln 351:1643, 1998)*	No therapy recommended. If within 2 wks of exposure, IVIG 0.02 mL per kg IM times 1 protective. Hep A vaccine equally effective as IVIG in randomized trial and is emerging as preferred Rx *(NEJM 357:1685, 2007)*.	40% of pts with chronic Hep C who developed superinfection with Hep A developed fulminant hepatic failure *(NEJM 338:286, 1998)*.

Hepatitis B—Chronic: For pts co-infected with HIV *see Table 12, Sanford Guide to HIV/AIDS Therapy 2011.*

Who to treat? Based on status of e antigen and viral quantification. Adapted from *Clin Gastro & Hepatology 4:936-962, 2006.* NIH Consensus Statement *(Ann Int Med 150:104, 2009)*.

	HBV DNA (IU/mL)[2]	ALT	Suggested Management
HBe Ag-Positive	≥20,000	Elevated or normal	Treat if ALT elevated[3] Treat if biopsy abnormal—even if ALT normal[3]
HBe Ag-Negative	≥2,000	Elevated or normal	Treat if ALT elevated[3] Treat if biopsy abnormal—even if ALT normal[3]
Documented cirrhosis (positive or negative HBe Ag)	≥2,000 and compensated cirrhosis	ALT not applicable	Treat with **adefovir** or **entecavir** long term[3]
	<2,000 and compensated cirrhosis	ALT not applicable	Observe or (**adefovir** or **entecavir** long term)[3]
	Decompensated cirrhosis; any HBV DNA level	ALT not applicable	Long term therapy with (**lamivudine** or **entecavir**) + **tenofovir**; waiting list for liver transplantation[3]. **Interferon and PEG-IFN contraindicated.**

[2] IU/mL equivalent to approximately 5.6 copies/mL; if patient treated, monitor every 6 mos if treated with adefovir; every 3 mos, if treated with lamivudine.
[3] Treatment duration varies with viral quantitation, presence/absence of cirrhosis & drug(s) used. *See Clin Gastro & Hepatology 4:936-962, 2006 for details.*
* *See page 2 for abbreviations.* NOTE: All dosage recommendations are for adults (unless otherwise indicated) and assume normal renal function.

TABLE 14A (3)

VIRUS/DISEASE	DRUG/DOSAGE	SIDE EFFECTS/COMMENTS
Hepatitis Viral Infections/Hepatitis B—Chronic *(continued)*		

For patients not infected with HIV: Tenofovir 300 mg po daily or **Entecavir** 0.5 mg daily. Alternative: **Adefovir** 10 mg po daily or **Lamivudine** 100 mg po daily.

- Treatment duration varies with viral quantitation, presence/absence of cirrhosis and drug(s) used. *See Clin Gastroenterol Hepatol 4:936-62, 2006.*
- Combination therapy with both agents *(Peterson, et al., AASLD 2009 Boston, October 30-November 1, 2009, Abstract 405)* or either agent + lamivudine for selected patients (those with cirrhosis; higher risk of poor response).
- Choose entecavir over tenofovir in those with renal insufficiency and those who had failed prior adefovir treatment; choose tenofovir over entecavir in those with normal renal function and those who had failed prior lamivudine therapy.

Comparison of Treatment Options for Chronic Hepatitis B (Patients **not** co-infected with HIV). **Note:** *See Table 14B* for more dosage details, adverse effects. Ref: *CID 51:1201, 2010.*

	Peg interferon alfa-2A	Lamivudine	Adefovir	Entecavir	Tenofovir
Dose:	180 mcg sc weekly	100 mg po daily	10 mg po daily	0.5 mg po daily	300 mg po daily
Parameter:					
Log10 ↓ in serum HBV DNA	4.5	No data	3.6	6.9	4.7-6.4 (HBeAg+)
HBV DNA below detection, %	25	57	21	67	81% (30% if ADF resistance)
% ALT normalizes	39	41-72	48	68	76%
% with improved histology	38	49-56	53	72	72%
Resistance develops	No	70% after 5 yrs	30% after 5 yrs	1% after 4 yrs	< 1% over 3 yrs

Hepatitis C (up to 3% of world infected, 4 million in U.S. Co-infection with HIV common—*see Sanford Guide to HIV/AIDS Therapy*).

VIRUS/DISEASE	DRUG/DOSAGE	SIDE EFFECTS/COMMENTS
Acute Usually asymptomatic (>75%). Can detect by PCR within 13 days; antibody in 36+ days *(CID 40:951, 2005)*.	Follow plasma HCV viral load by PCR: If clear within 3-4 mos., no treatment. If persists: PEG IFN ± ribavirin as below, albeit controversial *(NEJM 346:1091, 2002)*	15-40% clear infection within 6 mos *(JAMA 297:724, 2007)*. Sustained viral response with IFN alfa-2b therapy 32% vs. 4% with placebo, P 0.0007 *(Cochrane Database Sys & Rev CD000369, 2002)*. Alfa-INF alone effective in early infection *(CID 42;1673, 2006)*
Chronic *(See next page)*		

* *See page 2 for abbreviations.* NOTE: All dosage recommendations are for adults (unless otherwise indicated) and assume normal renal function.

TABLE 14A (4)

VIRUS/DISEASE	DRUG/DOSAGE	SIDE EFFECTS/COMMENTS
Hepatitis C *(continued)*		
Chronic: *NEJM 365:2444, 2006.*		
	Treat if: persistent elevated ALT/AST, + HCV RNA plasma viral load, fibrosis &/or inflam on biopsy.	• In U.S., 90% due to genotype 1. **Sustained viral response (SVR)** to 48-wk rx of genotype 1: 42–51%; SVR to 24-wk rx of genotype 2 or 3: 76–82%. Genotype 1, 4, 5, 6 infected patients who are IL-28 rs12979860 genotype ("CC" allele). "CT" and "TT" alleles 3-fold less responsive to IFN. • Avoid alcohol—accelerates HCV disease. • HIV accelerates HCV disease • *See Table 14B for drug adverse effects & cost.* Interferon alfa can cause serious depression. • Ribavirin is teratogenic & has dose-related hematologic toxicity. • For drugs in development, *see Hepatology 2009; 50:184-194.* • For genotypes 2 & 3, some use standard IFN; results similar & ↓ cost. • NOTE: High viral load = >800,000 IU/mL. Pts with HCV RNA levels <800,000 IU/mL have 15-35% better response rate. • Latinos with genotype 1 have worse SVR than non-Latinos *(NEJM 360:257, 2009)*. Pegylated Interferon alfa-2b 1.5 μg/kg sc less effective than alfa-2a 180 μg sc in head-to-head comparison *(Gastroenterology 138:108, 2010)*.
Genotypes 1, 4, 5 & 6	<u>**Pegylated interferon**</u> + <u>**Ribavirin**</u> **PEG IFN:** Either alfa-2a (Pegasys) 180 mcg subcut. 1x/wk **(Alternative) Alfa-2b** (PEG-INTRON) 1.5 mcg/kg subcut. 1x/wk **Weight / Ribavirin Dose:** <75 kg: 400 mg am & 600 mg pm; >75 kg: 600 mg am & 600 mg pm **Monitor response by quantification:** **HCV RNA / Result / Action** After 4 wks rx: <1 $\log_{10}$ ↓ IU/mL[4] → Discontinue therapy After 12 wks rx: <2 $\log_{10}$ ↓ IU/mL → Discontinue therapy >2 $\log_{10}$ ↓ IU/mL or undetectable → Treat 48 wks	
Genotype 2 or 3	**PEG IFN alfa-2a or 2b**—dose as for types 1 & 4 above + **Ribavirin** 400 mg po bid **Quant. HCV RNA / Result / Action** After 4 wks rx: Undetectable → Treat 12 wks *(NEJM 352:2609, 2005)* >1 $\log_{10}$ ↓ → Treat 24 wks *(See comment)*	**For Genotype 2 and 3** 12 wks of Rx less effective than 24 wks, except in those with very rapid response (< 1000 c/ml at 1 week) and those < 40 yrs old (if VL undetectable at day 29) *Hepatology 47:1837, 2008.* **For Genotype 4,** nitazoxanide 500 mg BID when added to either Peg-IFN Alfa-2 or Peg-IFN plus ribavirin more effective than Peg-IFN + ribavirin alone in SVR *(Gastroenterology 136:760,2009)*.
For prevention of acute and chronic infection, see *Table 15D, page 182.*		
Herpesvirus Infections		
Cytomegalovirus (CMV) Marked ↓ in HIV associated CMV infections & death with Highly Active Antiretroviral Therapy. Initial treatment should optimize ART.	Primary prophylaxis not generally recommended. Preemptive therapy in pts with ↑ CMV DNA titers in plasma & CD4 <100/mm³. Recommended by some: **valganciclovir** 900 mg po q24h *(CID 32: 783, 2001)*. Authors rec. primary prophylaxis be dc if response to ART with ↑ CD4 >100 for 6 mos. *(MMWR 53:98, 2004)*.	Risk for developing CMV disease correlates with quantity of CMV DNA in plasma: each $\log_{10}$ ↑ associated with 3.1-fold ↑ in disease *(JCI 101:497, 1998; CID 28:758, 1999)*.
Colitis, Esophagitis Dx by biopsy of ulcer base/edge *(Clin Gastro Hepatol 2:564, 2004)* with demonstration of CMV inclusions & other pathogen(s).	**Ganciclovir** as with retinitis except induction period extended for 3–6 wks. No agreement on use of maintenance; may not be necessary except after relapse. Responses less predictable than for retinitis. **Valganciclovir also likely effective.** Switch to oral valganciclovir when po tolerated & when symptoms not severe enough to interfere with absorption. Antiretroviral therapy is essential in long term suppression. Alternative: **Cidofovir** 5 mg/kg IV, qwk x 2 wks followed by administration q2 wks; MUST be administered with **probenecid** 2 gm po 3 hrs before each dose and further 1 gm doses 2 hrs and 8 hrs after completion of the cidofovir infusion. IV saline hydration is essential.	
Encephalitis, Ventriculitis: Treatment not defined, but should be considered the same as retinitis. Disease may develop while taking ganciclovir as suppressive therapy. *See Herpes 11 (Suppl. 12):95A, 2004.*		
Lumbosacral polyradiculopathy: diagnosis by CMV DNA in CSF	**Ganciclovir**, as with retinitis. **Foscarnet** 40 mg/kg IV q12h another option. Switch to **valganciclovir** when possible. Suppression continued until CD4 remains >100/mm³ for 6 mos. **Alternative: Cidofovir 5** mg/kg IV, qwk x 2 wks followed by administration q2 wks; MUST be administered with probenicid 2 gm po 3 hrs before each dose and further 1 gm doses 2 hrs and 8 hrs after completion of the cidofovir infusion. IV saline hydration is essential.	About 50% will respond; survival ↑ (5.4 wks to 14.6 wks) *(CID 27:345, 1998)*. Resistance can be demonstrated genotypically.
Mononeuritis multiplex	Not defined	Due to vasculitis & may not be responsive to antiviral therapy

[4] HCV RNA quantitation. By WHO international standard 800,000 IU/mL = 2 million copies/mL. Response to therapy based on $\log_{10}$ fall in IU/mL *(JAMA 297:724, 2007)*.

* *See page 2 for abbreviations.* NOTE: All dosage recommendations are for adults (unless otherwise indicated) and assume normal renal function.

TABLE 14A (5)

VIRUS/DISEASE	DRUG/DOSAGE		SIDE EFFECTS/COMMENTS
Herpesvirus Infections/Cytomegalovirus (CMV) *(continued)*			
Pneumonia— Seen predominantly in transplants (esp. bone marrow), **rare in HIV**. Treat only when histological evidence present in AIDS & other pathogens not identified. High rate of CMV reactivation in immunocompetent ICU patients; prolonged hospitalizations and increased mortality *(JAMA 300:413, 2008)*.	**Ganciclovir/valganciclovir**, as with retinitis. In bone marrow transplant pts, combination therapy with CMV immune globulin.		In bone marrow transplant pts, serial measure of pp65 antigen was useful in establishing early diagnosis of CMV interstitial pneumonia with good results if ganciclovir was initiated within 6 days of antigen positivity *(Bone Marrow Transplant 26:413, 2000)*. For preventive therapy, see *Table 15E*.
CMV Retinitis Most common cause of blindness in AIDS patients with <50/mm3 CD4 counts. 19/30 pts (63%) with inactive CMV retinitis who responded to HAART (↑ of ≥60 CD4 cells/mL) developed immune recovery vitreitis (vision ↓ & floaters with posterior segment inflammation —vitreitis, papillitis & macular changes) an average of 43 wks after rx started *(JID 179: 697, 1999)*. Corticosteroid rx ↓ inflammatory reaction of immune recovery vitreitis without reactivation of CMV retinitis, either periocular corticosteroids or short course of systemic steroid.	**For immediate sight-threatening lesions: Ganciclovir** intraocular implant & **valganciclovir** 900 mg po q24h. **For peripheral lesions: Valganciclovir** 900 mg po q12h x 14–21d, then 900 mg po q24h for maintenance therapy	**Ganciclovir** 5 mg/kg IV q12h x 14–21d, then **valganciclovir** 900 mg po q24h **OR** **Foscarnet** 60 mg/kg IV q8h or 90 mg/kg IV q12h x 14–21d then 90–120 mg/kg IV q24h **OR** **Cidofovir** 5 mg/kg IV x 2 wks, then 5 mg/kg every other wk; each dose should be administered with IV saline hydration & oral probenecid **OR** Repeated intravitreal injections with **fomivirsen** (for relapses only, not as initial therapy)	Differential diagnosis: HIV retinopathy, herpes simplex retinitis, varicella-zoster retinitis (rare, hard to diagnose). Valganciclovir po equal to GCV IV in induction of remission: *(NEJM 346:1119, 2002)*. Cannot use ganciclovir ocular implant alone as approx. 50% risk of CMV retinitis other eye at 6 mos. & 31% risk visceral disease. Risk ↓ with systemic rx but when contralateral retinitis does occur, ganciclovir-resistant mutation often present *(JID 189:611, 2004)*. **Concurrent systemic rx recommended!** Because of unique mode of action **fomivirsen** may have a role if isolates become resistant to other therapies. Retinal detachments 50–60% within 1 yr of dx of retinitis. *(Ophthal 111:2232, 2004)*. Equal efficacy of IV GCV & FOS. GCV avoids nephrotoxicity of FOS; FOS avoids bone marrow suppression of GCV. Although bone marrow toxicity may be similar to ganciclovir. **Oral valganciclovir should replace both.**
Pts who discontinue suppression therapy should undergo regular eye examination for early detection of relapses!	**Post treatment suppression** (Prophylactic) if CD4 count <100/mm³: **Valganciclovir** 900 mg po q24h.		Discontinue if CD4 >100/mm³ x 6 mos on ART.
CMV in Transplant patients: See *Table 15E*. Use of **valganciclovir** to prevent infections in CMV seronegative recipients who receive organs from a seropositive donor & in seropositive receivers has been highly effective *(Ln 365:2105, 2005); Pharm Ther 35:676, 2010*. Others suggest preemptive rx when pt develops CMV antigenemia or positive PCR post-transplant *(Transplant 79:85, 2005)*.			
Epstein Barr Virus (EBV)—Mononucleosis *(Ln ID 3:131, 2003)*	**No treatment.** Corticosteroids for tonsillar obstruction, CNS complications, or threat of splenic rupture.		Etiology of atypical lymphocytes: EBV, CMV, Hep A, Hep B, toxo, measles, mumps, drugs *(Int Pediatr 18:20, 2003)*.
HHV-6—Implicated as cause of roseola (exanthem subitum) & other febrile diseases of childhood *(NEJM 352:768, 2005)*. Fever & rash documented in transplant pts *(JID 179:311, 1999)*. Reactivation in 47% of 110 U.S. hematopoietic stem cell transplant pts assoc. with delayed monocytes & platelet engraftment *(CID 40:932, 2005)*. Recognized in assoc. with meningoencephalitis in immunocompetent adults. Diagnosis made by pos. PCR in CSF. ↓ viral copies in response to **ganciclovir** rx *(CID 40:890 & 894, 2005)*. Foscarnet therapy improved thrombotic microangiopathy *(Am J Hematol 76:156, 2004)*.			
HHV-7—ubiquitous virus (>90% of the population is infected by age 3 yrs). No relationship to human disease. Infects CD4 lymphocytes via CD4 receptor; transmitted via saliva.			
HHV-8—The agent of Kaposi's sarcoma, Castleman's disease, & body cavity lymphoma. Associated with diabetes in sub-Saharan Africa *(JAMA 299:2770,2008)*.	**No antiviral treatment.** Effective anti-HIV therapy may help.		Localized lesions: radiotherapy, laser surgery or intralesional chemotherapy. Systemic: chemotherapy. Castleman's disease responded to ganciclovir *(Blood 103:1632, 2004)* & valganciclovir *(JID 2006)*.

* *See page 2 for abbreviations.* NOTE: All dosage recommendations are for adults (unless otherwise indicated) and assume normal renal function.

TABLE 14A (6)

VIRUS/DISEASE	DRUG/DOSAGE	SIDE EFFECTS/COMMENTS
Herpes simplex virus (HSV Types 1 & 2)		
Bell's palsy H. simplex most implicated etiology. Other etiologic considerations: VZV, HHV-6, Lyme disease.	As soon as possible after onset of palsy: **Prednisone** 1 mg/kg po divided bid x 5 days then taper to 5 mg bid over the next 5 days (total of 10 days prednisone) Alternate: **Prednisone** (dose as above) + **Valacyclovir** 500 mg bid x 5 days	Prospective randomized double blind placebo controlled trial compared prednisolone vs acyclovir vs (prednisolone + acyclovir) vs placebo. Best result with prednisolone: 85% recovery with placebo, 96% recovery with prednisolone, 93% with combination of steroid & prednisolone *(NEJM 357:1598 & 1653, 2007)*. **Large meta-analysis confirms: Steroids alone, effective; antiviral drugs alone, not effective; steroids + antiviral drugs, no more effective than steroids alone** *(JAMA: 302: 985,2009)*.
Encephalitis (Excellent reviews: *CID 35: 254, 2002)*. UK experience *(EID 9:234, 2003; Eur J Neurol 12:331, 2005 ; Antiviral Res: 71:141-148, 2006)*	**Acyclovir** IV 10 mg/kg IV (infuse over 1 hr) q8h x 14–21 days. Up to 20 mg/kg q8h in children <12 yrs. Dose calculation in obese patients uncertain. To lessen risk of nephrotoxicity with larger doses, seems reasonable to infuse each dose over more than 1 hour.	HSV-1 is most common cause of sporadic encephalitis. Survival & recovery from neurological sequelae are related to mental status at time of initiation of rx. **Early dx and rx imperative**. Mortality rate reduced from >70% to 19% with acyclovir rx. PCR analysis of CSF for HSV-1 DNA is 100% specific & 75–98% sensitive. 8/33 (25%) CSF samples drawn before day 3 were neg. by PCR; neg. PCR assoc. with ↓ protein & <10 WBC per mm^3 in CSF *(CID 36:1335, 2003)*. All were + after 3 days. Relapse after successful rx reported in 7/27 (27%) children. Relapse was associated with a lower total dose of initial acyclovir rx (285 ± 82 mg per kg in relapse group vs. 462 ± 149 mg per kg, p <0.03) *(CID 30:185, 2000; Neuropediatrics 35:371, 2004)*.
Genital Herpes: *Sexually Transmitted Treatment Guidelines 2010: MMWR 59 (RR-12), 2010.*		
Primary (initial episode)	**Acyclovir** (Zovirax or generic) 400 mg po tid x 7–10 days OR	↓ by 2 days time to resolution of signs & symptoms, ↓ by 4 days time to healing of lesions, ↓ by 7 days duration of viral shedding. Does not prevent recurrences. For severe cases only: 5 mg per kg IV q8h times 5–7 days.
	Valacyclovir (Valtrex) 1000 mg po bid x 7-10 days OR	An ester of acyclovir, which is well absorbed, bioavailability 3–5 times greater than acyclovir.
	Famciclovir (Famvir) 250 mg po tid x 7–10 days	Metabolized to penciclovir, which is active component. Side effects and activity similar to acyclovir. **Famciclovir** 250 mg po tid **equal to acyclovir** 200 mg 5 times per day.
Episodic recurrences	**Acyclovir** 800 mg po tid **x 2 days** or 400 mg po tid **x 5 days** or **Famciclovir** 1000 mg bid **x 1 day** or 125 mg po bid x 5 days or **Valacyclovir** 500 mg po bid **x 3 days** or 1 gm po once daily **x 5 days** For HIV patients, *see Comment*	For episodic recurrences in HIV patients: **acyclovir** 400 mg po tid x 5-10 days or **famciclovir** 500 mg po bid x 5-10 days or **valacyclovir** 1 gm po bid x 5-10 days
Chronic daily suppression	**Suppressive therapy reduces the frequency of genital herpes recurrences by 70–80% among pts who have frequent recurrences (i.e., >6 recurrences per yr) & many report no symptomatic outbreaks.** **Acyclovir** 400 mg po bid , **or famciclovir** 250 mg po bid, **or valacyclovir** 1 gm po q24h; pts with <9 recurrences per yr could use 500 mg po q24h and then use valaciclovir 1 gm po q24h if breakthrough at 500 mg. For HIV patients, *see Comment*	For chronic suppression in HIV patients: **acyclovir** 400-800 mg po bid or tid or **famciclovir** 500 mg po bid or **valacyclovir** 500 mg po bid
Genital, immunocompetent		
Gingivostomatitis, primary (children)	**Acyclovir** 15 mg/kg po 5x/day x 7 days	Efficacy in randomized double-blind placebo-controlled trial *(BMJ 314:1800, 1997)*.
Keratoconjunctivitis and recurrent epithelial keratitis	**Trifluridine** (Viroptic), 1 drop 1% solution q2h (max. 9 drops per day) for max. of 21 days *(see Table 1A, page 12)*	In controlled trials, response % > idoxuridine. Suppressive rx with acyclovir (400 mg bid) reduced recurrences of ocular HSV from 32% to 19% *(NEJM 339:300, 1998)*.
Mollaret's recurrent "aseptic" meningitis (usually HSV-2) *(Ln 363:1772, 2004)*	No controlled trials of antiviral rx & resolves spontaneously. If therapy is to be given, **acyclovir** (15–30 mg/kg/day IV) or **valacyclovir** 1-2 gm po qid should be used.	Pos. PCR for HSV in CSF confirms dx *(EJCMID 23:560, 2004)*. Daily suppression rx might ↓ frequency of recurrence but no clinical trials. Oral Valacyclovir ref: *JAC 47:855, 2001*.

* *See page 2 for abbreviations.* NOTE: All dosage recommendations are for adults (unless otherwise indicated) and assume normal renal function.

TABLE 14A (7)

VIRUS/DISEASE	DRUG/DOSAGE	SIDE EFFECTS/COMMENTS
Herpes simplex virus (HSV Types 1 & 2) *(continued)*		
Mucocutaneous *(for genital see previous page)*		
Oral labial, "fever blisters":		
Normal host *See Ann Pharmacotherapy 38:705, 2004; JAC 53:703, 2004*	Start rx with prodrome symptoms (tingling/burning) before lesions show. **Drug** / **Dose** / **Sx Decrease** **Oral:** Valacyclovir — 2 gm po q12h x 1 day — ↓ 1 day Famciclovir[5] — 500 mg po bid x 7 days — ↓ 2 days Acyclovir[NFDA] — 400 mg po 5 x per day (q4h while awake) x 5 days) — ↓ ½ day **Topical:** Penciclovir 1% cream — q2h during day x 4 days — ↓ 1 day Acyclovir 5% cream[6] — 6x/day (q3h) x 7 days — ↓ ½ day	Penciclovir *(J Derm Treat 13:67, 2002; JAMA 277:1374, 1997; AAC 46: 2848, 2002)*. Docosanol *(J Am Acad Derm 45:222, 2001)*. Oral acyclovir 5% cream *(AAC 46:2238, 2002)*. Oral famciclovir *(JID 179:303, 1999)*. Topical fluocinonide (0.05% Lidex gel) q8h times 5 days in combination with famciclovir ↓ lesion size and pain when compared to famciclovir alone *(JID 181:1906, 2000)*.
Herpes Whitlow	*See Table 1A, page 25*	
Oral labial or genital: Immunocompromised (includes pts with AIDS) and critically ill pts in ICU setting/large necrotic ulcers in perineum or face. *(See Comment)*	**Acyclovir** 5 mg per kg IV (infused over 1 hr) q8h times 7 days (250 mg per M²) or 400 mg po 5 times per day times 14–21 days *(see Comment if suspect acyclovir-resistant)* **OR** **Famciclovir:** In HIV infected, 500 mg po bid for 7 days for recurrent episodes of genital herpes **OR** **Valacyclovir[NAI]:** In HIV-infected, 500 mg po bid for 5–10 days for recurrent episodes of genital herpes or 500 mg po bid for chronic suppressive rx.	**Acyclovir-resistant HSV: IV foscarnet** 90 mg/kg IV q12h x 7 days. Suppressive therapy with famciclovir (500 mg po bid), valacyclovir (500 mg po bid) or acyclovir (400-800 mg po bid) reduces viral shedding and clinical recurrences.
Pregnancy and genital H. simplex	Acyclovir safe even in first trimester. No proof that acyclovir at delivery reduces risk/severity of neonatal Herpes. In contrast, C-section in women with active lesions reduces risk of transmission. Ref. *Obstet Gyn 106:845, 2006.*	
Herpes simiae (Herpes B virus): **Monkey bite** *CID 35:1191, 2002*	**Postexposure prophylaxis:** Valacyclovir 1 gm po q8h times 14 days or acyclovir 800 mg po 5 times per day times 14 days. **Treatment of disease:** (1) CNS symptoms absent: Acyclovir 12.5–15 mg per kg IV q8h or ganciclovir 5 mg per kg IV q12h. (2) CNS symptoms present: Ganciclovir 5 mg per kg IV q12h	Fatal human cases of myelitis and hemorrhagic encephalitis have been reported following bites, scratches, or eye inoculation of saliva from monkeys. Initial sx include fever, headache, myalgias and diffuse adenopathy, incubation period of 2–14 days *(EID 9:246, 2003)*. In vitro ACV and ganciclovir less active than other nucleosides (penciclovir or 5-ethyldeoxyuridine may be more active; clinical data needed)*(AAC 51:2028, 2007)*.

[5] FDA approved only for HIV pts

[6] Approved for immunocompromised pts

* *See page 2 for abbreviations.* NOTE: All dosage recommendations are for adults (unless otherwise indicated) and assume normal renal function.

TABLE 14A (8)

VIRUS/DISEASE	DRUG/DOSAGE	SIDE EFFECTS/COMMENTS
Herpesvirus Infections *(continued)*		
Varicella-Zoster Virus (VZV)		
Varicella: Vaccination has markedly ↓ incidence of varicella & morbidity *(NEJM 352:450, 2005; NEJM 353:2377, 2005 & NEJM 356:1338, 2007)*. Guidelines for VZV vaccine *(MMWR 56(RR-4) 2007)*.		
Normal host (chickenpox) Child (2–12 years)	**In general, treatment not recommended.** Might use oral **acyclovir** for healthy persons at ↑ risk for moderate to severe varicella, i.e., >12 yrs of age; chronic cutaneous or pulmonary diseases; chronic salicylate rx (↑ risk of Reye syndrome), **acyclovir** dose: 20 mg/kg po qid x 5 days (start within 24 hrs of rash).	Acyclovir slowed development and ↓ number of new lesions and ↓ duration of disease in children: 9 to 7.6 days *(PIDJ 21:739, 2002)*. Oral dose of acyclovir in children should not exceed 80 mg per kg per day or 3200 mg per day.
Adolescents, young adults	**Acyclovir** 800 mg po 5x/day x 5–7 days (start within 24 hrs of rash) or **valacyclovir**[NFDA-I] 1000 mg po 3x/day x 5 days. **Famciclovir**[NAI] 500 mg po 3x/day probably effective but data lacking.	↓ duration of fever, time to healing, and symptoms *(AnIM 130:922, 1999)*.
Pneumonia or chickenpox in 3rd trimester of pregnancy	**Acyclovir** 800 mg po 5 times per day or 10 mg per kg IV q8h times 5 days. Risks and benefits to fetus and mother still unknown. Many experts recommend rx, especially in 3rd trimester. Some would add VZIG (varicella-zoster immune globulin).	Varicella pneumonia associated with 41% mortality in pregnancy Acyclovir ↓ incidence and severity *(JID 185:422, 2002)*. If varicella-susceptible mother exposed and respiratory symptoms develop within 10 days after exposure, start acyclovir
Immunocompromised host	**Acyclovir** 10–12 mg per kg (500 mg per M^2) IV (infused over 1 hr) q8h times 7 days	Disseminated 1° varicella infection reported during infliximab rx of rheumatoid arthritis *(J Rheum 31:2517, 2004)*. Continuous infusion of high-dose acyclovir (2 mg per kg per hr) successful in 1 pt with severe hemorrhagic varicella *(NEJM 336:732, 1997)*. Mortality high (43%) in AIDS pts *(Int J Inf Dis 6:6, 2002)*.
Prevention—Post-exposure prophylaxis Varicella deaths still occur in unvaccinated persons *(MMWR 56 (RR-4) 1-40, 2007)*	**CDC Recommendations for Prevention:** Since <5% of cases of varicella but >50% of varicella-related deaths occur in adults >20 yrs of age, the CDC recommends a more aggressive approach in this age group: **1st, varicella-zoster immune globulin** (VZIG) (125 units/10 kg (22 lbs) body weight IM up to a max. of 625 units; minimum dose is 125 units) is recommended for post-exposure prophylaxis in susceptible persons at greater risk for complications (immunocompromised such as HIV, malignancies, pregnancy, and steroid therapy) as soon as possible after exposure (<96 hrs). If varicella develops, initiate treatment quickly (<24 hrs of rash) with **acyclovir** as below. Some would rx presumptively with acyclovir in high-risk pts. **2nd**, susceptible adults should be vaccinated. Check antibody in adults with negative or uncertain history of varicella (10–30% will be Ab-neg.) and vaccinate those who are Ab-neg. **3rd**, susceptible children should receive vaccination. Recommended routinely before age 12–18 mos. but OK at any age.	

* *See page 2 for abbreviations.* NOTE: All dosage recommendations are for adults (unless otherwise indicated) and assume normal renal function.

TABLE 14A (9)

VIRUS/DISEASE	DRUG/DOSAGE	SIDE EFFECTS/COMMENTS
Herpesvirus Infections/Varicella-Zoster Virus (VZV) *(continued)*		
Herpes zoster (shingles) *(See NEJM 342:635, 2000 & 347:340, 2002)*		
Normal host Effective therapy most evident in pts >50 yrs. *(For treatment of post-herpetic neuralgia, see CID 36: 877, 2003)* 25-fold ↓ in zoster after immunization *(MMWR 48:R-6, 1999)* New vaccine ↓ herpes zoster & post-herpetic neuralgia *(NEJM 352: 2271, 2005; JAMA 292:157, 2006)*. Reviewed *in J Am Acad Derm 58:361, 2008.*	**[NOTE: Trials showing benefit of therapy: only in pts treated within 3 days of onset of rash]** **Valacyclovir** 1000 mg po tid times 7 days (adjust dose for renal failure)*(See Table 17)* **OR**	Valacyclovir ↓ post-herpetic neuralgia more rapidly than acyclovir in pts >50 yrs of age: median duration of zoster-associated pain was 38 days with valacyclovir and 51 days on acyclovir *(AAC 39:1546, 1995)*. Toxicity of both drugs similar *(Arch Fam Med 9:863, 2000)*.
	Famciclovir 500 mg tid x 7 days. Adjust for renal failure *(see Table 17)* **OR**	Time to healing more rapid. Reduced post-herpetic neuralgia (PHN) vs placebo in pts >50 yrs of age: duration of PHN with famciclovir 63 days, placebo 163 days. Famciclovir similar to acyclovir in reduction of acute pain and PHN *(J Micro Immunol Inf 37:75, 2004)*.
	Acyclovir 800 mg po 5 times per day times 7–10 days Add **Prednisone** in pts over 50 yrs old to decrease discomfort during acute phase of zoster. Does not decrease incidence of post-herpetic neuralgia. Dose: 30 mg po bid days 1–7, 15 mg bid days 8–14 and 7.5 mg bid days 15–21.	A meta-analysis of 4 placebo-controlled trials (691 pts) demonstrated that acyclovir accelerated by approx. 2-fold pain resolution by all measures employed and reduced post-herpetic neuralgia at 3 & 6 mos *(CID 22:341, 1996)*; med. time to resolution of pain 41 days vs 101 days in those >50 yrs. Prednisone added to acyclovir improved quality of life measurements (↓ acute pain, sleep, and return to normal activity) *(AnIM 125:376, 1996)*. In post-herpetic neuralgia, controlled trials demonstrated effectiveness of gabapentin, the lidocaine patch (5%) & opioid analgesic in controlling pain *(Drugs 64:937, 2004; J Clin Virol 29:248, 2004)*. Nortriptyline & amitriptyline are equally effective but nortriptyline is better tolerated *(CID 36:877, 2003)*. Role of antiviral drugs in rx of PHN unproven *(Neurol 64:21, 2005)* but 8 of 15 pt improved with IV acyclovir 10 mg/kg q 8 hrs x 14 days followed by oral valacyclovir 1 gm 3x a day for 1 month *(Arch Neur 63:940, 2006)*
Immunocompromised host Not severe	**Acyclovir** 800 mg po 5 times per day times 7 days. (**Options: Famciclovir** 750 mg po q24h or 500 mg bid or 250 mg 3 times per day times 7 days **OR valacyclovir** 1000 mg po tid times 7 days, though both are not FDA-approved for this indication)	If progression, switch to IV. RA pts on TNF-alpha inhibitors at high risk for VZV. Zoster more severe, but less post-herpetic neuralgia *(JAMA 301:737,2009)*.
Severe: >1 dermatome, trigeminal nerve or disseminated	**Acyclovir** 10–12 mg per kg IV (infusion over 1 hr) q8h times 7–14 days. In older pts, ↓ to 7.5 mg per kg. If nephrotoxicity and pt improving, ↓ to 5 mg per kg q8h.	A common manifestation of immune reconstitution following HAART in HIV-infected children *(J All Clin Immun 113:742, 2004)*. Rx must be begun within 72 hrs. Acyclovir-resistant VZV occurs in HIV+ pts previously treated with acyclovir. **Foscarnet** (40 mg per kg IV q8h for 14–26 days) successful in 4/5 pts but 2 relapsed in 7 and 14 days *(AnIM 115:19, 1991)*.

* *See page 2 for abbreviations.* NOTE: All dosage recommendations are for adults (unless otherwise indicated) and assume normal renal function.

TABLE 14A (10)

Influenza (A & B)

- Refs: *http://www.cdc.gov/flu/weekly; http://www.cdc.gov/flu/professionals/antivirals/recommendations.htm*
- Guidelines: *ACIP (MMWR 60 (RR-1): Jan 21, 2011); IDSA (CID 48:1003–1032, 2009).*
- **Novel A H1N1 Swine Flu** emerged in Spring 2009. *(Science 325:197, 2009).* **Rapid Test for influenza may be falsely negative in over 50% of cases of Swine Flu. During epidemic, treatment should be started based on symptoms alone.** Antiviral therapy cost-effective without viral testing in febrile pt with typical symptoms during influenza season *(CID 49:1090, 2009).*
- Vaccine info *(http://www.cdc.gov/h1n1flu/recommendations.htm).*
- **Oseltamivir: Caution: potential for confusion in dosing oral suspension** *(NEJM 361:1912, 2009).*
- **Pathogenic avian influenza (H5N1)** emerged in poultry (mainly chickens & ducks) in East & Southeast Asia. As of August 30, 2006, 246 laboratory confirmed cases reported in 10 countries with 144 deaths *(see www.cdc.gov/flu/avian).* Human-to-human transmission reported; most have had direct contact with poultry. Mortality highest in young age 10-19 (73%) vs. 56% overall and associated with high viral load and cytokine storm *(Nature Medicine 12:1203, 2006).* **Human isolates resistant to amantadine/rimantadine.** Oseltamivir therapy recommended if avian H5N1 suspected. ↑ dose & duration of oseltamivir necessary for maximum effect in mouse model *(JID 192:665, 2005; Nature 435:419, 2005).*

Virus/Disease	Susceptible to (Recommended Drug/Dosage):	Resistant to:	Side Effects/Comments
Novel A/H1N1 (Swine)	**Oseltamivir** 75 mg po bid times 5 days (also approved for rx of children age 1–12 yrs, dose 2 mg per kg up to a total of 75 mg bid times 5 days)* **or** **Zanamivir** 2 inhalations (5 mg each) bid for 5 days. *In morbidly obese patient, increase dose of oseltamivir to 150 mgs po bid. For patients who are severely ill with influenza, consideration may be given to use of oseltamivir at higher doses (150 mg bid) and for extended courses (eg, ≥ 10 days) *(MMWR 58:749, 2009);* Safety of high doses not established in pregnancy (http://www.who.int/csr/resources/publications/swineflu/clinical_management_h1n1.pdf).	Amantadine and rimantadine (100%)	**Caution:** do not reconstitute zanamivir powder for use in nebulizers or mechanical ventilators ***(MedWatch report of death).*** **For severe, life-threatening disease consider compassionate use IV Peramivir** (Biocryst/Shinoygi: investigational) 600 mg IV daily for a minimum of 5 days. For access to compassionate use call 205-989-3262 or website: http://www.biocryst.com/e_ind. Peramivir is an investigational IV neuraminidase inhibitor with activity against influenza A and B, including H1N1 Swine. In phase III studies a single IV dose (300 or 600 mg) was non-inferior to oseltamivir (75 mg bid x 5 days), time to symptom resolution was 78, 81 and 81.8 hrs, respectively. In a second non-comparative study of pts at high risk for complications of influenza, using daily IV peramivir, the median time to alleviation of symptoms in all 37 pts was 68.6 hrs.
A/H1N1 (Seasonal)	**Zanamivir** 2 inhalations (5 mg each) bid for 5 days.	Oseltamivir (99.4% resistant)	**Peramivir IV** alternative agent for serious infection (as above). Pts with COPD or asthma, **potential risk of bronchospasm with zanamivir.** All ↓ duration of symptoms by approx. 50% (1–2 days) if given within 30–36 hrs after onset of symptoms. Benefit influenced by duration of symptoms before rx; initiation of oseltamivir within 1st 12 hrs after fever onset ↓ total median illness duration by 74.6 hrs *(JAC 51:123, 2003).* ↓ risk of pneumonia *(Curr Med Res Opin 21:761, 2005).*
A/H3N2	**Oseltamivir** 75 mg po bid times 5 days (also approved for rx of children age 1–12 yrs, dose 2 mg per kg up to a total of 75 mg bid times 5 days) or **Zanamivir** (as above)	Amantadine/ rimantadine (100% resistant)	**Peramivir** alternative agent for serious infection (as above).
B	**Oseltamivir or Zanamivir** (as above)	No data	**Peramivir** alternative agent for serious infection (as above).

* *See page 2 for abbreviations.* NOTE: All dosage recommendations are for adults (unless otherwise indicated) and assume normal renal function.

TABLE 14A (11)

Influenza (A & B) *(continued)*

Virus/Disease	Susceptible to (Recommended Drug/Dosage):	Resistant to:	Side Effects/Comments
H5N1 (Avian)	**Oseltamivir or Zanamivir** (as above)	Amantadine/ rimantadine	**Peramivir** alternative agent for serious infection (as above). Report of increasing resistance in up to 18% of children with H5N1 treated with oseltamivir and less responsive H5N1 virus in several patients. Less resistance to zanamivir so far.
Prevention : Influenza A & B	Give vaccine and if ≥13 yrs age, consider **oseltamivir** 75 mg po q24h or **zanamivir** 2 inhalations (5 mg each) once daily for 5 days for the two weeks following vaccination or for the duration of peak influenza in community or for outbreak control in high-risk populations if vaccination cannot be administered *(CID 2009; 48:1003–1032)*. Avoid Oseltamivir if seasonal H1N1 infection predominates with Oseltamivir resistant strain. (Consider for similar populations as immunization recommendations.)		Immunization contraindicated if hypersensitivity to chicken eggs.

VIRUS/DISEASE	DRUG/DOSAGE	SIDE EFFECTS/COMMENTS
Measles While measles in the US is at the lowest rates ever (55/100,000) much higher rates reported in developing countries *(CID 42:322, 2006)*. Imported measles in US on the rise *(MMWR 57: 169,2008)*. High attack rates in the unvaccinated *(CID 47:1143,2008)*. Concern about lack of vaccine effectiveness in developing countries *(Lancet 373:1543, 2009)*.		
Children	No therapy or **vitamin A** 200,000 units po daily times 2 days	Vitamin A may ↓ severity of measles.
Adults	No rx or **ribavirin** IV: 20–35 mg per kg per day times 7 days	↓ severity of illness in adults *(CID 20:454, 1994)*.
Metapneumovirus (HMPV) A paramyxovirus isolated from pts of all ages, with mild bronchiolitis/bronchospasm to pneumonia. Can cause lethal pneumonia in HSCT pts *(Ann Intern Med 144:344, 2006)*	**No proven antiviral therapy** (intravenous ribavirin used anecdotally with variable results)	Human metapneumovirus isolated from 6-21% of children with RTIs *(NEJM 350:443, 2004)*. Dual infection with RSV assoc. with severe bronchiolitis *(JID 191:382, 2005)*. Nucleic acid test now approved to detect 12 respiratory viruses *(xTAG Respiratory Viral Panel, Luminex Molecular Diagnostics)*.
Monkey pox (orthopox virus) *(see LnID 4:17, 2004)* Outbreak from contact with ill prairie dogs. Source likely imported Gambian giant rats *(MMWR 42:642, 2003)*.	**No proven antiviral therapy**. Cidofovir is active in vitro & in mouse model *(AAC 46:1329, 2002; Antiviral Res 57:13, 2003)* *(Potential new drugs Virol J 4:8, 2007)*	Incubation period of 12 days, then fever, headache, cough, adenopathy, & a vesicular papular rash that pustulates, umbilicates, & crusts on the head, trunk, & extremities. Transmission in healthcare setting rare *(CID 40:789, 2005; CID 41:1742, 2005; CID 41;1765, 2005)*.
Norovirus (Norwalk-like virus, or NLV) Vast majority of outbreaks of non-bacterial gastroenteritis.	**No antiviral therapy.** Replete volume. Transmission by contaminated food, fecal-oral contact with contaminated surfaces, or fomites.	Sudden onset of nausea, vomiting, and/or watery diarrhea lasting 12–60 hours. Ethanol-based hand rubs effective *(J Hosp Inf 60:144, 2005)*.
Papillomaviruses: Warts **External Genital Warts**	***Patient applied:*** **Podofilox** (0.5% solution or gel): apply 2x/day x 3 days, 4th day no therapy, repeat cycle 4x; OR **Imiquimod** 5% cream: apply once daily hs 3x/wk for up to 16 wks. **Provider administered:** Cryotherapy with liquid nitrogen; repeat q1-2 wks; OR **Podophyllin resin** 10-25% in tincture of benzoin. Repeat weekly as needed; OR **Trichloroacetic acid** (TCA): repeat weekly as needed; OR surgical removal.	**Podofilox**: Inexpensive and safe (pregnancy safety not established). Mild irritation after treatment. **Imiquimod:** Mild to moderate redness & irritation. Topical imiquimod effective for treatment of vulvar intraepithelial neoplasms *(NEJM 358:1465, 2008)*. Safety in pregnancy not established. **Cryotherapy:** blistering and skin necrosis common. **Podophyllin resin:** Must air dry before treated area contacts clothing. Can irritate adjacent skin. **TCA:** caustic. Can cause severe pain on adjacent normal skin. Neutralize with soap or sodium bicarbonate.

* *See page 2 for abbreviations.* NOTE: All dosage recommendations are for adults (unless otherwise indicated) and assume normal renal function.

TABLE 14A (12)

VIRUS/DISEASE	DRUG/DOSAGE	SIDE EFFECTS/COMMENTS
Papillomaviruses: Warts/External Genitial Warts *(continued)*		
Warts on cervix	Need evaluation for evolving neoplasia	Gynecological consult advised.
Vaginal warts	Cryotherapy with liquid nitrogen or **TCA**	
Urethral warts	Cryotherapy with liquid nitrogen or **Podophyllin resin** 10-25% in tincture of benzoin	
Anal warts	Cryotherapy with liquid nitrogen or **TCA** or surgical removal	Advise anoscopy to look for rectal warts.
Skin papillomas	**Topical α-lactalbumin. Oleic acid** (from human milk) applied 1x/day for 3 wks	↓ lesion size & recurrence vs placebo (p <0.001) *(NEJM 350:2663, 2004)*. Further studies warranted.
Parvo B19 Virus (Erythrovirus B19). *Review: NEJM 350:586, 2004. Wide range of manifestation.* **Treatment options for common symptomatic infections:**		
Erythema infectiosum	Symptomatic treatment only	Diagnostic tools: IgM and Igb antibody titers. Perhaps better: blood parvovirus PCR. Dose of IVIG not standardized; suggest 400 mg/kg IV of commercial IVIG for 5 or 10 days or 1000 mg/kg IV for 3 days. Most dramatic anemias in pts with pre-existing hemolytic anemia. Bone marrow shown erythrocyte maturation arrest with giant pronormoblasts.
Arthritis/arthralgia	Nonsteroidal anti-inflammatory drugs (NSAID)	
Transient aplastic crisis	Transfusions and oxygen	
Fetal hydrops	Intrauterine blood transfusion	
Chronic infection with anemia	**IVIG** and transfusion	
Chronic infection without anemia	Perhaps **IVIG**	
Papovavirus/Polyomavirus		
Progressive multifocal leukoencephalopathy (PML) Serious demyelinating disease due to JC virus in immunocompromised pts.	No specific therapy for JC virus. Two general approaches: 1. In HIV pts: HAART. Cidofovir may be effective. 2. Stop or decrease immunosuppressive therapy.	Failure of treatment with interferon alfa-2b, cytarabine and topotecan. Immunosuppressive natalizumab temporarily removed from market due to reported associations with PML. Mixed reports on cidofovir. Most likely effective in pts with HAART experience.
BK virus induced nephropathy in immunocompromised pts and hemorrhagic cystitis	Decrease immunosuppression if possible. Suggested antiviral therapy based on anecdotal data. If progressive renal dysfunction: 1. **Fluoroquinolone** first; 2. **IVIG** 500 mg/kg IV; 3. **Leflunomide** 100 mg po daily x 3 days, then 10-20 mg po daily; 4. **Cidofovir** only if refractory to all of the above *(see Table 14B for dose)*.	Use PCR to monitor viral "load" in urine and/or plasma. Report of cidofovir as potentially effective for BK hemorrhagic cystitis *(CID 49:233, 2009)*.
Rabies *(see Table 20B, page 198; see MMWR 54: RR-3:1, 2005, CDC Guidelines for Prevention and Control 2006, MMWR/55/RR-5,2006)*		
Rabid dogs account for 50,000 cases per yr worldwide. Most cases in the U.S. are cryptic, i.e., no documented evidence of bite or contact with a rabid animal *(CID 35:738, 2003)*. 70% assoc. with 2 rare bat species *(EID 9:151, 2003)*. An organ donor with early rabies infected 4 recipients (2 kidneys, liver & artery) who all died of rabies avg. 13 days after transplant *(NEJM 352:1103, 2005)*.	**Mortality 100% with only survivors those who receive rabies vaccine before the onset of illness/symptoms** *(CID 36:61, 2003)*. A 15-year-old female who developed rabies 1 month post-bat bite survived after drug induction of coma (+ other rx) for 7 days; did not receive immunoprophylaxis *(NEJM 352:2508, 2005)*.	Corticosteroids ↑ mortality rate and ↓ incubation time in mice. Therapies that have failed after symptoms develop include rabies vaccine, rabies immunoglobulin, rabies virus neutralizing antibody, ribavirin, alfa interferon, & ketamine.

* *See page 2 for abbreviations.* NOTE: All dosage recommendations are for adults (unless otherwise indicated) and assume normal renal function.

TABLE 14A (13)

VIRUS/DISEASE	DRUG/DOSAGE	SIDE EFFECTS/COMMENTS
Respiratory Syncytial Virus (RSV) Major cause of morbidity in neonates/infants. Nucleic acid test now approved to detect 12 respiratory viruses (*xTAG Respiratory Viral Panel, Luminex Molecular Diagnostics*).	Hydration, supplemental oxygen. Routine use of ribavirin not recommended. Ribavirin therapy associated with small increases in O_2 saturation. No consistent decrease in need for mech. ventilation or ICU stays. High cost, aerosol administration & potential toxicity (*Red Book of Pediatrics, 2006*).	In adults, RSV accounted for 10.6% of hospitalizations for pneumonia, 11.4% for COPD, 7.2% for asthma & 5.4% for CHF in pts >65 yrs of age (*NEJM 352:1749, 2005*). RSV caused 11% of clinically important respiratory illnesses in military recruits (*CID 41:311, 2005*). Palivizumab (Synagis) 15 mg/kg IM once per month November-April. Timing of coverage may need to be adjusted in some regions based on reported cases in the region, as opposed to using fixed dosing schedules (*Pediatrics 126:e116, 2010*).
Prevention of RSV in: (1) Children <24 mos. old with chronic lung disease of prematurity (formerly broncho-pulmonary dysplasia) requiring supplemental O_2 or (2) Premature infants (<32 wks gestation) and <6 mos. old at start of RSV season or (3) Children with selected congenital heart diseases	**Palivizumab** (Synagis) 15 mg per kg IM q month Nov.-April. *Ref: Red Book of Pediatrics, 2006.*	Expense argues against its use, but in 2004 approx. 100,000 infants received drug annually in U.S. (*PIDJ 23:1051, 2004*). Significant reduction in RSV hospitalization among children with congenital heart disease (*Expert Opin Biol Ther. 7:1471-80, 2007*)
Rhinovirus (Colds) *See Ln 361:51, 2003* Found in 1/2 of children with community-acquired pneumonia; role in pathogenesis unclear (*CID 39:681, 2004*). High rate of rhinovirus identified in children with significant lower resp tract infections (*Ped Inf Dis 28:337, 2009*)	No antiviral rx indicated (*Ped Ann 34:53, 2005*). Symptomatic rx: • ipratropium bromide nasal (2 sprays per nostril tid) • clemastine 1.34 mg 1–2 tab po bid–tid (OTC). Avoid zinc products (*see Comment*).	Sx relief: ipratropium nasal spray ↓ rhinorrhea and sneezing vs placebo (*AnIM 125:89, 1996*). Clemastine (an antihistamine) ↓ sneezing, rhinorrhea but associated with dry nose, mouth & throat in 6–19% (*CID 22:656, 1996*). Oral **pleconaril** given within 24 hrs of onset reduced duration (1 day) & severity of "cold symptoms" in DBPCT (p < .001) (*CID 36:1523, 2003*). Echinacea didn't work (*CID 38:1367, 2004 & 40:807, 2005*)—put it to rest! Public health advisory advising that three over-the-counter cold remedy products containing zinc (e.g., Zicam) should not be used because of multiple reports of permanent anosmia (*www.fda.gov/Safety/MedWatch/SafetyInformation/SafetyAlertsforHumanMedicalProducts/ucm166996.htm*).
Rotavirus: Leading recognized cause of diarrhea-related illness among infants and children world-wide and kills ½ million children annually.	No antiviral rx available; oral hydration life-saving. In one study, **Nitazoxanide 7.5 mg/kg 2x/d x 3 days** reduced duration of illness from 75 to 31 hrs in Egyptian children. Impact on rotavirus or other parameters not measured. (*Lancet 368:100 & 124, 2006*) Too early to recommend routine use (*Lancet 368:100, 2006*)	Two live-attenuated vaccines highly effective (85 and 98%) and safe in preventing rotavirus diarrhea and hospitalization (*NEJM 354; 1 & 23, 2006*). ACIP recommends either of the two vaccines, RV1 or RV5, for infants (*MMWR 58(RR02). 1, 2009*).
SARS-CoV: *See page 145*		
Smallpox (*NEJM 346:1300, 2002*)	Smallpox vaccine (if within 4 days of exposure) + cidofovir (dosage uncertain but likely similar to CMV (5 mg/kg IV once weekly for 2 weeks followed by once weekly dosing. Must be used with hydration and Probenecid; *contact CDC: 770-488-7100*)	
Contact vaccinia (*JAMA 288:1901, 2002*)	From vaccination: Progressive vaccinia—vaccinia immune globulin may be of benefit. To obtain immune globulin, contact CDC: 770-488-7100. (*CID 39:759, 776 & 819, 2004*)	
West Nile virus: *See page 146*		

* *See page 2 for abbreviations.* NOTE: All dosage recommendations are for adults (unless otherwise indicated) and assume normal renal function.

TABLE 14B – ANTIVIRAL DRUGS (NON-HIV)

DRUG NAME(S) GENERIC (TRADE)	DOSAGE/ROUTE IN ADULTS*	COMMENTS/ADVERSE EFFECTS
CMV *(See Sanford Guide to HIV/AIDS Therapy)*		
Cidofovir (Vistide)	5 mg per kg IV once weekly for 2 weeks, then once every other week. **Properly timed IV prehydration with normal saline & Probenecid must be used with each cidofovir infusion:** 2 gm po 3 hrs before each dose and further 1 gm doses 2 & 8 hrs after completion of the cidofovir infusion. Renal function (serum creatinine and urine protein) must be monitored prior to each dose *(see pkg insert for details)*. Contraindicated if creatinine >1.5 mg/dL, CrCl ≤55 mL/min or urine protein ≥100 mg/dL.	**Adverse effects: Nephrotoxicity;** dose-dependent proximal tubular injury (Fanconi-like syndrome): proteinuria, glycosuria, bicarbonaturia, phosphaturia, polyuria (nephrogenic diabetic insipidus, *Ln 350:413, 1997*), acidosis, ↑ creatinine. Concomitant saline prehydration, probenecid, extended dosing intervals allow use but still highly nephrotoxic. Other toxicities: nausea 69%, fever 58%, alopecia 27%, myalgia 16%, probenecid hypersensitivity 16%, neutropenia 29%. Iritis and uveitis reported; also ↓ intraocular pressure. **Black Box warning.** Renal impairment can occur after ≤2 doses. Contraindicated in pts receiving concomitant nephrotoxic agents. Monitor for ↓ WBC. In animals, carcinogenic, teratogenic, causes ↓ sperm and ↓ fertility. FDA indication only CMV retinitis in HIV pts. **Comment:** Recommended dosage, frequency or infusion rate must not be exceeded. Dose must be reduced or discontinued if changes in renal function occur during rx. For ↑ of 0.3–0.4 mg per dL in serum creatinine, cidofovir dose must be ↓ from 5 to 3 mg per kg; discontinue cidofovir if ↑ of 0.5 mg per dL above baseline or 3+ proteinuria develops (for 2+ proteinuria, observe pts carefully and consider discontinuation).
Foscarnet (Foscavir)	Induction: 90 mg per kg IV, over 1.5-2 hours, q12h **OR** 60 mg per kg, over 1 hour, q8h Maintenance: 90 –120 mg per kg IV, over 2 hours, q24h Dosage adjustment with renal dysfunction *(see Table 17)*.	Use infusion pump to control rate of administration. **Adverse effects: Major toxicity is renal impairment (1/3 of patients)** --↑ creatinine, proteinuria, nephrogenic diabetes insipidus, ↓K+, ↓Ca++, ↓ Mg++. Toxicity ↑ with other nephrotoxic drugs [ampho B, aminoglycosides or pentamidine (especially severe ↓ Ca++)]. Adequate hydration may ↓ toxicity. Other: headache, mild (100%); fatigue (100%), nausea (80%), fever (25%). CNS: seizures. Hematol: ↓ WBC, ↓ Hgb. Hepatic: liver function tests ↑. Neuropathy. Penile and oral ulcers.
Ganciclovir (Cytovene)	IV: 5 mg per kg q12h times 14 days (induction) 5 mg per kg IV q24h or 6 mg per kg 5 times per wk (maintenance) Dosage adjust. with renal dysfunction *(see Table 17)*	**Adverse effects: Black Box warnings:** cytopenias, carcinogenicity/teratogenicity & aspermia in animals. Absolute neutrophil count dropped below 500 per mm³ in 15%, thrombocytopenia 21%, anemia 6%. Fever 48%. GI 50%: nausea, vomiting, diarrhea, abdominal pain 19%, rash 10%. Retinal detachment 11% (likely due to underlying diseases). Confusion, headache, psychiatric disturbances and seizures. Neutropenia may respond to granulocyte colony stimulating factor (G-CSF or GM-CSF). Severe myelosuppression may be ↑ with coadministration of zidovudine or azathioprine. 32% dc/interrupted rx, principally for neutropenia. Avoid extravasation.
	Oral: 1.0 gm tid with food (fatty meal) (250 mg & 500 mg cap)	Hematologic less frequent than with IV. Granulocytopenia 18%, anemia 12%, thrombocytopenia 6%. GI, skin same as with IV. Retinal detachment 8%.
Ganciclovir (Vitrasert)	Intraocular implant, 4.5 mg	**Adverse effects:** Late retinal detachment (7/30 eyes). Does not prevent CMV retinitis in good eye or visceral dissemination. **Comment:** Replacement every 6 months recommended.
Valganciclovir (Valcyte)	900 mg (two 450 mg tabs) po bid times 21 days for induction, followed by 900 mg po q24h. Take with food. Dosage adjustment for renal dysfunction *(See Table 17A)*.	A prodrug of ganciclovir with better bioavailability than oral ganciclovir: 60% with food. **Adverse effects:** Similar to ganciclovir.
Herpesvirus (non-CMV)		
Acyclovir (Zovirax or generic)	Doses: *see Table 14A for various indications* 400 mg or 800 mg tab 200 mg cap Suspension 200 mg per 5 mL Ointment or cream 5% IV injection Dosage adjustment for renal dysfunction *(See Table 17A)*.	**po:** Generally well-tolerated with occ. diarrhea, vertigo, arthralgia. Less frequent rash, fatigue, insomnia, fever, menstrual abnormalities, acne, sore throat, muscle cramps, lymphadenopathy. **IV:** Phlebitis, caustic with vesicular lesions with IV infiltration, CNS (1%): lethargy, tremors, confusion, hallucinations, delirium, seizures, coma—all reversible Renal (5%): ↑ creatinine, hematuria. With high doses may crystallize in renal tubules → obstructive uropathy (rapid infusion, dehydration, renal insufficiency and ↑ dose ↑ risk). Adequate pre-hydration may prevent such nephrotoxicity. Hepatic: ↑ ALT, AST. Uncommon: neutropenia, rash, diaphoresis, hypotension, headache, nausea.

* *See page 2 for abbreviations. NOTE: All dosage recommendations are for adults (unless otherwise indicated) and assume normal renal function.*

TABLE 14B (2)

DRUG NAME(S) GENERIC (TRADE)	DOSAGE/ROUTE IN ADULTS*	COMMENTS/ADVERSE EFFECTS
Herpesvirus (non-CMV) *(continued)*		
Famciclovir (Famvir)	125 mg, 250 mg, 500 mg tabs Dosage depends on indication: *(see label and Table 14A)*.	Metabolized to penciclovir. **Adverse effects:** similar to acyclovir, included headache, nausea, diarrhea, and dizziness but incidence does not differ from placebo. May be taken without regard to meals. Dose should be reduced if CrCl <60 mL per min *(see package insert & Table 14A, page 150 & Table 17, page 194)*. May be taken with or without food.
Penciclovir (Denavir)	Topical 1% cream	Apply to area of recurrence of herpes labialis with start of sx, then q2h while awake times 4 days. Well tolerated.
Trifluridine (Viroptic)	Topical 1% solution: 1 drop q2h (max. 9 drops/day) until corneal re-epithelialization, then dose is ↓ for 7 more days (one drop q4h for at least 5 drops/day), not to exceed 21 days total rx.	Mild burning (5%), palpebral edema (3%), punctate keratopathy, stromal edema. For HSV keratoconjunctivitis or recurrent epithelial keratitis.
Valacyclovir (Valtrex)	500 mg, 1 gm tabs Dosage depends on indication and renal function *(see label, Table 14A & Table 17A)*	An ester pro-drug of acyclovir that is well-absorbed, bioavailability 3–5 times greater than acyclovir. **Adverse effects** similar to acyclovir *(see JID 186:540, 2002)*. Thrombotic thrombocytopenic purpura/hemolytic uremic syndrome reported in pts with advanced HIV disease and transplant recipients participating in clinical trials at doses of 8 gm per day.
Hepatitis		
Adefovir dipivoxil (Hepsera)	10 mg po q24h (with normal CrCl); *see Table 17A if renal impairment.* 10 mg tab	Adefovir dipivoxil is a prodrug of adefovir. It is an acyclic nucleotide analog with activity against hepatitis B (HBV) at 0.2–2.5 mM (IC_{50}). *See Table 9* for Cmax & T½. Active against YMDD mutant lamivudine-resistant strains and in vitro vs. entecavir- resistant strains. To minimize resistance, package insert recommends using in combination with lamivudine for lamivudine-resistant virus; consider alternative therapy if viral load remains > 1,000 copies/mL with treatment. Primarily renal excretion—adjust dose. No food interactions. Generally few side effects, but **Black Box warning** regarding lactic acidosis/hepatic steatosis with nucleoside analogs and severe exacerbation of hepB on discontinuing therapy; monitoring required after discontinuation. At 10 mg per day potential for delayed nephrotoxicity. Monitor renal function, esp. with pts with pre-existing or other risks for renal impairment. Pregnancy Category C. Hepatitis may exacerbate when treatment discontinued; Up to 25% of pts developed ALT ↑ 10 times normal within 12 wks; usually responds to re-treatment or self-limited, but hepatic decompensation has occurred.
Entecavir (Baraclude)	0.5 mg q24h. If refractory or resistant to lamivudine or telbivudine: 1 mg per day Tabs: 0.5 mg & 1 mg. Oral solution: 0.05 mg/mL. Administer on an empty stomach.	A nucleoside analog active against HBV including lamivudine-resistant mutants. Minimal adverse effects reported: headache, fatigue, dizziness, & nausea reported in 22% of pts. Alopecia, anaphylactoid reactions reported. Potential for lactic acidosis and exacerbation of hepB at discontinuation (**Black Box warning**) as above. Do not use as single anti-retroviral agent in HIV co-infected pts; M134 mutation can emerge *(NEJM 356:2614, 2007)*. Adjust dosage in renal impairment *(see Table 17, page 194)*.
Interferon alfa is available as alfa-2a (Roferon-A), **alfa-2b** (Intron-A)	For hepC, usual Roferon-A and Intron-A doses are 3 million international units 3x weekly subQ.	Depending on agent, available in pre-filled syringes, vials of solution, or powder. **Black Box warnings:** include possibility of causing or aggravating serious neuropsychiatric effects, autoimmune disorders, ischemic events, infection. Withdraw therapy if any of these suspected. **Adverse effects:** Flu-like syndrome is common, esp. during 1st wk of rx: fever 98%, fatigue 89%, myalgia 73%, headache 71%. **GI:** anorexia 46%, diarrhea 29%. CNS: dizziness 21%. Hemorrhagic or ischemic stroke. Rash 18%, may progress to Stevens Johnson or exfoliative dermatitis. Profound fatigue & psychiatric symptoms in up to ½ of pts *(J Clin Psych 64:708, 2003)* (depression, anxiety, emotional lability & agitation); consider prophylactic antidepressant in pts with history. Alopecia. ↑ TSH, autoimmune thyroid disorders with ↓- or ↑- thyroidism. Hematol: ↓ WBC 49%, ↓ Hgb 27%, ↓ platelets 35%. Post-marketing reports of antibody-mediated pure red cell aplasia in patients receiving interferon/ribavirin with erythropoiesis-stimulating agents. Acute reversible hearing loss &/or tinnitus in up to 1/3 *(Ln 343:1134, 1994)*. Optic neuropathy (retinal hemorrhage, cotton wool spots, ↓ in color vision) reported *(AIDS 18:1805, 2004)*. Doses may require adjustment (or dc) based on individual response or adverse events, and can vary by product, indication (eg, HCV or HBV) and mode of use (mono- or combination-rx). (Refer to labels of individual products and to ribavirin if used in combination for details of use.)
PEG interferon alfa-2b (PEG-Intron)	0.5–1.5 mcg/kg subQ q wk	
Pegylated-40k interferon alfa-2a (Pegasys)	180 mcg subQ q wk	

* See page 2 for abbreviations. NOTE: All dosage recommendations are for adults (unless otherwise indicated) and assume normal renal function.

TABLE 14B (3)

DRUG NAME(S) GENERIC (TRADE)	DOSAGE/ROUTE IN ADULTS*	COMMENTS/ADVERSE EFFECTS
Hepatitis *(continued)*		
Lamivudine (3TC) (Epivir-HBV)	Hepatitis B dose: 100 mg po q24h Dosage adjustment with renal dysfunction *(see label)*. Tabs 100 mg and oral solution 5 mg/mL.	**Black Box warnings:** caution, dose is lower than HIV dose, so must exclude co-infection with HIV before using this formulation; lactic acidosis/hepatic steatosis; severe exacerbation of liver disease can occur on dc. YMDD-mutants resistant to lamivudine may emerge on treatment. **Adverse effects:** *See Table 14D*.
Ribavirin (Rebetol, Copegus)	For use with an interferon for hepatitis C. Available as 200 mg caps and 40 mg/mL oral solution (Rebetol) or 200 mg and 400 mg tabs (Copegus) *(See Comments regarding dosage)*.	**Black Box warnings:** ribavirin monotherapy of HCV is ineffective; hemolytic anemia may precipitate cardiac events; teratogenic/ embryocidal (**Preg Category X**). Drug may persist for 6 mo, avoid pregnancy for at least 6 mo after end of rx of women *or their partners*. Only approved for pts with Ccr > 50 mL/min. Also should not be used in pts with severe heart disease or some hemoglobinopathies. ARDS reported *(Chest 124:406, 2003)*. **Adverse effects:** hemolytic anemia (may require dose reduction or dc), dental/periodontal disorders, and all adverse effects of concomitant interferon used *(see above)*. Postmarketing: retinal detachment, ↓ hearing, hypersensitivity reactions. See *Table 14A* for specific regimens, but dosing depends on: interferon used, weight, HCV genotype, and is modified (or dc) based on side effects (especially degree of hemolysis, with different criteria in those with/without cardiac disease). For example, initial Rebetrol dose with Intron A (interferon alfa-2b) is wt-based: 400 mg am & 600 mg pm for ≤ 75 kg, and 600 mg am & 600 mg pm for wt > 75 kg, but with Pegintron approved dose is 400 mg am & 400 mg pm with meals. Doses and duration of Copegus with peg-interferon alfa-2a are less in pts with genotype 2 or 3 (800 mg per day divided into 2 doses, for 24 wks) than with genotypes 1 or 4 (1000 mg per day divided into 2 doses for wt < 75 kg and 1200 mg per day divided into 2 doses for ≥ 75 kg for 48 wks); in HIV/HCV co-infected pts, dose is 800 mg per day regardless of genotype. *(See individual labels for details, including initial dosing and criteria for dose modification in those with/without cardiac disease.)*
Telbivudine (Tyzeka)	600 mg orally q24h, without regard to food. Dosage adjustment with renal dysfunction, Ccr < 50 mL/min *(see label)*. 600 mg tabs; 100 mg per 5 mL solution.	An oral nucleoside analog approved for Rx of Hep B. It has ↑ rates of response and superior viral suppression than lamivudine *(NEJM 357:2576, 2007)*. **Black Box warnings** regarding lactic acidosis/hepatic steatosis with nucleosides and potential for severe exacerbation of HepB on dc. Generally well-tolerated with ↓ mitochondrial toxicity vs other nucleosides and no dose limiting toxicity observed *(Ann Pharmacother 40:472, 2006; Medical Letter 49:11, 2007)*. Myalgias, myopathy and rhabdomyolysis reported. Peripheral neuropathy. Genotypic resistance rate was 4.4% by one yr, ↑ to 21.5% by 2 yrs of rx of eAg+ pts. Selects for YMDD mutation like lamivudine. Combination with lamivudine was inferior to monotherapy *(Hepatology 45:507, 2007)*.

Influenza A. Treatment and prophylaxis of influenza has become more complicated. Many circulating strains are resistant to adamantanes (amantadine & rimantidine), while others are resistant to the neuraminidase inhibitor, oseltamivir, but susceptible to adamantane. Resistance to the neuraminidase inhibitor, zanamivir, is very rare, but there are limitations to the use of this inhalation agent. In this rapidly evolving area, close attention to guidance from public health authorities is warranted. In patients severely ill with influenza, combination therapy, higher than usual doses of oseltamivir and/or longer than usual treatment courses may be considered in appropriate circumstances *(MMWR 58: 749-752, 2009; NEJM 358:261-273, 2008)*.

DRUG NAME(S) GENERIC (TRADE)	DOSAGE/ROUTE IN ADULTS*	COMMENTS/ADVERSE EFFECTS
Amantadine (Symmetrel) **or Rimantadine** (Flumadine)	**Amantadine** 100 mg caps, tabs; 50 mg/mL oral solution & syrup. Treatment or prophylaxis: 100 mg bid; or 100 mg daily if age ≥65 y; dose reductions with Ccr starting at ≤50 mL/min. **Rimantadine** 100 mg tabs, 50 mg/5 mL syrup. Treatment or prophylaxis: 100 mg bid, or 100 mg daily in elderly nursing home pts, or severe hepatic disease, or Ccr ≤10 mL/min. For children, rimantadine only approved for prophylaxis.	**Side-effects/toxicity:** CNS (nervousness, anxiety, difficulty concentrating, and lightheadedness). Symptoms occurred in 6% on rimantadine vs 14% on amantadine. They usually ↓ after 1st week and disappear when drug dc. GI (nausea, anorexia). Some serious side-effects—delirium, hallucinations, and seizures—are associated with high plasma drug levels resulting from renal insufficiency, esp. in older pts, those with prior seizure disorders, or psychiatric disorders. Activity restricted to influenza A viruses.

* *See page 2 for abbreviations. NOTE: All dosage recommendations are for adults (unless otherwise indicated) and assume normal renal function.*

TABLE 14B (4)

DRUG NAME(S) GENERIC (TRADE)	DOSAGE/ROUTE IN ADULTS*	COMMENTS/ADVERSE EFFECTS
Influenza A and B—For both drugs, initiate within 48 hrs of symptom onset		
Zanamivir (Relenza) For pts ≥ 7 yrs of age (treatment) or ≥ 5 yrs (prophylaxis)	Powder is inhaled by specially designed inhalation device. Each blister contains 5 mg zanamivir. **Treatment:** oral inhalation of 2 blisters (10 mg) bid for 5 days. **Prophylaxis:** oral inhalation of 2 blisters (10 mg) once daily for 10 days (household outbreak) to 28 days (community outbreak).	Active by inhalation against neuraminidase of both influenza A and B and inhibits release of virus from epithelial cells of respiratory tract. Approx. 4–17% of inhaled dose absorbed into plasma. Excreted by kidney but with low absorption, dose reduction not necessary in renal impairment. Minimal side-effects: <3% cough, sinusitis, diarrhea, nausea and vomiting. **Reports of respiratory adverse events in pts with or without h/o airways disease, should be avoided in pts with underlying respiratory disease.** Allergic reactions and neuropsychiatric events have been reported. **Caution: do not reconstitute zanamivir powder for use in nebulizers or mechanical ventilators** (MedWatch report of death). Zanamivir for iv administration is available for compassionate use through an emergency IND application that can be accessed at: *http://www.fda.gov/Drugs/DevelopmentApprovalProcess/HowDrugsareDevelopedandApproved/ApprovalApplications/InvestigationalNewDrugINDApplication/default.htm*
Oseltamivir (Tamiflu) For pts ≥ 1 yr (treatment or prophylaxis)	For adults: **Treatment**, 75 mg po bid for 5 days; 150 mg po bid has been used for critically ill or morbidly obese patients but this dose is not FDA-approved. **Prophylaxis**, 75 mg po once daily for 10 days to 6 wk. *(See label for pediatric weight-based dosing.)* Adjust doses for Ccr ≤30 mL/min. 30 mg, 45 mg, 75 mg caps; powder for oral suspension.	Well absorbed (80% bioavailable) from GI tract as ethyl ester of active compound GS 4071. T½ 6–10 hrs; excreted unchanged by kidney. Adverse effects include diarrhea, nausea, vomiting, headache. Nausea ↓ with food. Rarely, severe skin reactions (toxic epidermal necrolysis, Stevens-Johnson syndrome, erythema multiforme). **Delirium** & abnormal behavior reported *(CID 48:1003, 2009)*.
Respiratory Syncytial Virus (RSV)		
Palivizumab (Synagis) Used for prevention of RSV infection in high-risk children	15 mg per kg IM q month throughout RSV season Single dose 100 mg vial	A monoclonal antibody directed against the F glycoprotein on surface of virus; side-effects are uncommon, occ. ↑ ALT. Anaphylaxis $<1/10^5$ pts; acute hypersensitivity reaction <1/1000. Postmarketing reports: URI, otitis media, fever, ↓ plts, injection site reactions. Preferred over polyclonal immune globulin in high risk infants & children.
Warts *(See CID 28:S37, 1999)* Regimens are from drug labels specific for external genital and/or perianal condylomata acuminata only *(see specific labels for indications, regimens, age limits)*.		
Interferon alfa-2b (IntronA)	Injection of 1 million international units into base of lesion, thrice weekly on alternate days for up to 3 wks. Maximum 5 lesions per course.	Interferons may cause "flu-like" illness and other systemic effects. 88% had at least one adverse effect. **Black box warning:** alpha interferons may cause or aggravate neuropsychiatric, autoimmune, ischemic or infectious disorders.
Interferon alfa-N3 (Alferon N)	Injection of 0.05 mL into base of each wart, up to 0.5 mL total per session, twice weekly for up to 8 weeks.	Flu-like syndrome and hypersensitivity reactions. Contraindicated with allergy to mouse IgG, egg proteins, or neomycin.
Imiquimod (Aldara)	5% cream. Thin layer applied at bedtime, washing off after 6-10 hr, thrice weekly to maximum of 16 wks.	Erythema, itching & burning, erosions. Flu-like syndrome, increased susceptibility to sunburn (avoid UV).
Podofilox (Condylox)	0.5% gel or solution twice daily for 3 days, no therapy for 4 days; can use up to 4 such cycles.	Local reactions—pain, burning, inflammation in 50%. Can ulcerate. Limit surface area treated as per label.
Sinecatechins (Veregen)	15% ointment. Apply 0.5 cm strand to each wart three times per day until healing but not more than 16 weeks.	Application site reactions, which may result in ulcerations, phimosis, meatal stenosis, superinfection.

* *See page 2 for abbreviations. NOTE: All dosage recommendations are for adults (unless otherwise indicated) and assume normal renal function.*

TABLE 14C – AT A GLANCE SUMMARY OF SUGGESTED ANTIVIRAL AGENTS AGAINST TREATABLE PATHOGENIC VIRUSES

Virus	ANTIVIRAL AGENT													
	Acyclovir	Amantadine	Adefovir Entecavir Lamivudine Tenofovir	Cidofovir	Famciclovir	Foscarnet	Ganciclovir	αInterferon Or PEG INF	Oseltamivir	Ribavirin	Rimantadine	Valacyclovir	Valganciclovir	Zanamivir
Adenovirus	-	-	-	+	-	-	±	-	-	-	-	-	±	-
BK virus	-	-	-	+	-	-	-	-	-	-	-	-	-	-
Cytomegalo-virus	±	-	-	+++	±	+++	+++	-	-	-	-	±	+++	-
Hepatitis B	-	-	+++	-	-	-	-	+++	-	±	-	-	-	-
Hepatitis C	-	-	-	-	-	-	-	+++*	-	+++*	-	-	-	-
Herpes simplex virus	+++	-	-	++	+++	++	++	-	-	-	-	+++	++	-
Influenza A Influenza B	-	±**	-	-	-	-	-	- -	+++*** ++	-	±**	-	-	+++ ++
JC Virus	-	-	-	+	-	-	-	-	-	-	-	-	-	-
Respiratory Syncytial Virus	-	-	-	-	-	-	-	-	-	+	-	-	-	-
Varicella-zoster virus	+	-	-	+	++	++	+	-	-	-	-	+++	+	-

* 1st line rx = an IFN + Ribavirin ** not CDC recommended due to high prevalence of resistance *** High level resistance H1N1 (non-swine) in 2008; Swine H1N1 susceptible.

- = no activity; ± = possible activity; + = active, 3rd line therapy (least active clinically)
++ = Active, 2nd line therapy (less active clinically); +++ = Active, 1st line therapy (usually active clinically)

TABLE 14D – ANTIRETROVIRAL THERAPY IN TREATMENT-NAÏVE ADULTS (HIV/AIDS)

(See the 2011 Sanford Guide to HIV/AIDS Therapy, Table 6, for additional information regarding treatment and complications of antiretroviral agents)

The U.S. Dept of Health & Human Services (DHHS) updated guidelines for treatment of adults and adolescents with HIV-1 infection in January 2011, *see http://www.aidsinfo.nih.gov/contentfiles/AdultandAdolescentGL.pdf*. These, and guidelines for pediatric patients and pregnant women, can be found at www.aidsinfo.nih.gov. Note that **immune reconstitution syndromes (IRIS)** may result from initiation of any ART and may require medical intervention. For additional explanation and other acceptable alternatives relating to these tables, *see www.aidsinfo.nih.gov*.

The following concepts guide therapy:

- **The goal of rx is to inhibit maximally viral replication, allowing re-establishment & persistence of an effective immune response that will prevent or delay HIV-related morbidity.**
- **Fully undetectable levels of virus (< 50 c/mL) is the target of therapy for ALL patients, regardless of stage of disease or number / type of prior regimens.**
- **The lower the viral RNA can be driven, the lower the rate of accumulation of drug resistance mutations & the longer the therapeutic effect will last.**
- **To achieve maximal & durable suppression of viral RNA, combinations of potent antiretroviral agents are required, as is a high degree of adherence to the chosen regimens.**
- **Resistance testing should be performed prior to initiation of the first regimen and prior to any change in regimen when viral load is > 500 - 1000 c/ml (while the patient is still on the ailing regimen)**
- **Treatment regimens must be tailored to the individual as well as to the virus. Antiretroviral drug toxicities can compromise adherence in the short term & can cause significant negative health effects over time. Carefully check for specific risks to the individual, for interactions between the antiretrovirals selected & between those & concurrent drugs, & adjust doses as necessary for body weight, for renal or hepatic dysfunction, & for possible pharmacokinetic interactions.**

A. **When to start therapy?** *(see www.aidsinfo.nih.gov* for additional indications: pregnancy, nephropathy, HBV co-infection requiring rx)

HIV Symptoms	CD4 cells/µL	Start Treatment	Comment
Yes	Any	Yes	
No	< 500	Yes	
No	≥ 500	Yes*	* Most pts with CD4 count > 350 cells/µL are likely to benefit from ARV therapy *(see discussion in www.aidsinfo.nih.gov)*. Treatment is indicated for any patient, especially those with Hepatitis B co-infection, HIV associated renal disease, and pregnant women. Several recent cohort studies have shown mortality benefit with starting therapy in any patient regardless of CD4 cell count *(NAACCORD, NEJM, 360:1815, 2009)*. IAS-USA Guidelines suggest considering ART in all patients regardless of CD4 count *(JAMA 2010 www.iasusa.org)*.

B. **Acute HIV Infection.** The benefits of ART in acute HIV infection are uncertain, but may include improved immunological response to the virus and decreased potential for transmission. However, treatment also exposes the patient to risks of drug adverse events, and the optimal duration of rx is unknown. Therefore, treatment is considered optional and is best undertaken in a research setting. Optimal regimens in this setting have not yet been defined. An observational study of acute or early HIV-1 infection showed comparable results from either PI-based or NNRTI-based regimens *(CID 42:1024, 2006)*, although some feel that the higher barrier to resistance of PIs might be advantageous *(www.iasusa.org)*.

TABLE 14D (2)

C. **Approach to constructing ARV regimens for treatment naïve adults.** *(Guidelines for the Use of Antiretroviral Agents in HIV-1-Infected Adults and Adolescents at www.aidsinfo.nih.gov. See that document for explanations, qualifications and further alternatives.)*

Design a regimen consisting of
[either an NNRTI ***OR*** a Protease Inhibitor ***OR*** an Integrase Inhibitor] ***PLUS*** [a dual-NRTI component]

- See section D of this table for specific regimens and tables which follow for drug characteristics, usual doses, adverse effects and additional details
- Selection of components will be influenced by many factors, such as
  - Co-morbidities (e.g., lipid effects of PIs, liver or renal disease, etc)
  - Pregnancy (e.g., avoid efavirenz—pregnancy class D)
  - HIV status (e.g., avoid nevirapine in women with CD4 > 250 and men with CD4 > 400)
  - Results of viral resistance testing
  - Potential drug interactions or adverse drug effects; special focus on tolerability (even low grade side effects can profoundly effect adherence).
  - Convenience of dosing

Co-formulations increase convenience, but sometimes prescribing the two constituents individually is preferred, as when dose-adjustments are needed for renal disease.

Preferred components by class (alphabetical order)

NNRTI	Protease Inhibitor	Integrase Inhibitor	Dual-NRTI
Efavirenz	Atazanavir + ritonavir or Darunavir + ritonavir once daily	Raltegravir	Tenofovir + Emtricitabine(co-formulated)

Alternative components by class

NNRTI	Protease Inhibitor	Integrase Inhibitor	Dual-NRTI
Nevirapine	Atazanavir or Fosamprenavir or Fosamprenavir + ritonavir (once or twice-daily regimen) or Lopinavir + ritonavir (co-formulated, once or twice-daily regimen)		Abacavir + Lamivudine (co-formulated; for pts who test neg for HLA-B5701) or Didanosine + (emtricitabine or lamivudine) or Zidovudine + lamivudine (co-formulated)

D. **During pregnancy. Expert consultation mandatory.** Timing of rx initiation & drug choice must be individualized. Viral resistance testing should be performed. Long-term effects of agents unknown. Certain drugs hazardous or contraindicated. *(See Table 8A of the Sanford Guide to HIV/AIDS Therapy)*. For additional information & alternative options, see *www.aidsinfo.nih.gov*. For regimens to prevent perinatal transmission, *see Table 8A of the Sanford Guide to HIV/AIDS Therapy*. *See JID 193:1191, 2006* re pre-term delivery with PIs.

a.	(Zidovudine + Lamivudine) + Nevirapine	(300 + 150) + 200	(Combination-Combivir 1 tab bid) + 1 tab bid fed or fasting [after 14-day lead-in period of 1 tab q24h]	4	See especially nevirapine **Black Box warnings**—among others ↑ risk of **potentially fatal hepatotoxicity** in women with CD4 >250. Avoid in this group unless benefits clearly > risks; monitor intensively if drug must be used. **Nevirapine contraindicated in Childs Pugh B & C liver disease.**
b.	(Zidovudine + Lamivudine) + Lopinavir + ritonavir	(300 + 150) + 200/50	(Combination—Combivir 1 tab bid) + 2 tabs bid without regard to food	6	Optimal dose in 3rd trimester unknown. May need to monitor levels as ↑ dose may be required. Once-daily dosing of lopinavir/ritonavir not recommended.

TABLE 14D (3)

E. **Selected Characteristics of Antiretroviral Drugs**

1. **Selected Characteristics of Nucleoside or Nucleotide Reverse Transcriptase Inhibitors (NRTIs)**
All agents have Black Box warning: Risk of lactic acidosis/hepatic steatosis. Also, labels note risk of fat redistribution/accumulation with ARV therapy. For combinations, see warnings for component agents.

Generic/Trade Name	Pharmaceutical Prep.	Usual Adult Dosage & Food Effect	% Absorbed, po	Serum T½, hrs	Intracellular T½, hrs	Elimination	Major Adverse Events/Comments (*See Table 14E*)
Abacavir (ABC; Ziagen)	300 mg tabs or 20 mg/ml oral solution	300 mg po bid or 600 mg po q24h. Food OK	83	1.5	20	Liver metab., renal excretion of metabolites, 82%	**Hypersensitivity reaction:** fever, rash, N/V, malaise, diarrhea, abdominal pain, respiratory symptoms. (Severe reactions may be ↑ with 600 mg dose.) **Do not rechallenge!** Report to 800-270-0425. **Test HLA-B*5701 before use. *See Comment Table 14E.*** Studies raise concerns re ABC/3TC regimens in pts with VL ≥ 100,000 (www3.niaid.nih.gov/news/newsreleases/2008/actg5202bulletin.htm). Recent report suggests possible ↑ risk of cardiac event in pts with other cardiac risk factors *(Ln 371:1417, 2008; updated CROI abst LB 44, 2009).*
Abacavir/lamivudine/zidovudine (Trizivir)	Film-coated tabs: ABC 300 mg + 3TC 150 mg + ZDV 300 mg	1 tab po bid (not recommended for wt <40 kg or CrCl <50 mL/min or impaired hepatic function)	*(See individual components)*				*(See Comments for individual components)* Note: **Black Box warnings** for ABC hypersensitivity reaction & others. Should only be used for regimens intended to include these 3 agents. Black Box warning— limited data for VL >100,000 copies/mL. Not recommended as initial therapy because of inferior virologic efficacy.
Didanosine (ddI; Videx or Videx EC)	125, 200, 250, 400 enteric-coated caps; 100, 167, 250 mg powder for oral solution;	≥60 kg. Usually 400 mg enteric-coated po q24h 0.5 hr before or 2 hrs after meal. Do not crush. <60 kg: 250 mg EC po q24h. Food ↓ levels. *See Comment*	30–40	1.5	25–40	Renal excretion, 50%	**Pancreatitis,** peripheral neuropathy, lactic acidosis & hepatic steatosis (rare but life-threatening, esp. combined with stavudine in pregnancy). Retinal, optic nerve changes. **The combination ddI + TDF is generally avoided, but if used,** reduce dose of ddI-EC from 400 mg to 250 mg EC q24h (or from 250 mg EC to 200 mg EC for adults <60 kg). **Monitor for ↑ toxicity & possible ↓ in efficacy of this combination; may result in ↓ CD4.** Possible increased risk of cardiovascular disease *(Ln 371:1417, 2008).*

TABLE 14D (4)

Generic/Trade Name	Pharmaceutical Prep.	Usual Adult Dosage & Food Effect	% Absorbed, po	Serum T½, hrs	Intracellular T½, hrs	Elimination	Major Adverse Events/Comments *(See Table 14E)*
Emtricitabine (FTC, Emtriva)	200 mg caps; 10 mg per mL oral solution.	200 mg po q24h. Food OK	93 (caps), 75 (oral sol'n)	Approx. 10	39	Renal excretion 86%, minor bio-transformation, 14% excretion in feces	Well tolerated; headache, nausea, vomiting & diarrhea occasionally, skin rash rarely. Skin hyperpigmentation. Differs only slightly in structure from lamivudine (5-fluoro substitution). **Exacerbation of Hep B reported in pts after stopping FTC.** Monitor at least several months after stopping FTC in Hep B pts; some may need anti-HBV therapy.
Emtricitabine/tenofovir disoproxil fumarate (Truvada)	Film-coated tabs: FTC 200 mg + TDF 300 mg	1 tab po q24h for CrCl ≥50 ml/min. Food OK	93/25	10/17	—	Primarily renal/renal	*See Comments for individual agents* **Black Box warning—Exacerbation of HepB after stopping FTC;** but preferred therapy for those with Hep B.
Emtracitabine/tenofovir/efavirenz (Atripla)	Film-coated tabs: FTC 200 mg + TDF 300 mg + efavirenz 600 mg	1 tab po q24h on an empty stomach, preferably at bedtime. Do not use if CrCl <50 ml/min		*(See individual components)*			Not recommended for pts <18yrs. *(See warnings for individual components).* **Exacerbation of Hep B** reported in pts discontinuing component drugs; some may need anti-HBV therapy (preferred anti-Hep B therapy). **Pregnancy category D-** may cause fetal harm. Avoid in pregnancy or in women who may become pregnant.
Lamivudine (3TC; Epivir)	150, 300 mg tabs; 10 mg/ml oral solution	150 mg po bid or 300 mg po q24h. Food OK	86	5–7	18	Renal excretion, minimal metabolism	**Use HIV dose, not Hep B dose.** Usually well-tolerated. **Risk of exacerbation of Hep B after stopping 3TC.** Monitor at least several months after stopping 3TC in Hep B pts; some may need anti-HBV therapy.
Lamivudine/abacavir (Epzicom)	Film-coated tabs: 3TC 300 mg + abacavir 600 mg	1 tab po q24h. Food OK Not recommended for CrCl <50 ml/min or impaired hepatic function	86/86	5–7/1.5	16/20	Primarily renal/ metabolism	*See Comments for individual agents.* **Note abacavir hypersensitivity Black Box warnings** (severe reactions may be somewhat more frequent with 600 mg dose) and 3TC Hep B warnings. Test HLA-B*5701 before use.
Lamivudine/ zidovudine (Combivir)	Film-coated tabs: 3TC 150 mg + ZDV 300 mg	1 tab po bid. Not recommended for CrCl <50 ml/min or impaired hepatic function Food OK	86/64	5-7/ 0.5-3	—	Primarily renal/ metabolism with renal excretion of glucuronide	*See Comments for individual agents* See ***Black Box warning***—exacerbation of Hep B in pts stopping 3TC

TABLE 14D (5)

Generic/Trade Name	Pharmaceutical Prep.	Usual Adult Dosage & Food Effect	% Absorbed, po	Serum T½, hrs	Intracellular T½, hrs	Elimination	Major Adverse Events/Comments (*See Table 14E*)
Stavudine (d4T; Zerit)	15, 20, 30, 40 mg capsules; 1 mg per mL oral solution	≥60 kg: 40 mg po bid <60 kg: 30 mg po bid Food OK	86	1.2–1.6	3.5	Renal excretion, 40%	Not recommended by DHHS as initial therapy because of adverse reactions. **Highest incidence of lipoatrophy, hyperlipidemia, & lactic acidosis of all NRTIs.** Pancreatitis. Peripheral neuropathy. *(See didanosine comments.)*
Tenofovir disoproxil fumarate (TDF; Viread)—a nucleotide	300 mg tabs	CrCl ≥50 ml/min: 300 mg po q24h. Food OK; high-fat meal ↑ absorption	39 (with food) 25 (fasted)	17	>60	Renal excretion	Headache, N/V. **Cases of renal dysfunction reported:** Check renal function before using. Dose reductions necessary if CrCL < 50 mL/min. Avoid concomitant nephrotoxic agents. One study found ↑ renal dysfunction at 48-wk in pts receiving TDF with a PI (mostly lopinavir/ritonavir) than with a NNRTI *(JID 197:102, 2008)*. Must adjust dose of ddI (↓) if used concomitantly but best to avoid this combination *(see ddI Comments)*. Atazanavir & lopinavir/ritonavir ↑ tenofovir concentrations: monitor for adverse effects. **Black Box warning—exacerbations of Hep B reported after stopping tenofovir.** Monitor several months after stopping TDF in Hep B pts; some may need anti-HBV Rx.
Zidovudine (ZDV, AZT; Retrovir)	100 mg caps, 300 mg tabs; 10 mg per mL IV solution; 10 mg/mL oral syrup	300 mg po q12h. Food OK	64	1.1	11	Metabolized to glucuronide & excreted in urine	Bone marrow suppression, GI intolerance, headache, insomnia, malaise, myopathy.

2. **Selected Characteristics of Non-Nucleoside Reverse Transcriptase Inhibitors (NNRTIs)**

Generic/Trade Name	Pharmaceutical Prep.	Usual Adult Dosage & Food Effect	% Absorbed, po	Serum T½, hrs	Elimination	Major Adverse Events/Comments
Delavirdine (Rescriptor)	100, 200 mg tabs	400 mg po three times daily. Food OK	85	5.8	Cytochrome P450 (3A inhibitor). 51% excreted in urine (<5% unchanged), 44% in feces	Rash severe enough to stop drug in 4.3%. ↑ AST/ALT, headaches. **Use of this agent is not recommended.**

TABLE 14D (6)

Generic/Trade Name	Pharmaceutical Prep.	Usual Adult Dosage & Food Effect	% Absorbed, po	Serum T½, hrs	Elimination	Major Adverse Events/Comments
Efavirenz (Sustiva) **(Pregnancy Category D)**	50, 100, 200 mg capsules; 600 mg tablet	600 mg po q24h at bedtime, without food. Food may ↑ serum conc., which can lead to ↑ in risk of adverse events. Pts with Hep C-induced cirrhosis & HIV: standard dose may be excessive *(JAC 65:2445, 2010)*.	42	40–55 *See Comment*	Cytochrome P450 2B6 (3A mixed inducer/ inhibitor). 14–34% of dose excreted in urine as glucuronidated metabolites, 16–61% in feces	Rash severe enough to dc use of drug in 1.7%. High frequency of diverse CNS AEs: somnolence, dreams, confusion, agitation. Serious psychiatric symptoms. Certain CYP2B6 polymorphisms may predict exceptionally high plasma levels with standard doses *(CID 45:1230, 2007)*. False-pos. cannabinoid screen. **Pregnancy Category D—may cause fetal harm—avoid in pregnant women or those who might become pregnant.** (Note: No single method of contraception is 100% reliable). Very long tissue T½. **If rx to be discontinued, stop efavirenz 1–2 wks before stopping companion drugs.** Otherwise, risk of developing efavirenz resistance, as after 1–2 days only efavirenz in blood &/or tissue. Some authorities bridge this gap by adding a PI to the NRTI backbone if feasible after efavirenz is discontinued. *(CID 42:401, 2006)*
Etravirine (Intelence)	100, 200 mg tabs	200 mg twice daily after a meal	Unknown (↓ systemic exposure if taken fasting)	41	Metabolized by CYP 3A4 (inducer) & 2C9, 2C19 (inhibitor). Excreted into feces (> 90%), mostly unchanged drug.	For pts with HIV-1 resistant to NNRTIs & others. Active in vitro against most such isolates. Rash common, but rarely can be severe. Potential for multiple drug interactions. Generally, multiple mutations are required for high-level resistance *(See Sanford HIV Guide, Table 3 for details)*. Because of interactions, do not use with boosted tipranavir, unboosted PIs, or other NNRTIs.
Nevirapine (Viramune)	200 mg tabs; 50 mg per 5 mL oral suspension	200 mg po q24h x14 days & then 200 mg po bid *(see Comments & **Black Box warning**)* Food OK	>90	25–30	Cytochrome P450 (3A4, 2B6) inducer; 80% of dose excreted in urine as glucuronidated metabolites, 10% in feces	**Black Box warning—fatal hepatotoxicity.** Women with CD4 >250 esp. vulnerable, inc. pregnant women. Avoid in this group unless benefits clearly > risks *(www.fda.gov/ cder drug/advisory/nevirapine.htm)*. If used, intensive monitoring required. Men with CD4 >400 also at ↑ risk. Rash severe enough to stop drug in 7%, **severe or life-threatening skin reactions** in 2%. Do not restart if any suspicion of such reactions. 2 wk dose escalation period may ↓ skin reactions. As with efavirenz, because of long T½, consider continuing companion agents for several days if nevirapine is discontinued. **Nevirapine is contraindicated in pts with Childs Pugh B & C liver disease.**

TABLE 14D (7)

3. **Selected Characteristics of Protease Inhibitors (PIs).**

All PIs: Glucose metabolism: new diabetes mellitus or deterioration of glucose control; fat redistribution; possible hemophilia bleeding; hypertriglyceridemia or hypercholesterolemia. Exercise caution re: potential drug interactions & contraindications. QTc prolongation has been reported in a few pts taking PIs; some PIs can block HERG channels in vitro *(Lancet 365:682, 2005)*

Generic/Trade Name	Pharmaceutical Prep.	Usual Adult Dosage & Food Effect	% Absorbed, po	Serum T½, hrs	Elimination	Major Adverse Events/Comments *(See Table 14E)*
Atazanavir (Reyataz)	100, 150, 200, 300 mg capsules	400 mg po q24h with food. Ritonavir-boosted dose (atazanavir 300 mg po q24h + ritonavir 100 mg po q24h), with food, is recommended for ARV rx-experienced pts. The boosted dose is also used when combined with either efavirenz 600 mg po q24h or TDF 300 mg po q24h. If used with buffered ddI, take with food 2 hrs pre or 1 hr post ddI.	Good oral bioavailability; food enhances bioavailability & ↓ pharmacokinetic variability. Absorption ↓ by antacids, H_2-blockers, proton pump inhibitors. Avoid unboosted drug with PPIs/H2-blockers. Boosted drug can be used with or > 10 hr after H2-blockers or > 12 hr after a PPI, as long as limited doses of the acid agents are used *(see 2008 drug label changes)*.	Approx. 7	Cytochrome P450 (3A4, 1A2 & 2C9 inhibitor) & UGT1A1 inhibitor, 13% excreted in urine (7% unchanged), 79% excreted in feces (20% unchanged)	Lower potential for ↑ lipids. Asymptomatic unconjugated hyperbilirubinemia common; jaundice especially likely in Gilbert's syndrome *(JID 192:1381, 2005)*. Headache, rash, GI symptoms. Prolongation of PR interval (1st degree AV block) reported. Caution in pre-existing conduction system disease. Efavirenz & tenofovir ↓ atazanavir exposure: use atazanavir/ritonavir regimen; also, atazanavir ↑ tenofovir concentrations—watch for adverse events. In rx-experienced pts taking TDF and needing H2 blockers, atazanavir 400 mg with ritonavir 100 mg can be given; do not use PPIs. Rare reports of renal stones
Darunavir (Prezista)	400 mg, 600 mg tablets	[Rx-experienced (+ at least one Dar-resistance assoc substitution): 600 mg darunavir + 100 mg ritonavir] po bid with food Rx-naive and -experienced (but no Dar-resistance assoc substitution): [800 mg darunavir + 100 mg ritonavir] po q24h with food (naive patients).	82% absorbed (taken with ritonavir). Food ↑ absorption.	Approx 15 hr (with ritonavir)	Metabolized by CYP3A and is a CYP3A inhibitor	Once daily dosing regimen mostly in 1st line therapy. Contains sulfa moiety. Rash, nausea, headaches seen. Coadmin of certain drugs cleared by CYP3A is contraindicated *(see label)*. Use with caution in pts with hepatic dysfunction. (Recent FDA warning about occasional hepatic dysfunction early in the course of treatment). Monitor carefully, esp. first several months and with pre-existing liver disease. May cause hormonal contraception failure.

TABLE 14D (8)

Generic/Trade Name	Pharmaceutical Prep.	Usual Adult Dosage & Food Effect	% Absorbed, po	Serum T½, hrs	Elimination	Major Adverse Events/Comments *(See Table 14E)*
Fosamprenavir (Lexiva)	700 mg tablet, 50 mg/ml oral suspension	1400 mg (two 700 mg tabs) po bid **OR** with ritonavir: [1400 mg fosamprenavir (2 tabs) + ritonavir 200 mg] po q24h **OR** [1400 mg fosamprenavir (2 tabs) + ritonavir 100 mg] po q24h **OR** [700 mg fosamprenavir (1 tab) + ritonavir 100 mg] po bid	Bioavailability not established. Food OK	7.7 Amprenavir	Hydrolyzed to amprenavir, then acts as cytochrome P450 (3A4 substrate, inhibitor, inducer)	Amprenavir prodrug. Contains sulfa moiety. Potential for serious drug interactions *(see label)*. Rash, including Stevens-Johnson syndrome. Once daily regimens: (1) not recommended for PI-experienced pts, (2) additional ritonavir needed if given with efavirenz *(see label)*. Boosted twice daily regimen is recommended for PI-experienced pts.
Indinavir (Crixivan)	100, 200, 400 mg capsules Store in original container with desiccant	Two 400 mg caps (800 mg) po q8h, without food or with light meal. Can take with enteric-coated Videx. [If taken with ritonavir (e.g., 800 mg indinavir + 100 mg ritonavir po q12h), no food restrictions]	65	1.2–2	Cytochrome P450 (3A4 inhibitor)	**Maintain hydration. Nephrolithiasis,** nausea, inconsequential ↑ of indirect bilirubin (jaundice in Gilbert syndrome), ↑ AST/ALT, headache, asthenia, blurred vision, metallic taste, hemolysis. ↑ urine WBC (>100/hpf) has been assoc. with nephritis/medullary calcification, cortical atrophy.
Lopinavir + ritonavir (Kaletra)	(200 mg lopinavir + 50 mg ritonavir), and (100 mg lopinavir + 25 mg ritonavir) tablets. Tabs do not need refrigeration. Oral solution: (80 mg lopinavir + 20 mg ritonavir) per mL. Refrigerate, but can be kept at room temperature (≤77 °F) x2 mos.	(400 mg lopinavir + 100 mg ritonavir)—2 tabs po bid. Higher dose may be needed in non-rx-naïve pts when used with efavirenz, nevirapine, or unboosted fosamprenavir. [Dose adjustment in concomitant drugs may be necessary; *see Table 22B]*	No food effect with tablets.	5–6	Cytochrome P450 (3A4 inhibitor)	Nausea/vomiting/diarrhea (worse when administered with zidovudine), ↑ AST/ALT, pancreatitis. Oral solution 42% alcohol. Lopinavir + ritonavir can be taken as a single daily dose of 4 tabs (total 800 mg lopinavir + 200 mg ritonavir), except in treatment-experienced pts or those taking concomitant efavirenz, nevirapine, amprenavir, or nelfinavir.
Nelfinavir (Viracept)	625, 250 mg tabs; 50 mg/gm oral powder	Two 625 mg tabs (1250 mg) po bid, with food	20–80 Food ↑ exposure & ↓ variability	3.5–5	Cytochrome P450 (3A4 inhibitor)	Diarrhea. Coadministration of drugs with life-threatening toxicities & which are cleared by CYP3A4 is contraindicated. Not recommended in initial regimens because of inferior efficacy. Prior concerns about EMS now resolved. Acceptable choice in pregnant women.

TABLE 14D (9)

Generic/Trade Name	Pharmaceutical Prep.	Usual Adult Dosage & Food Effect	% Absorbed, po	Serum T½, hrs	Elimination	Major Adverse Events/Comments *(See Table 14E)*
Ritonavir (Norvir)	100 mg capsules; 600 mg per 7.5 mL solution. Refrigerate caps but not solution. Room temperature for 1 mo. is OK.	Full dose not recommended *(see comments)* **With rare exceptions, used exclusively to enhance pharmacokinetics of other PIs, using lower ritonavir doses.**	Food ↑ absorption	3–5	Cytochrome P450. Potent 3A4 & 2D6 inhibitor	Nausea/vomiting/diarrhea, extremity & circumoral paresthesias, hepatitis, pancreatitis, taste perversion, ↑ CPK & uric acid. **Black Box warning—** potentially fatal drug interactions. Many drug interactions—*see Table 22A – Table 22B*
Saquinavir (Invirase—hard gel caps or tabs) **+ ritonavir**	Saquinavir 200 mg caps, 500 mg film-coated tabs; ritonavir 100 mg caps	[2 tabs saquinavir (1000 mg) + 1 cap ritonavir (100 mg)] po bid with food	Erratic for saquinavir alone. Much more reliably absorbed when boosted with ritonavir.	1–2	Cytochrome P450 (3A4 inhibitor)	Nausea, diarrhea, headache, ↑ AST/ ALT. Avoid rifampin with saquinavir + ritonavir: ↑ hepatitis risk. **Black Box warning**—Invirase to be used only with ritonavir. **New Warning** regarding prolongation of QTc when SQV used as hard gel (Invirase formulation).
Tipranavir (Aptivus)	250 mg caps. Refrigerate unopened bottles. Use opened bottles within 2 mo. 100 mg/mL solution	[500 mg (two 250 mg caps) + ritonavir 200 mg] po bid with food. <u>Solution:</u> Adults: 5 mL oral solution with 200 mg ritonavir twice daily Pediatrics: (age 2-18 yrs). Calculate dose based on body weight or BSA.	May be taken with or without food, ↓ with Al^{+++} & mg^{++} antacids.	5.5-6	Cytochrome 3A4 but with ritonavir most of drug is eliminated in feces.	Contains sulfa moiety. **Black Box warning—reports of fatal/nonfatal intracranial hemorrhage, hepatitis, fatal hepatic failure.** Use cautiously in liver disease, esp. hepB, hepC; contraindicated in Child-Pugh class B-C. Monitor LFTs. Coadministration of certain drugs contraindicated *(see label)*. **For treatment-experienced pts or for multiple-PI resistant virus.** Do not use tipranavir and etravirine together owing to 76% reduction in etravirine levels.

4. **Selected Characteristics of Fusion Inhibitors**

Generic/Trade Name	Pharmaceutical Prep.	Usual Adult Dosage	% Absorbed	Serum T½ hrs	Elimination	Major Adverse Events/Comments ***(See Table 14E)***
Enfuvirtide (T20, Fuzeon)	Single-use vials of 90 mg/mL when reconstituted. Vials should be stored at room temperature. Reconstituted vials can be refrigerated for 24 hrs only.	90 mg (1 ml) subcut. bid. Rotate injection sites, avoiding those currently inflamed.	84	3.8	Catabolism to its constituent amino acids with subsequent recycling of the amino acids in the body pool. Elimination pathway(s) have not been performed in humans. Does not alter the metabolism of CYP3A4, CYP2D6, CYP1A2, CYP2C19 or CYP2E1 substrates.	Local reaction site reactions 98%, 4% discontinue; erythema/induration ~80–90%, nodules/cysts ~80%. **Hypersensitivity reactions reported** (fever, rash, chills, N/V, ↓ BP, &/or ↑ AST/ALT)—do not restart if occur. Including background regimens, peripheral neuropathy 8.9%, insomnia 11.3%, ↓ appetite 6.3%, myalgia 5%, lymphadenopathy 2.3%, eosinophilia ~10%. ↑ incidence of bacterial pneumonias: Alone offers little benefit to a failing regimen *(NEJM 348:2249, 2003)*.

TABLE 14D (10)

5. **Selected Characteristics of CCR-5 Co-receptor Antagonists**

Generic/ Trade name	Pharmaceutical Prep. (Avg. Wholesale Price)	Usual Adult Dosage (po) & Food Effect	% Absorbed po	Serum T½, hrs	Elimination	Major Adverse Effects/Comments
Maraviroc (Selzentry)	150 mg, 300 mg film-coated tabs	Without regard to food: 150 mg bid if concomitant meds include CYP3A inhibitors including PIs (except tipranavir/ritonavir) and delavirdine (with/without CYP3A inducers) 300 mg bid without significantly interacting meds including NRTIs, tipranavir/ritonavir, nevirapine 600 mg bid if concomitant meds include CYP3A inducers, including efavirenz, (without strong CYP3A inhibitors)	Est. 33% with 300 mg dosage	14-18	CYP3A and P-glycoprotein substrate. Metabolites (via CYP3A) excreted feces > urine.	**Black Box Warning-Hepatotoxicity,** may be preceded by rash, ↑ eos or IgE. NB: no hepatoxicity was noted in MVC trials. Data lacking in hepatic/ renal insufficiency; ↑ concern with either could ↑ risk of ↓ BP. Approved for use in ARV naive patients and in treatment- experienced patients with multi-resistant strains. Document CCR-5-tropic virus before use, as treatment failures assoc. with appearance of CXCR-4 or mixed-tropic virus.

6. **Selected Characteristics of Integrase Inhibitors**

Generic/ Trade name	Pharmaceutical Prep. (Avg. Wholesale Price)	Usual Adult Dosage (po) & Food Effect	% Absorbed po	Serum T½, hrs	Elimination	Major Adverse Effects/Comments
Raltegravir (Isentress)	400 mg film-coated tabs	400 mg po bid, without regard to food	Unknown	~ 9	Glucuronidation via UGT1A1, with excretion into feces and urine. (Therefore does NOT require ritonavir boosting)	For treatment experienced pts with multiply-resistant virus. Generally well-tolerated. Nausea, diarrhea, headache, fever similar to placebo. CK ↑ & rhabdomyolysis reported, with unclear relationship to drug. Watch for worsening of depression.

TABLE 14E– ANTIRETROVIRAL DRUGS AND ADVERSE EFFECTS (HIV/AIDS)
(www.aidsinfo.nih.gov)

See also www.aidsinfo.nih.gov; for combinations, see individual components

DRUG NAME(S): GENERIC (TRADE)	MOST COMMON ADVERSE EFFECTS	MOST SIGNIFICANT ADVERSE EFFECTS
Nucleoside Reverse Transcriptase Inhibitors (NRTI) (Black Box warning for all nucleoside/nucleotide RTIs: lactic acidosis/hepatic steatosis, potentially fatal. Also carry Warnings that fat redistribution has been observed)		
Abacavir (Ziagen)	Headache 7–13%, nausea 7–19%, diarrhea 7%, malaise 7-12%	**Black Box warning-Hypersensitivity reaction (HR)** in 8% with malaise, fever, GI upset, rash, lethargy & respiratory symptoms most commonly reported; myalgia, arthralgia, edema, paresthesia less common. **Discontinue immediately if HR suspected. Rechallenge contraindicated; may be life-threatening. HLA-B*5701 allele** predicts ↑ risk of HR in Caucasian pop.; excluding pts with B*5701 markedly ↓'d HR incidence *(NEJM 358:568, 2008; CID 46:1111-1118, 2008)*. DHHS guidelines recommend testing for B*5701 and use of abacavir-containing regimens only if HLA-B*5701 negative; Vigilance essential in all groups. Possible increased risk of MI under study *(www.fda.gov/CDER)*.
Didanosine (ddI) (Videx)	Diarrhea 28%, nausea 6%, rash 9%, headache 7%, fever 12%, hyperuricemia 2%	**Pancreatitis 1–9%. Black Box warning—Cases of fatal & nonfatal pancreatitis** have occurred in pts receiving ddI, especially when used in combination with d4T or d4T + hydroxyurea. Fatal lactic acidosis in pregnancy with ddI + d4T. Peripheral neuropathy in 20%, 12% required dose reduction. Rarely, retinal changes. Possible increased risk of MI under study *(www.fda.gov/CDER)*. Non-cirrhotic portal hypertension with ddI use has been reported to the FDA.
Emtricitabine (FTC) (Emtriva)	Well tolerated. Headache, diarrhea, nausea, rash, skin hyperpigmentation	Potential for lactic acidosis (as with other NRTIs). Also **in Black Box—severe exacerbation of hepatitis B on stopping drug reported—monitor clinical/labs for several months after stopping in pts with hepB.** Anti-HBV rx may be warranted if FTC stopped.
Lamivudine (3TC) (Epivir)	Well tolerated. Headache, nausea, diarrhea, abdominal pain, insomnia. Pancreatitis more common in pediatrics (15%).	**Black Box warning.** Make sure to use HIV dosage, not Hep B dosage. **Exacerbation of hepatitis B on stopping drug. Patients with hepB who stop lamivudine require close clinical/lab monitoring for several months.** Anti-HBV rx may be warranted if 3TC stopped.
Stavudine (d4T) (Zerit)	Diarrhea, nausea, vomiting, headache	**Peripheral neuropathy** 15–20%. Pancreatitis 1%. Appears to produce lactic acidosis more commonly than other NRTIs. **Black Box warning—Fatal & nonfatal pancreatitis with d4T + ddI ± hydroxyurea. Fatal lactic acidosis/steatosis in pregnant women receiving d4T + ddI.** Motor weakness in the setting of lactic acidosis mimicking the clinical presentation of Guillain-Barré syndrome (including respiratory failure) (rare).
Zidovudine (ZDV, AZT) (Retrovir)	Nausea 50%, anorexia 20%, vomiting 17%, **headache 62%.** Also reported: asthenia, insomnia, myalgias, nail pigmentation. Macrocytosis expected with all dosage regimens.	**Black Box warning—hematologic toxicity, myopathy. Anemia** (<8 gm, 1%), granulocytopenia (<750, 1.8%). Anemia may respond to epoetin alfa if endogenous serum erythropoietin levels are ≤500 milliUnits/mL. Possible increased toxicity if used with ribavirin.
Nucleotide Reverse Transcriptase Inhibitor (NtRTI) (Black Box warning for all nucleoside/nucleotide RTIs: lactic acidosis/hepatic steatosis, potentially fatal. Also carry Warnings that fat redistribution has been observed)		
Tenofovir disoproxil fumarate (TDF) (Viread)	Diarrhea 11%, nausea 8%, vomiting 5%, flatulence 4% (generally well tolerated)	**Black Box Warning—Severe exacerbations of hepatitis B reported in pts who stop tenofovir.** Monitor carefully if drug is stopped; anti-HBV rx may be warranted if TDF stopped. May cause decreased bone mineral density. Consider monitoring bone density in pts at risk. Reports of Fanconi syndrome & **renal injury induced by tenofovir** *(CID 37:e174, 2003; J AIDS 35:269, 2004; CID 42:283 2006)*. Fanconi syndrome and diabetes insipidus reported with TDF + ddI *(AIDS Reader 19:114, 2009)*. Modest decline in Ccr with TDF may be greater than with other NRTIs *(CID 40:1194, 2005)*. Monitor creatinine clearance and serum phosphate, especially carefully in those with pre-existing renal dysfunction. **Dose reduce to every 48 hrs if CrCl<50 cc/min.** Decline in renal function may be more rapid in pts receiving TDF with a PI vs. TDF with an NNRTI *(JID 197:102, 2008)*.

TABLE 14E (2)

DRUG NAME(S): GENERIC (TRADE)	MOST COMMON ADVERSE EFFECTS	MOST SIGNIFICANT ADVERSE EFFECTS
Non-Nucleoside Reverse Transcriptase Inhibitors (NNRTI)		
Delavirdine (Rescriptor)	Nausea, diarrhea, vomiting, headache	**Skin rash** has occurred in 18%; can continue or restart drug in most cases. Stevens-Johnson syndrome & erythema multiforme have been reported rarely. ↑ in liver enzymes in <5% of patients.
Efavirenz (Sustiva)	**CNS side-effects 52%;** symptoms include dizziness, insomnia, somnolence, impaired concentration, psychiatric sx, & abnormal dreams; symptoms are worse after 1st or 2nd dose & improve over 2–4 weeks; discontinuation rate 2.6%. Rash 26% (vs. 17% in comparators); often improves with oral antihistamines; discontinuation rate 1.7%. Can cause false-positive urine test results for cannabinoid with CEDIA DAU multi-level THC assay.	**Caution:** CNS effects may impair driving and other hazardous activities. Serious neuropsychiatric symptoms reported, including severe depression (2.4%) & suicidal ideation (0.7%). Elevation in liver enzymes; hepatic failure has been reported. **Teratogenicity reported in primates; pregnancy category D—may cause fetal harm, avoid in pregnant women or those who might become pregnant** *(see Table 8A of The Sanford Guide to HIV/AIDS Therapy 2010)*. NOTE: No single method of contraception is 100% reliable. Barrier + 2nd method of contraception advised, continued 12 weeks after stopping EFV. Contraindicated with certain drugs metabolized by CYP3A4 ; potential for CYP-mediated drug interactions. Slow metabolism in those homozygous for the CYP-2B6 G516T allele resulting in exaggerated toxicity and intolerance. This allele much more common in blacks and women *(CID 42:408, 2006)*. Has been associated with severe Vitamin D deficiency *(AIDS 24:1923, 2010)*. Because of long T½, stopping drug may require special considerations, including adequate conception for 12 wks after discontinuation *(see Table 6A, Sanford HIV Guide)*.
Etravirine (Intelence)	Rash 9%, generally mild to moderate and spontaneously resolving; 2% dc clinical trials for rash. More common in women. Peripheral neuropathy.	Hypersensitivity or severe rash (erythema multiforme, toxic epidermal necrosis or Stevens-Johnson) reported. Monitor liver enzymes. Potential for CYP-mediated drug interactions.
Nevirapine (Viramune)	**Rash 37%:** usually occurs during 1st 6 wks of therapy. Follow recommendations for 14-day lead-in period to ↓ risk of rash *(see Table 14D)*. Women experience 7-fold ↑ in risk of severe rash *(CID 32:124, 2001)*. 50% resolve within 2 wks of dc drug & 80% by 1 month. 6.7% discontinuation rate.	**Black Box warning—Severe life-threatening skin reactions reported:** Stevens-Johnson syndrome, toxic epidermal necrolysis, & hypersensitivity reaction or drug rash with eosinophilia & systemic symptoms (DRESS) *(ArIM 161:2501, 2001)*. For severe rashes, dc drug immediately & do not restart. In a clinical trial, the use of prednisone ↑ the risk of rash. **Black Box warning—Life-threatening hepatotoxicity reported,** 2/3 during the first 12 wks of rx. Overall 1% develop hepatitis. Pts with pre-existing ↑ in ALT or AST &/or history of chronic Hep B or C ↑ susceptible *(Hepatol 35:182, 2002)*. Women with CD4 >250, including pregnant women, at ↑ risk. Avoid in this group unless no other option. Men with CD4 >400 also at ↑ risk. Monitor pts intensively (clinical & LFTs), esp. during the first 12 wks of rx. If clinical hepatotoxicity, severe skin or hypersensitivity reactions occur, dc drug & never rechallenge.
Protease inhibitors (PI) Abnormalities in glucose metabolism, dyslipidemias, fat redistribution syndromes are potential problems. Pts taking PI may be at increased risk for developing osteopenia/osteoporosis. Spontaneous bleeding episodes have been reported in HIV+ pts with hemophilia being treated with PI. Rheumatoid complications have been reported with use of PIs *(An Rheum Dis 61:82, 2002)*. Potential of some PIs for QTc prolongation has been suggested *(Lancet 365:682, 2005)*. **Caution for all PIs**—Coadministration with certain drugs dependent on CYP3A for elimination & for which ↑ levels can cause serious toxicity may be contraindicated. As with other classes, rx may result in immune reconstitution syndrome.		
Atazanavir (Reyataz)	Asymptomatic unconjugated hyperbilirubinemia in up to 60% of pts, jaundice in 7–9% (especially with Gilbert syndrome *(JID 192: 1381, 2005)*). Moderate to severe events: Diarrhea 1–3%, nausea 6–14%, abdominal pain 4%, headache 6%, rash 5–7%.	Prolongation of PR interval (1st degree AV block) reported; rarely 2° AV block. QTc increase and torsades reported *(CID 44:e67, 2007)*. Acute interstitial nephritis *(Am J Kid Dis 44:E81, 2004)* and urolithiasis (atazanavir stones) reported *(AIDS 20:2131, 2006; NEJM 355:2158, 2006)*. Potential increase transaminases in pts co-infected with HBV or HCV. Severe hyperbilirubinemia associated with UGT1A1*28 allele and MDR G2677T/A variation *(CID 51:101, 2010)*. Severe skin reactions have been reported.
Darunavir (Prezista)	With background regimens, headache 15%, nausea 18%, diarrhea 20%. Rash in 17% of treated; abdominal pain, vomiting, 3% discontinuation.	Hepatitis in 0.5%. Reports of liver injury, some fatal. Use caution in pts with HBV or HCV co-infections or other hepatic dysfunction. Monitor for clinical symptoms and LFTs. Stevens-Johnson syndrome, erythema multiforme. Potential for major drug interactions. May cause failure of hormonal contraceptives. Contains sulfa moiety.
Fosamprenavir (Lexiva)	Skin rash ~ 20% (moderate or worse in 3–8%), nausea, headache, diarrhea.	Rarely Stevens-Johnson syndrome, hemolytic anemia. Pro-drug of amprenavir. Contains sulfa moiety. Angioedema and nephrolithiasis reported in post-marketing experience.

TABLE 14E (3)

DRUG NAME(S): GENERIC (TRADE)	MOST COMMON ADVERSE EFFECTS	MOST SIGNIFICANT ADVERSE EFFECTS
Protease inhibitors *(continued)*		
Indinavir (Crixivan)	↑ in indirect bilirubin 10–15% (≥2.5 mg/dl), with overt jaundice especially likely in those with Gilbert syndrome *(JID 192: 1381, 2005)*. Nausea 12%, vomiting 4%, diarrhea 5%. Paronychia of big toe reported *(CID 32:140, 2001)*.	**Kidney stones.** Due to indinavir crystals in collecting system. Nephrolithiasis in 12% of adults, higher in pediatrics. Minimize risk with good hydration (at least 48 oz. water/day) *(AAC 42:332, 1998)*. Tubulointerstitial and hepatic failure, nephritis/renal cortical atrophy reported in association with asymptomatic ↑ urine WBC. Severe hepatitis reported. Hemolytic anemia reported.
Lopinavir/Ritonavir (Kaletra)	**GI: diarrhea** 14–24%, nausea 2–16%. More diarrhea with q24h dosing.	Lipid abnormalities in up to 20–40%. Hepatitis, with hepatic decompensation; caution especially in those with pre-existing liver disease. Prolonged PR and QTc intervals reported. Pancreatitis, including fatalities. Inflammatory edema of legs *(AIDS 16:673, 2002)*. Stevens-Johnson syndrome & erythema multiforme reported. Note high concentration in oral solution.
Nelfinavir (Viracept)	Mild to moderate **diarrhea** 20%. Oat bran tabs, calcium, or oral anti-diarrheal agents (e.g., loperamide, diphenoxylate/ atropine sulfate) can be used to manage diarrhea.	Potential for severe drug interactions. Powder contains phenylalanine.
Ritonavir (Norvir) (With rare exceptions, only use is to enhance levels of other anti-retrovirals, because of ↑ toxicity/ interactions with full-dose ritonavir)	**GI:** bitter aftertaste ↓ by taking with chocolate milk, Ensure, or Advera; nausea 23%, ↓ by initial dose esc (titration) regimen; vomiting 13%; diarrhea 15% Circumoral paresthesias 5–6%. ↑ dose >100 mg bid assoc. with ↑ GI side-effects & ↑ in lipid abnormalities.	Hepatic failure *(AnIM 129:670, 1998)*. **Black Box warning** relates to many important drug-drug interactions—inhibits P450 CYP3A & CYP2D6 —may be life-threatening. Rarely Stevens-Johnson syndrome, anaphylaxis. Primary A-V block (and higher) and pancreatitis have been reported.
Saquinavir (Invirase: hard cap, tablet)	**Diarrhea,** abdominal discomfort, nausea, headache	**Black Box Warning—Use Invirase only with ritonavir.** Avoid garlic capsules (may reduce SQV levels) and use cautiously with proton-pump inhibitors (increased SQV levels significant; may lead to increased GI sx, triglycerides, DVT). May cause severe skin reactions. Avoid Rifampin due to risk of severe hepatotoxicity. Avoid in patients with ↑ QTc or taking drugs that cause ↑ QTc.
Tipranavir (Aptivus)	Nausea & vomiting, diarrhea, abdominal pain. Rash in 8-10%, more common in women, & 33% in women taking ethinyl estradiol. Discontinue drug if skin rash develops. Major lipid effects.	**Black Box Warning—associated with hepatitis & fatal hepatic failure.** Risk of hepatotoxicity increased in hepB or hepC co-infection. **Associated with fatal/nonfatal intracranial hemorrhage (can inhibit platelet aggregation).** Caution in those with bleeding risks. Potential for major drug interactions. Contains sulfa moiety and Vitamin E.
Fusion Inhibitor		
Enfuvirtide (T20, Fuzeon)	Local injection site reactions (98% at least 1 local ISR, 4% dc because of ISR) (pain & discomfort, induration erythema, nodules & cysts, pruritus, & ecchymosis). Diarrhea 32%, nausea 23%, fatigue 20%.	↑ Rate of bacterial pneumonia (6.7 pneumonia events/100 pt yrs), **hypersensitivity reactions** ≤1% (rash, fever, nausea & vomiting, chills, rigors, hypotension, & ↑ serum liver transaminases); can occur with reexposure.
CCR5 Co-receptor Antagonists		
Maraviroc (Selzentry)	With ART background: cough 13%, fever 12%, rash 10%, abdominal pain 8%. Also, dizziness, myalgia, arthralgias. ↑ Risk of URI, HSV infection.	**Black box warning-Hepatotoxicity.** May be preceded by allergic features. Stevens-Johnson syndrome reported. Use with caution in pt with HepB or C. Cardiac ischemia/infarction in 1.3%. May cause ↓ BP, syncope. Significant interactions with CYP3A inducers/inhibitors. Long-term risk of malignancy unknown.
Integrase Inhibitors		
Raltegravir (Isentress)	Diarrhea, headache, nausea. LFT ↑ may be more common in pts co-infected with HBV or HCV.	Hypersensitivity can occur. ↑ CK with myopathy or rhabdomyolysis reported *(AIDS 22:1382, 2008)*. Increase in preexisting depression reported in 4 pts; all could continue raltegravir after adjustment of psych meds *(AIDS 22: 1890,2008)*. Stevens-Johnson syndrome reported post-marketing.

TABLE 15A – ANTIMICROBIAL PROPHYLAXIS FOR SELECTED BACTERIAL INFECTIONS*

CLASS OF ETIOLOGIC AGENT/DISEASE/CONDITION	PROPHYLAXIS AGENT/DOSE/ROUTE/DURATION	COMMENTS
Group B streptococcal disease (GBS), neonatal: Approaches to management [CDC Guidelines, *MMWR 59 (RR-10):1, 2010*]:		
Pregnant women—intrapartum antimicrobial prophylaxis procedures: 1. Screen all pregnant women with vaginal & rectal swab for GBS at 35–37 wks gestation (unless other indications for prophylaxis exist: GBS bacteriuria during this pregnancy or previously delivered infant with invasive GBS disease; even then cultures may be useful for susceptibility testing). Use transport medium; GBS survive at room temp. up to 96 hrs. **Rx during labor if swab culture positive.** 2. Rx during labor if previously delivered infant with invasive GBS infection, or if any GBS bacteriuria during this pregnancy. 3. Rx if GBS status unknown but if any of the following are present: (a) delivery at <37 wks gestation [see *MMWR 59 (RR-10): 1, 2010 algorithm* for threatened preterm delivery]; or (b) duration of ruptured membranes ≥18 hrs; or (c) intrapartum temp. ≥100.4°F (≥38.0°C). 4. Rx if positive intra-partum NAAT for GBS during pregnancy. 5. Rx not indicated if: negative vaginal/rectal cultures at 35-37 wks gestation or C-section performed before onset of labor with intact amniotic membranes.		**Prophylactic regimens during labor**: **Penicillin G** 5 million Units IV (load) then 2.5-3 million Units IV q4h until delivery. Alternative rx: **Ampicillin** 2 gm IV (load) then 1 gm IV q4h until delivery. ***Penicillin-allergic:*** • **Pts NOT at high risk for anaphylaxis:** Cefazolin 2 gm IV initial dose, then 1 gm q8h. • Pts at high risk for anaphylaxis: □ GBS susceptible to erythromycin and clindamyci nor susceptible to clinda (D-zone testing): **Clindamycin** 900 mg IV q8h. □ **Vancomycin** for pts at high risk for Pen anaphylaxis when alternative to clindamycin or erythromycin needed (e.g., GBS resistant or of unknown susceptibility to clindamycin/erythromycin). Continue treatment until delivery.
Neonate of mother given prophylaxis	Careful observation of signs & symptoms. 95% of infants will show clinical signs of infection during the 1st 24 hrs whether mother received intrapartum antibiotics or not *(Pediatrics 106:244, 2000)*. For gestational age <35 wks or intrapartum antibiotics <4 hrs, lab evaluation (CBC, diff, blood culture) & ≥48 hr observation recommended. See algorithm: *MMWR 59 (RR-10):1, 2010*.	
Preterm, premature rupture of the membranes in Group B strep-negative women	(IV **ampicillin** 2 gm q6h + IV **erythromycin** 250 mg q6h) for 48 hrs followed by po **amoxicillin** 250 mg q8h + po **erythromycin** base 333 mg q8h for 5 days. Decreases infant morbidity. *(JAMA 278:989, 1997)* *(Note:* May require additional antibiotics for therapy of specific existing infections*)*	Antibiotic rx reduced infant respiratory distress syndrome (50.6% to 40.8%, p = 0.03), necrotizing enterocolitis (5.8% to 2.3%, p = 0.03) and prolonged pregnancy (2.9 to 6.1 days, p < 0.001) vs placebo. In 1 large study (4809 pts), po erythromycin rx improved neonatal outcomes vs placebo (11.2% vs 14.4% poor outcomes, p=0.02 for single births) but not co-AM-CL or both drugs in combination (both assoc. with ↑ necrotizing enterocolitis) *(Ln 357:979, 2001)*. *(See ACOG discussion, Ob Gyn 102:875, 2003; Practice Bulletin in ObGyn 109:1007, 2007; Rev Obstet Gynecol 1:11, 2008; J Obstet Gynecol Can 31:863 & 868, 2009)*.
Post-splenectomy bacteremia. Likely agents: Pneumococci (90%), meningococci , H. influenzae type b. Bacteremia due to Enterobacteriaceae, S. aureus, Capnocytophaga spp. and rarely P. aeruginosa described. Also at ↑ risk for fatal malaria, severe babesiosis. Ref: *RedBookOnline, 2009. Amer Acad Pediatrics.*	**Immunizations:** Ensure admin. of pneumococcal vaccine, H. influenzae B, & quadrivalent meningococcal vaccines at recommended times. In addition, asplenic children with sickle cell anemia, thalassemia, & perhaps others, daily antimicrobial prophylaxis until at least age 5—*see Comments and Sickle-cell disease (below)*. Sepsis due to susceptible organisms may occur despite daily prophylaxis *(JClinPath 54:214, 2001)*.	Antimicrobial prophylaxis until age 5: Amox 20 mg/kg/day or Pen V-K 125 mg bid. Over age 5: Consider Pen V-K 250 mg bid for at least 1 yr in children post-splenectomy. Some recommend prophylaxis for a minimum of 3 yrs or until at least age 18. Maintain immunizations plus self-administer AM-CL with any febrile illness while seeking physician assistance. For self-administered therapy, cefuroxime axetil can be used in the penicillin-allergic pt who is not allergic to cephalosporins; alternatively, respiratory FQ can be considered in beta lactam-allergic pt in appropriate populations. Pen. allergy: TMP-SMX or clarithro are options, but resistance in *S. pneumo* may be significant in some areas, particularly among pen-resistant isolates.
Sexual Exposure		
Sexual assault survivor [likely agents and risks, see *MMWR 59 (RR-10):1, 2010]*.	(**Ceftriaxone** 125 mg IM) + (**metronidazole** 2 gm po single dose) + [(**azithromycin** 1 gm po single dose) or (**doxycycline** 100 mg po bid times 7 days)] *[See MMWR 59 (RR-10):1, 2010]*.	Obtain expert advice re: forensic exam & specimens, pregnancy, physical trauma, psychological support. If decision is to proceed with spec. collection, at initial exam: Test for gonococci & chlamydia, wet mount for T. vaginalis (& culture vaginal swab). Serologic evaluation for syphilis, Hep B, HIV, others as appropriate. Initiate post-exposure protocols for HIV & hepatitis B as appropriate *(see Table 15D)*. Follow-up exam for STD at 1–2 wks. Retest syphilis & HIV serology at 6, 12, 24 wks if negative earlier.
Sexual contacts, likely agents: N. gonorrhoeae, C. trachomatis	[(**Ceftriaxone** 125 mg IM once) or (**cefixime** 400 mg po once)] for GC, *plus* [(**doxycycline** 100 mg bid, po times 7 days) or (**azithromycin** 1 gm po once)], for Chlamydia	Be sure to check for syphilis since all regimens may not eradicate incubating syphilis. Consider also T. vaginalis. Identify & rx contacts as appropriate to suspected STD *[see MMWR 59 (RR-10):1, 2010 for other etiologies & rx options]*. Evaluate for HIV/HBV risks *(See Table 15D)*.

TABLE 15A (2)

CLASS OF ETIOLOGIC AGENT/DISEASE/CONDITION	PROPHYLAXIS AGENT/DOSE/ROUTE/DURATION	COMMENTS
Sexual Exposure *(continued)*		
Syphilis exposure		Presumptive rx for exposure within 3 mos., as tests may be negative. *See Table 1A, page 22.* If exposure occurred > 90 days prior, establish dx or treat empirically *(MMWR 59 (RR-10): 1, 2010).*
Sickle-cell disease. Likely agent: S. pneumoniae *(see post-splenectomy, above)* Ref.: *2009 Red Book Online, Amer Acad Pediatrics*	Children <5 yrs: **Penicillin V** 125 mg po bid ≥5 yrs: **Penicillin V** 250 mg po bid. (Alternative in children: Amoxicillin 20 mg per kg per day)	Start prophylaxis by 2 mos. *(Pediatrics 106:367, 2000)*; continue until at least age 5. When to d/c must be individualized. Age-appropriate vaccines, including pneumococcal, Hib, influenza, meningococcal. Treating infections, consider possibility of penicillin non-susceptible pneumococci.

TABLE 15B – ANTIBIOTIC PROPHYLAXIS TO PREVENT SURGICAL INFECTIONS IN ADULTS*

(CID 38:1706, 2004; Am J Surg 189:395, 2005)

General Comments:

- To be optimally effective, antibiotics must be started within 2 hrs of surgical incision *(NEJM 326:281, 1992)*, preferably ≤ 1 hr before incision for most agents except vancomycin and quinolones *(JAC 58:645, 2006; CID 38:1706, 2004)*.
- Most applications employ a single preoperative dose *(Treat Guide Med Lett 7:47, 2009)*.
- For procedures lasting > 2 half-lives of prophylactic agent, intraoperative supplementary dose(s) may be required *(see CID 38:1706, 2004 for schedule)*.
- Standard regimens may give relatively low tissue levels in pts with high BMI, but implications of this are not clear *(see Surgery 136:738, 2004 for cefazolin; EurJClin Pharm 54:632, 1998 for vancomycin; CID 38:1706, 2004 for wt-based dosing)*.
- In most cases, prophylaxis is not extended beyond 24 hrs *(CID 38:1706, 2004)*.
- Prophylaxis does carry risk: e.g., C. difficile colitis *(CID 46:1838, 2008)*.
- Active screening for S. aureus nasal colonization and application of chlorhexidine washes and intranasal mupirocin has been reported as a strategy that decreases surgical site infection in an area of low MRSA prevalence *(NEJM 362:9, 2010)*.

Use of Vancomycin:

- For many common prophylaxis indications, vancomycin is considered an alternative to β-lactams in pts allergic to or intolerant of the latter.
- Vancomycin use may be justifiable in centers where rates of post-operative infection with methicillin-resistant staphylococci are high, or in pts at high risk for these.
- Unlike β-lactams in common use, vancomycin has no activity against gram-negative organisms. **When gram-negative bacteria are a concern following specific procedures, it may be necessary or desirable to add a second agent with appropriate in vitro activity.** This can be done using cefazolin with vancomycin in the non-allergic pt, or in pts intolerant of β-lactams using vancomycin with another gram-negative agent (e.g., aminoglycoside, fluoroquinolone, possibly aztreonam, if pt not allergic; local resistance patterns and pt factors would influence choice).
- Infusion of vancomycin, especially too rapidly, may result in hypotension or other manifestations of histamine release syndrome *(J CardiothorVascAnesth 5:574, 1991)*.

TYPE OF SURGERY	PROPHYLAXIS	COMMENTS
Cardiovascular Surgery Antibiotic prophylaxis in cardiovascular surgery has been proven beneficial only in the following procedures: • Reconstruction of abdominal aorta • Procedures on the leg that involve a groin incision • Any vascular procedure that inserts prosthesis/foreign body • Lower extremity amputation for ischemia • Cardiac surgery • Permanent Pacemakers *(Circulation 121:458, 2010)*	**Cefazolin** 1–2 gm IV as a single dose or q8h for 1–2 days or **cefuroxime** 1.5 gm IV as a single dose or q12h for total of 6 gm or **vancomycin** 1 gm IV as single dose or q12h for 1–2 days. Consider **intranasal mupirocin** evening before, day of surgery & bid for 5 days post-op in pts with pos. nasal culture for S. aureus. Mupirocin resistance has been encountered *(CID 49:935, 2009)*.	Single infusion just before surgery probably as effective as multiple doses. Not needed for cardiac catheterization. For prosthetic heart valves, customary to stop prophylaxis either after removal of retrosternal drainage catheters or just a 2nd dose after coming off bypass. Vancomycin may be preferable in hospitals with ↑ freq of MRSA or in high-risk pts *(CID 38: 1555, 2004)*, or those colonized with MRSA *(CID 38:1706, 2004)*; however, does not cover gm-neg. bacilli, therefore would add cefazolin. Meta-analysis failed to demonstrate overall superiority of vancomycin over β-lactam prophylaxis for cardiac surgery *(CID 38: 1357, 2004)*. Intranasal mupirocin ↓ sternal wound infections from S. aureus in 1850 pts; used historical controls *(An Thor Surg 71:1572, 2001)*; in another trial, t ↓ nosocomial S. aureus infections only in nasal carriers *(NEJM 346:1871, 2002)*. One study of 0.12% chlorhexidine gluconate gel to nares and oral rinse showed ↓ deep surg site and lower resp infections *(JAMA 296:2460, 2006)*.

TABLE 15B (2)

TYPE OF SURGERY	PROPHYLAXIS	COMMENTS
Gastric, Biliary and Colonic Surgery		
Gastroduodenal/Biliary		
Gastroduodenal, includes percutaneous endoscopic gastrostomy (high-risk only; *see Comments*). Biliary, includes laparoscopic cholecystectomy (high-risk only; *see Comments*).	**Cefazolin** or **cefoxitin** or **cefotetan** or **cefuroxime** 1.5 gm IV as a single dose (some give additional doses q12h for 2–3 days).	Gastroduodenal: High-risk is marked obesity, obstruction, ↓ gastric acid or ↓ motility. Meta-analysis supports use in percutaneous endoscopic gastrostomy *(Am J Gastro 95:3133, 2000)*. Biliary high-risk: age >70, acute cholecystitis, non-functioning gallbladder, obstructive jaundice or common duct stones. With cholangitis, treat as infection, not prophylaxis *(See Table 1A, page 15)*. (For guidelines of American Soc of Gastrointestinal Endoscopy, *see Gastroint Endosc 67:791, 2008)*.
Endoscopic retrograde cholangiopancreatography Controversial: No benefit from single dose piperacillin in randomized placebo-controlled trial, *AnIM 125:442, 1996* *(see Comment)*	No rx without obstruction. If obstruction: **Ciprofloxacin** 500–750 mg po 2 hrs prior to procedure or **PIP-TZ** 4.5 gm IV 1 hr prior to procedure	Most studies show that **achieving adequate drainage** will prevent postprocedural cholangitis or sepsis and no further benefit from prophylactic antibiotics; greatest benefit likely when complete drainage cannot be achieved. Meta-analysis suggested antibiotics may ↓ bacteremia, but not sepsis/cholangitis *(Endoscopy 31:718, 1999)*. Oral CIP as effective as cephalosporins in 2 studies & less expensive but quinolone resistance increasing *(CID 23:380, 1996)*. *See Gastroint Endosc 67:791, 2008* for Amer Soc Gastroint Endosc recommendations.
Colorectal	Oral antibiotics for elective surgery *(see Comments)* **Parenteral regimens** (emergency or elective): [**Cefazolin** 1-2 gm IV + **metronidazole** 0.5 gm IV] or **cefoxitin** or **cefotetan** 1-2 gm IV (if available) or **AM-SB** 3 gm IV or **ERTA** 1 gm IV *(NEJM 355:2640, 2006* study found ertapenem more effective than cefotetan, but associated with non-significant ↑ risk of C. difficile).	**Oral regimens: Neomycin** + **erythromycin** Pre-op day: (1) 10 am 4L polyethylene glycol electrolyte solution (Colyte, GoLYTELY) po over 2 hr. (2) Clear liquid diet only. (3) 1 pm, 2 pm & 11 pm, neomycin 1 gm + erythro base 1 gm po. (4) NPO after midnight. Alternative regimens have been less well studied; GoLYTELY 1–6 pm, then neomycin 2 gm po + metronidazole 2 gm po at 7 pm & 11 pm. Oral regimen as effective as parenteral; parenteral in addition to oral not required but often used *(AmJSurg 189:395, 2005)*. Many used both parenteral + oral regimens for elective procedures *(AmJSurg 189:395, 2005)*, but recent ↓ enthusiasm for mechanical bowel preparation. Meta-analysis did not support mech bowel prep in preventing anastomotic leaks with elective colorectal surg *(Cochr Database Syst Rev 1:CD001544, 2009)*.
Ruptured viscus: *See Peritoneum/Peritonitis, Secondary, Table 1A, page 45.*		
Head and Neck Surgery *(Ann Otol Rhinol Laryngol 101 Suppl: 16, 1992)*		
Cefazolin 2 gm IV (Single dose)(some add **metronidazole** 500 mg IV *(Treat Guide Med Lett 7:47, 2009)* **OR** **Clindamycin** 600-900 mg IV (single dose) + **gentamicin** 1.5 mg/kg IV (single dose)*(See Table 10D for weight-based dose calculation)*.		Antimicrobial prophylaxis in head & neck surg appears efficacious only for procedures involving oral/ pharyngeal mucosa (e.g., laryngeal or pharyngeal tumor) but even with prophylaxis, wound infection rate can be high *(Head Neck 23:447, 2001)*. Uncontaminated head & neck surg does not require prophylaxis.
Neurosurgical Procedures [Prophylaxis not effective in ↓ infection rate with intracranial pressure monitors in retrospective analysis of 215 pts *(J Neurol Neurosurg Psych 69:381, 2000)*]		
Clean, non-implant; e.g., craniotomy	**Cefazolin** 1-2 gm IV once. Alternative: **vanco** 1 gm IV once	Reference: *Ln 344:1547, 1994*
Clean, contaminated (cross sinuses, or naso/oropharynx)	**Clindamycin** 900 mg IV (single dose)	British recommend amoxicillin-clavulanate 1.2 gm IV[NUS] or (cefuroxime 1.5 gm IV + metronidazole 0.5 gm IV)
CSF shunt surgery:	**Cefazolin** 1-2 gm IV once. Alternative: **vanco** 1 gm IV once.	Meta-analysis suggests benefit *(Cochrane Database 3: CD 005365)*. Randomized study in a hospital with high prevalence of infection due to methicillin-resistant staphylococci showed vancomycin was more effective than cefazolin in preventing CSF shunt infections *(J Hosp Infect 69:337, 2008)*.

TABLE 15B (3)

TYPE OF SURGERY	PROPHYLAXIS	COMMENTS
Obstetric/Gynecologic Surgery *(See ACOG Practice Bulletin in Obstet & Gyn 113:1180, 2009 for additional procedures and alternatives).*		
Vaginal or abdominal hysterectomy	**Cefazolin** 1–2 gm or **cefoxitin** 1–2 gm or **cefotetan** 1–2 gm or **cefuroxime** 1.5 gm all IV 30 min. before surgery.	1 study found cefotetan superior to cefazolin *(CID 20:677, 1995)*. For prolonged procedures, doses can be repeated q4–8h for duration of procedure. Ampicillin-sulbactam is considered an acceptable alternative *(CID 43:322, 2006)*. Treat pts with bacterial vaginosis pre-op.
Cesarean section for premature rupture of membranes or active labor	**Cefazolin** 1-2 gm IV *(See Comments)*.	Prophylaxis decreases risk of endometritis and wound infection. Traditional approach had been to administer antibiotics after cord is clamped to avoid exposing infant to antibiotic. However, recent studies suggest that administering prophylaxis before the skin incision results in fewer surgical site infections *(Obstet Gynecol 115:187, 2010; Amer J Obstet Gynecol 199:301.e1 and 310:e1, 2008)* and endometritis *(Amer J Obstet Gynecol 196:455.e1, 2007)*.
Surgical Abortion (1st trimester)	1st trimester: **Doxycycline** 300 mg po, as 100 mg 1 hr before procedure + 200 mg post-procedure.	Meta-analysis showed benefit of antibiotic prophylaxis in all risk groups. One regimen was doxy 100 mg orally 1 hr before procedure, then 200 mg after procedure *(Ob Gyn 87:884, 1996)*.
Orthopedic Surgery		
Hip arthroplasty, spinal fusion	Same as cardiac	Customarily stopped after "Hemovac" removed. NSIPP workgroup recommends stopping prophylaxis within 24 hrs of surgery *(CID 38:1706, 2004)*.
Total joint replacement (other than hip)	**Cefazolin** 1–2 gm IV pre-op (± 2nd dose) or **vancomycin** 1 gm IV	NSIPP workgroup recommends stopping prophylaxis within 24 hrs of surgery *(CID 38:1706, 2004)*. Recent study in total knee arthroplasty found dosing cefuroxime 1.5 gm just prior to tourniquet release (+ 2nd dose 6 hr after surgery) was not inferior to dosing before inflation (+ 2nd dose) *(CID 46:1009, 2008)*.
Open reduction of closed fracture with internal fixation	**Ceftriaxone** 2 gm IV or IM once	3.6% (ceftriaxone) vs 8.3% (for placebo) infection found in Dutch trauma trial *(Ln 347:1133, 1996)*. Several alternative antimicrobials can ↓ risk of infection *(Cochrane Database Syt Rev 2001: CD 000244)*.
Prophylaxis to protect prosthetic joints from hematogenous infection related to distant procedures (patients with plates, pins and screws only are not considered to be at risk)	• In 2003, the American Academy of Orthopedic Surgeons (AAOS), in conjunction with the American Dental Association and the American Urological Association, developed *Advisory Statements* on the use of antibiotic prophylaxis to prevent infection of implanted joint prostheses for procedures that may cause bacteremia. *(J Am Dental Assn 134:895, 2003; J Urol 169:1796, 2003)*. These documents stratified procedures for risk of bacteremia, described patient factors that might place joints at ↑ risk of infection (incl. all pts in first 2 years after insertion), and offered antibiotic options. (See also *Med Lett 47:59, 2005* and review in *Infect Dis Clin N Amer 19:931, 2005*). • A February 2009 *Information Statement* from the AAOS listed patient factors that may ↑ risk of infection, but recommended that antibiotic prophylaxis *be considered* for any invasive procedure that may cause bacteremia in all patients with a joint replacement *(http://aaos.org/about/papers/advistmt/1033.asp)*. • The editors believe that the latter approach is excessively broad and exposes many to the risks of antibiotics without definite evidence of benefit. As pointed out in guidelines for prevention of endocarditis, transient bacteremias occur with routine daily activities (*Circulation 2007; 116:1736*). • A recent prospective, case-control study concluded that antibiotic prophylaxis for dental procedures *did not* decrease the risk of hip or knee prosthesis infection (*Clin Infect Dis 50:8, 2010*). • For patients with prosthetic joints, infections involving tissue to be manipulated surgically should be treated before surgery whenever possible. Prophylaxis with an anti-staphylococcal β-lactam or vancomycin (according to susceptibility of the organism) for procedures involving tissues colonized by staphylococci would be appropriate, as these organisms are common causes of prosthetic joint infections. In other circumstances, decisions must be based on individual judgment; for now, the 2003 documents cited above appear to provide the best information on which to base such decisions.	
Peritoneal Dialysis Catheter Placement	**Vancomycin** single 1 gm IV dose 12 hrs prior to procedure	Effectively reduced peritonitis during 14 days post-placement in 221 pts: vanco 1%, cefazolin 7%, placebo 12% (p=0.02) *(Am J Kidney Dis 36:1014, 2000)*.

TABLE 15B (4)

TYPE OF SURGERY	PROPHYLAXIS	COMMENTS
Urologic Surgery/Procedures • *See Best Practice Policy Statement* of Amer. Urological Assoc. (AUA) *(J Urol 179:1379, 2008)* for detailed recommendations on specific procedures/circumstances. • Selection of agents targeting urinary pathogens may require modification based on local resistance patterns; ↑ TMP-SMX and/or fluoroquinolone (FQ) resistance among enteric gram-negative bacteria is a concern.		
Cystoscopy	• Prophylaxis generally not necessary if urine is sterile (however, AUA recommends FQ or TMP-SMX for those with several potentially adverse host factors (e.g., advanced age, immunocompromised state, anatomic abnormalities, etc.) • Treat patients with UTI prior to procedure using an antimicrobial active against pathogen isolated	
Cystoscopy with manipulation	Ciprofloxacin 500 mg po (TMP-SMX 1 DS tablet po may be an alternative in populations with low rates of resistance)	Procedures mentioned include ureteroscopy, biopsy, fulguration, TURP, etc. Treat UTI with targeted therapy before procedure if possible.
Transrectal prostate biopsy	Ciprofloxacin 500 mg po 12 hrs prior to biopsy and repeated 12 hrs after 1st dose	Bacteremia 7% with CIP vs 37% with gentamicin *(JAC 39:115, 1997)*. Levofloxacin 500 mg 30-60 min before procedure was effective in low risk pts; additional doses were given for ↑ risk *(J Urol 168:1021, 2002)*. Serious bacteremias due to FQ-resistant organisms have been encountered in patients receiving FQ prophylaxis. Clinicians should advise patients to immediately report symptoms suggesting infection. Pre-operative prophylaxis should be determined on an institutional basis based on susceptibility profiles of prevailing organisms.
Other		
Breast surgery, herniorrhaphy	**Cefazolin** 1-2 gm IV pre-op	Benefits of prophylaxis for clean surgical procedures not clear *(Treat Guide MedLett 7:47, 2009)*. Antibiotics may reduce risk of surgical site infection in breast cancer surgery (studies not examining immediate reconstruction), but great variability in regimens selected *(Cochrane Database Syst Rev 2006; (2): CD 005360)*. For inguinal hernia repair, one analysis found prophylaxis to be beneficial in repairs with mesh *(J Hosp Infect 62: 427, 2006)*, while another concluded that antibiotics may reduce risk of infection in pooled population or in those repaired with prosthetic material (mesh), but that the data were not sufficiently strong to make firm recommendations for or against their use universally *(Cochrane Database Syst Rev 2007; (3): CD 003769)*.

TABLE 15C – ANTIMICROBIAL PROPHYLAXIS FOR THE PREVENTION OF BACTERIAL ENDOCARDITIS IN PATIENTS WITH UNDERLYING CARDIAC CONDITIONS*

In 2007, the American Heart Association guidelines for the prevention of bacterial endocarditis were updated. The resulting document (*Circulation 2007; 116:1736-1754 and http://circ.ahajournals.org/cgi/reprint/116/15/1736*), which was also endorsed by the Infectious Diseases Society of America, represents a significant departure from earlier recommendations.

- Antibiotic prophylaxis for dental procedures is now directed at individuals who are likely to suffer the most devastating consequences should they develop endocarditis. Prophylaxis to prevent endocarditis is no longer specified for gastrointestinal or genitourinary procedures. The following is adapted from and reflects the new AHA recommendations. *See original publication for explanation and precise details.*

SELECTION OF PATIENTS FOR ENDOCARDITIS PROPHYLAXIS				
FOR PATIENTS WITH ANY OF THESE HIGH-RISK CARDIAC CONDITIONS ASSOCIATED WITH ENDOCARDITIS:	**WHO UNDERGO DENTAL PROCEDURES INVOLVING:**	**WHO UNDERGO INVASIVE RESPIRATORY PROCEDURES INVOLVING:**	**WHO UNDERGO INVASIVE PROCEDURES OF THE GI OR GU TRACTS:**	**WHO UNDERGO PROCEDURES INVOLVING INFECTED SKIN AND SOFT TISSUES:**
Prosthetic heart valves Previous infective endocarditis Congenital heart disease with any of the following: • Completely repaired cardiac defect using prosthetic material (Only for 1st 6 months) • Partially corrected but with residual defect near prosthetic material • Uncorrected cyanotic congenital heart disease • Surgically constructed shunts and conduits Valvulopathy following heart transplant	Any manipulation of gingival tissue, dental periapical regions, or perforating the oral mucosa. **PROPHYLAXIS RECOMMENDED‡** *(see Dental Procedures Regimens table below)* (Prophylaxis is *not* recommended for routine anesthetic injections (unless through infected area), dental x-rays, shedding of primary teeth, adjustment of orthodontic appliances or placement of orthodontic brackets or removable appliances.)	Incision of respiratory tract mucosa **CONSIDER PROPHYLAXIS** *(see Dental Procedures Regimens table)* Or For treatment of established infection **PROPHYLAXIS RECOMMENDED** *(see Dental Procedures Regimens table for oral flora, but include anti-staphylococcal coverage when S. aureus is of concern)*	PROPHYLAXIS is no longer recommended solely to prevent endocarditis **but the following approach is reasonable:** For patients with enterococcal UTIs • treat before elective GU procedures • include enterococcal coverage in peri-operative regimen for non-elective procedures[†] For patients with existing GU or GI infections or those who receive peri-operative antibiotics to prevent surgical site infections or sepsis • it is reasonable to include agents with anti-enterococcal activity in peri-operative coverage[†].	Include coverage against staphylococci and β-hemolytic streptococci in treatment regimens

[†] Agents with anti-enterococcal activity include penicillin, ampicillin, amoxicillin, piperacillin, vancomycin and others. Check susceptibility if available. (*See Table 5 for highly resistant organisms.*)
‡ 2008 AHA/ACC focused update of guidelines on valvular heart disease use term "is reasonable" to reflect level of evidence (*Circulation 118:887, 2008*).

PROPHYLACTIC REGIMENS FOR DENTAL PROCEDURES		
SITUATION	**AGENT**	**REGIMEN[1]**
Usual oral prophylaxis	Amoxicillin	Adults 2 gm, children 50 mg per kg; orally, 1 hour before procedure
Unable to take oral medications	Ampicillin[2]	Adults 2 gm, children 50 mg per kg; IV or IM, within 30 min before procedure.
Allergic to penicillins	Cephalexin[3] OR	Adults 2 gm, children 50 mg per kg; orally, 1 hour before procedure
	Clindamycin OR	Adults 600 mg, children 20 mg per kg; orally, 1 hour before procedure
	Azithromycin or clarithromycin	Adults 500 mg, children 15 mg per kg; orally, 1 hour before procedure
Allergic to penicillins and unable to take oral medications	Cefazolin[3] OR	Adults 1 gm, children 50 mg per kg; IV or IM, within 30 min before procedure
	Clindamycin	Adults 600 mg, children 20 mg per kg; IV or IM, within 30 min before procedure

[1] Children's dose should not exceed adult dose. AHA document lists all doses as 30-60 min before procedure.
[2] AHA lists cefazolin or ceftriaxone (at appropriate doses) as alternatives here.
[3] Cephalosporins should not be used in individuals with immediate-type hypersensitivity reaction (urticaria, angioedema, or anaphylaxis) to penicillins or other β-lactams. AHA proposes ceftriaxone as potential alternative to cefazolin; and other 1st or 2nd generation cephalosporin in equivalent doses as potential alternatives to cephalexin.

TABLE 15D – MANAGEMENT OF EXPOSURE TO HIV-1 AND HEPATITIS B AND C*

OCCUPATIONAL EXPOSURE TO BLOOD, PENILE/VAGINAL SECRETIONS OR OTHER POTENTIALLY INFECTIOUS BODY FLUIDS OR TISSUES WITH RISK OF TRANSMISSION OF HEPATITIS B/C AND/OR HIV-1 (E.G., NEEDLESTICK INJURY)

Free consultation for occupational exposures, call (PEPline) 1-888-448-4911. *[Information also available at www.aidsinfo.nih.gov]*

General steps in management:

1. Wash clean wounds/flush mucous membranes immediately (use of caustic agents or squeezing the wound is discouraged; data lacking regarding antiseptics).
2. Assess risk by doing the following: (a) Characterize exposure; (b) Determine/evaluate source of exposure by medical history, risk behavior, & testing for hepatitis B/C, HIV; (c) Evaluate and test exposed individual for hepatitis B/C & HIV.

Hepatitis B Occupational Exposure

Exposed Person[§]	Exposure Source		
	HBs Ag+	**HBs Ag–**	**Status Unknown or Unavailable for Testing[†]**
Unvaccinated	Give HBIG 0.06 mL per kg IM & initiate HB vaccine	Initiate HB vaccine	Initiate HB vaccine
Vaccinated (antibody status unknown)	Do anti-HBs on exposed person: If titer ≥10 milli-International units per mL, no rx If titer <10 milli-International units per mL, give HBIG + 1 dose HB vaccine**	No rx necessary	Do anti-HBs on exposed person: If titer ≥10 milli-International units per mL, no rx If titer <10 milli-International units per mL, give 1 dose of HB vaccine**

[§] Persons previously infected with HBV are immune to reinfection and do not require postexposure prophylaxis.

For known vaccine series responder (titer ≥10 milli-International units per mL), monitoring of levels or booster doses not currently recommended. Known non-responder (<10 milli-International units per mL) to 1° series HB vaccine & exposed to either HBsAg+ source or suspected high-risk source—rx with HBIG & re-initiate vaccine series **or** give 2 doses HBIG 1 month apart. For non-responders after a 2nd vaccine series, 2 doses HBIG 1 month apart is preferred approach to new exposure.

[†] If known high risk source, treat as if source were HBsAG positive

** Follow-up to assess vaccine response or address completion of vaccine series.

Hepatitis B Non-Occupational Exposure *[see MMWR 54 (RR11 and RR16), 2006; MMWR 59 (RR-10):1, 2010]*

Post-exposure prophylaxis is recommended for persons with discrete nonoccupational exposure to blood or body fluids. Exposures include percutaneous (e.g., bite, needlestick or mucous membrane exposure to HBsAG-positive blood or sterile body fluids), sexual or needle-sharing contact of an HBsAG-positive person, or a victim of sexual assault or sexual abuse by a perpetrator who is HBsAg-positive. If immunoprophylaxis is indicated, it should be initiated ideally within 24 h of exposure. Postexposure prophylaxis is unlikely to be effective if administered more than 7 days after a parenteral exposure or 14 days after a sexual exposure. The hepatitis B vaccine series should be completed regardless. The same guidelines for management of occupational exposures can also be used for nonoccupational exposures. For a previously vaccinated person (i.e., written documentation of being vaccinated) and no documentation of postvaccination titers with a discrete exposure to a HBsAG-positive source, it also is acceptable to administer a booster dose of hepatitis B vaccine without checking titers. No treatment is required for a vaccinated person exposed to a source of unknown HBsAG status.

Hepatitis C Exposure

Determine antibody to hepatitis C for both exposed person &, if possible, exposure source. If source + or unknown and exposed person negative, follow-up HCV testing for HCV RNA (detectable in blood in 1-3 weeks) and HCV antibody (90% who seroconvert will do so by 3 months) is advised. **No recommended prophylaxis;** immune serum globulin not effective. Monitor for early infection, as therapy may ↓ risk of progression to chronic hepatitis. Persons who remain viremic 8-12 weeks after exposure should be treated with a course of pegylated interferon *(Gastro 130:632, 2006 and Hpt 43:923, 2006). See Table 14A*. Case-control study suggested risk factors for occupational HCV transmission include percutaneous exposure to needle that had been in artery or vein, deep injury, male sex of HCW, & was more likely when source VL >6 log10 copies/mL

TABLE 15D (2)

HIV: Occupational exposure management *[Adapted from CDC recommendations, MMWR 54 (RR9), 2005, available at www.cdc.gov/mmwr/indrr_2005.html]*

- The decision to initiate post-exposure prophylaxis (PEP) for HIV is a clinical judgment that should be made in concert with the exposed healthcare worker (HCW). It is based on:
  1. Likelihood of the source patient having HIV infection: ↑ with history of high-risk activity—injection drug use, sexual activity with known HIV+ person, unprotected sex with multiple partners (either hetero- or homosexual), receipt of blood products 1978–1985. ↑ with clinical signs suggestive of advanced HIV (unexplained wasting, night sweats, thrush, seborrheic dermatitis, etc.).
  2. Type of exposure (approx. 1 in 300–400 needlesticks from infected source will transmit HIV).
  3. Limited data regarding efficacy of PEP *(Cochrane Database Syst Rev. Jan 24;(1):CD002835, 2007)*.
  4. Significant adverse effects of PEP drugs & potential for drug interactions.

  Substances considered potentially infectious include: blood, tissues, semen, vaginal secretions, CSF, synovial, pleural, peritoneal, pericardial and amniotic fluids; and other visibly bloody fluids. Fluids normally considered low risk for transmission, unless visibly bloody, include: urine, vomitus, stool, sweat, saliva, nasal secretions, tears and sputum.
- If source person is **known positive for HIV** or **likely to be infected** and **status of exposure warrants PEP,** antiretroviral drugs should be started **immediately.** If source person is HIV antibody negative, drugs can be stopped **unless source is suspected of having acute HIV infection.** The HCW should be re-tested at **3–4 weeks, 3 & 6 months whether PEP is used or not** (the vast majority of seroconversions will occur by 3 months; delayed conversions after 6 months are exceedingly rare). Tests for HIV RNA should not be used for dx of HIV infection in HCW because of false-positives (esp. at low titers) & these tests are only approved for established HIV infection [a possible exception is if pt develops signs of acute HIV (mononucleosis-like) syndrome within the 1st 4–6 wks of exposure when antibody tests might still be negative.]
- PEP for HIV is usually given for **4 wks** and monitoring of adverse effects recommended: baseline **complete blood count, renal and hepatic panel** to be **repeated at 2 weeks.** 50–75% of HCW on PEP demonstrate mild side-effects (nausea, diarrhea, myalgias, headache, etc.) but in up to ½ severe enough to discontinue PEP. Consultation with infectious diseases/ HIV specialist valuable when questions regarding PEP arise. **Seek expert help in special situations, such as pregnancy, renal impairment, treatment-experienced source.**

3 Steps to HIV Post-Exposure Prophylaxis (PEP) After Occupational Exposure: *[Latest CDC recommendations available at www.aidsinfo.nih.gov]*

Step 1: Determine the exposure code (EC)

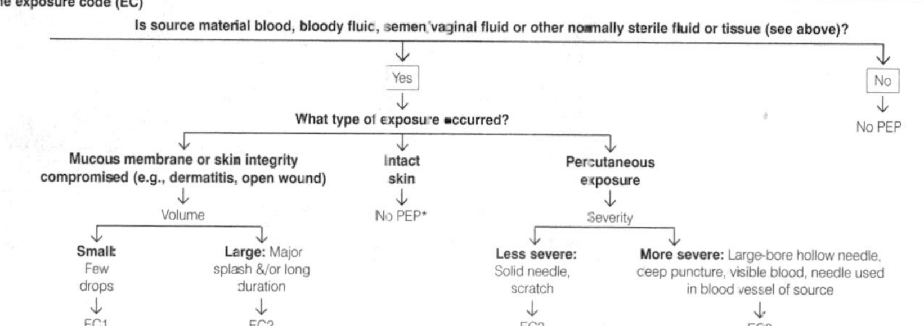

* *Exceptions can be considered when there has been prolonged, high-volume contact.*

TABLE 15D (3)

3 Steps to HIV Post-Exposure Prophylaxis (PEP) After Occupational Exposure *(continued)*

Step 2: Determine the HIV Status Code (HIV SC)

What is the HIV status of the exposure source?

- **HIV negative** → No PEP
- **HIV positive**
  - **Low titer exposure:** asymptomatic & high CD4 count, low VL (<1500 copies per mL) → HIV SC 1
  - **High titer exposure:** advanced AIDS, primary HIV, high viral load or low CD4 count → HIV SC 2
- **Status unknown** → HIV SC unknown
- **Source unknown** → HIV SC unknown

Step 3: Determine Post-Exposure Prophylaxis (PEP) Recommendation

EC	HIV SC	PEP
1	1	Consider basic regimen[a]
1	2	Recommend basic regimen[a,b]
2	1	Recommend basic regimen[b]
2	2	Recommend expanded regimen
3	1 or 2	Recommend expanded regimen
1, 2, 3	Unknown	If exposure setting suggests risks of HIV exposure, consider basic regimen[c]

[a] Based on estimates of ↓ risk of infection after mucous membrane exposure in occupational setting compared with needlestick.
[b] Or, consider expanded regimen[1].
[c] In high risk circumstances, consider expanded regimen[1] on case-by-case basis.

Around the clock, urgent expert consultation available from: National Clinicians' Post-Exposure Prophylaxis Hotline (PEPline) at 1-888-448-4911 (1-888-HIV-4911) and on-line at http://www.ucsf.edu/hivcntr

Regimens: (Treat for 4 weeks; monitor for drug side-effects every 2 weeks)

Basic regimen: ZDV + 3TC, or **FTC + TDF**, or as an alternative **d4T + 3TC.**

Expanded regimen: Basic regimen + one of the following: lopinavir/ritonavir *(preferred)*, or *(as alternatives)* atazanavir/ritonavir or fosamprenavir/ritonavir. Efavirenz can be considered (except in pregnancy or potential for pregnancy—**Pregnancy Category D**), but CNS symptoms might be problematic. [**Do not use nevirapine;** serious adverse reactions including hepatic necrosis reported in healthcare workers.]

Other regimens can be designed. If possible, use antiretroviral drugs for which resistance is unlikely based on susceptibility data or treatment history of source pt (if known). Seek expert consultation if ART-experienced source or in pregnancy or potential for pregnancy.

NOTE: Some authorities feel that an expanded regimen should be employed whenever PEP is indicated. Expanded regimens are likely to be advantageous with ↑ numbers of ART-experienced source pts or when there is doubt about exact extent of exposures in decision algorithm. Mathematical model suggests that under some conditions, completion of full course basic regimen is better than prematurely discontinued expanded regimen. However, while expanded PEP regimens have ↑ adverse effects, there is not necessarily ↑ discontinuation.

POST-EXPOSURE PROPHYLAXIS FOR NON-OCCUPATIONAL EXPOSURES TO HIV-1

[Adapted from CDC recommendations, MMWR 54 (RR2), 2005, available at www.cdc.gov/mmwr/indrr 2005.html]

Because the risk of transmission of HIV via sexual contact or sharing needles by injection drug users may reach or exceed that of occupational needlestick exposure, it is reasonable to consider PEP in persons who have had a non-occupational exposure to blood or other potentially infected fluids (e.g., genital/rectal secretions, breast milk) from an HIV+ source. Risk of HIV acquisition per exposure varies with the act (for needle sharing and receptive anal intercourse, ≥0.5%; approximately 10-fold lower with insertive vaginal or anal intercourse, 0.05–0.07%). Overt or occult traumatic lesions may ↑ risk in survivors of sexual assault.

For pts at risk of HIV acquisition through non-occupational exposure to HIV+ source material having occurred ≤72 hours before evaluation, DHHS recommendation is to treat for 28 days with an antiretroviral **expanded regimen**, using preferred regimens [efavirenz *(not in pregnancy or pregnancy risk—**Pregnancy Category D**)* + (3TC or FTC) + (ZDV or TDF)] **or** [lopinavir/ritonavir + (3TC or FTC) + ZDV] or one of several alternative regimens *[see Table 14D & MMWR 54(RR-2):1, 2005]*. Failures of prophylaxis have been reported, and may be associated with longer interval from exposure to start of PEP; this supports prompt initiation of PEP if it is to be used.

Areas of uncertainty: (1) expanded regimens are not proven to be superior to 2-drug regimens, (2) while PEP not recommended for exposures >72 hours before evaluation, it may possibly be effective in some cases, (3) when HIV status of source patient is unknown, decision to treat and regimen selection must be individualized based on assessment of specific circumstances.

Evaluate for exposures to Hep B, Hep C *(see Occupational PEP above)*, and bacterial sexually-transmitted diseases *(see Table 15A)* and treat as indicated. DHHS recommendations for sexual exposures to HepB and bacterial pathogens are available in *MMWR 55(RR-11), 2006*. Persons who are unvaccinated or who have not responded to full HepB vaccine series should receive hepB immune globulin preferably within 24-hours of percutaneous or mucosal exposure to blood or body fluids of an HBsAg-positive person, along with hepB vaccine, with follow-up to complete vaccine series. Unvaccinated or not-fully-vaccinated persons exposed to a source with unknown HepBsAg-status should receive vaccine and complete vaccine series. See *MMWR 55(RR-11), 2006* for details and recommendations in other circumstances.

TABLE 15E – PREVENTION OF SELECTED OPPORTUNISTIC INFECTIONS IN HUMAN HEMATOPOIETIC CELL TRANSPLANTATION (HCT) OR SOLID ORGAN TRANSPLANTATION (SOT) IN ADULTS WITH NORMAL RENAL FUNCTION.

General comments: Medical centers performing transplants will have detailed protocols for the prevention of opportunistic infections which are appropriate to the infections encountered, patients represented and resources available at those sites. Regimens continue to evolve and protocols adopted by an institution may differ from those at other centers. Care of transplant patients should be guided by physicians with expertise in this area. The above recommendations are adopted from 2009 HCT guidelines referenced below.

References:

For HCT: Expert guidelines endorsed by the IDSA, updating earlier guidelines *(MMWR 49 (RR-10):1, 2000)* in: *Biol Blood Marrow Transpl 15:1143, 2009*. These guidelines provide recommendations for prevention of additional infections not discussed in this table and provide more detailed information on the infections included here.

For SOT: Recommendations of an expert panel of The Transplantation Society for management of CMV in solid organ transplant recipients in: *Transplantation 89:779, 2010*. Timeline of infections following SOT in: *Amer J Transpl 9 (suppl 4):S3, 2009*.

OPPORTUNISTIC INFECTION	TYPE OF TRANSPLANT	PROPHYLACTIC REGIMENS
CMV (Recipient + **or** Donor +/Recipient –)	SOT	**Prophylaxis approach:** • **Kidney, kidney/pancreas, pancreas:** Valganciclovir 450 mg or 900 mg po q24h for 3-6 months. Ref for low dose: *Pharm Ther 35:676, 2010*. Alternative: Ganciclovir iv or po. • **Liver:** Ganciclovir 5 mg/kg iv q24h or Ganciclovir 1 gm po tid for 3-6 months. Valganciclovir[NAI] 900 mg po q24h not FDA approved for this indication, but is widely used and recommended as an alternative. • **Lung:** Ganciclovir 5 mg/kg iv q24h (some give this dose bid for 5-7 days initially, before switching to q24h) or Valganciclovir[NAI] 900 mg po q24h for ≥ 6 months. Some add CMV immune globulin in selected cases. • **Heart:** Ganciclovir 5 mg/kg iv q24h or Ganciclovir 1 gm po tid or Valganciclovir 900 mg po q24h for 3-6 months. Some add CMV immune globulin in selected cases. • **Intestine:** Ganciclovir 5 mg/kg iv q24h or Ganciclovir 1 gm po tid or Valganciclovir 900 mg po q24h for ≥ 6 months. Some add CMV immune globulin in selected cases. **Pre-emptive therapy:** for kidney, liver, pancreas, heart, monitor weekly for viremia (by PCR or antigenemia) for at least 3 months post transplant. If viremia detected, begin treatment doses of Ganciclovir 5 mg/kg iv bid or Valganciclovir 900 mg po bid. Continue treatment until clearing of test for viremia, but for not less than 2 weeks. At that point, either switch to secondary prophylaxis or resume pre-emptive approach. **Comments:** • Expert panel recommendations from which the above are adopted favor prophylaxis approach in highest risk recipients of SOT (*Transplantation 89:779, 2010*). • With anti-viral prophylaxis, onset of CMV disease appearing later; maintain vigilance for possible late-onset CMV disease and treat accordingly. • Anti-lymphocyte therapies increase risk of CMV and may require extension or re-institution of prophylaxis or pre-emptive approach. • CMV immune globulin regimens for lung, heart, liver or pancreas SOT: 150 mg/kg within 72 h of transplant and at 2, 4, 6 and 8 weeks; then 100 mg/kg at weeks 12 and 16.
	HCT	**Pre-emptive therapy:** monitor ≥ once weekly from day 10 to 100 for CMV viremia by PCR or CMV-antigenemia, and start treatment if positive. • **Allogeneic:** Ganciclovir 5 mg/kg iv bid for 7-14 days (induction) then once daily (maintenance) until negative viral tests (minimum treatment 3 weeks total course of induction + maintenance). • **Autologous:** Ganciclovir 5 mg/kg iv bid 7 days (induction), then once daily (maintenance) until negative viral tests (minimum treatment 2 weeks total course). Oral Valganciclovir[NAI] (900 mg po bid induction, then 900 mg po once daily for maintenance) has been used in place of iv Ganciclovir, but is not approved for this indication. • Continue screening after completion of each course. **OR, alternatively:** **Prophylaxis approach:** from engraftment to day 100, Ganciclovir 5 mg/kg iv bid for 5-7 days (induction), then 5 mg/kg once daily (maintenance). **Late CMV reactivation:** certain HCT recipients require screening for CMV reactivation (and pre-emptive treatment) beyond 100 days (for details, see *Biol Blood Marrow Transpl 15:1143, 2009*).

TABLE 15E (2)

OPPORTUNISTIC INFECTION	TYPE OF TRANSPLANT	PROPHYLACTIC REGIMENS
Hepatitis B	SOT	For anti-viral agents with activity against HBV, see *Table 14A, page 146*. For discussion of HBV hyperimmune globulin in liver transplantation, see *J Viral Hepatitis (Suppl 1): 27, 2007*. Regimens to prevent re-infection after transplantation are evolving *(Liver Transplantation 14 (suppl 2): S23, 2008)*.
	HCT	Patients who are anti-Hbc positive and anti-Hbs positive, but without evidence of active viral replication, can be monitored for ↑LFTs and presence of +HBV-DNA, and given pre-emptive therapy at that time. Alternatively, prophylactic anti-viral therapy can be given, commencing before transplant. (*See guidelines for other specific situations: Biol Blood Marrow Transpl 15:1143, 2009.*) These guidelines recommend Lamivudine 100 mg po q24h as an anti-viral.
Herpes simplex	SOT	Acyclovir 400 mg po bid, starting early post-transplant *(Clin Microbiol Rev 10:86, 1997)*
	HCT	Acyclovir 250 mg per meter-squared iv q12h **or** Acyclovir 400 mg to 800 mg po bid, from conditioning to engraftment or resolution or mucositis. For those requiring prolonged suppression of HSV, the higher dose (Acyclovir 800 mg po bid) is recommended to minimize the risk of emerging resistance.
Aspergillus spp.	SOT	Lung/heart-lung transplant: optimal mgmt unknown. Aerosolized lipid Ampho B + oral anti-aspergillus agent used *(Amer J Transpl 4 (Suppl 10:110, 2004)*.
	HCT	Posaconazole 200 mg po tid approved for prophylaxis of invasive infection due to Aspergillus spp. and Candida spp. in high-risk, severely immunocompromised patients (eg, HCT with GVHD). In comparative trial in patients with GVHD, Posaconazole was similar to Fluconazole in preventing invasive fungal infections, but was more effective in preventing invasive Aspergillus infection *(NEJM 356:335, 2007)* Retrospective analysis suggests that Voriconazole[NAI] would have efficacy in steroid-treated patients with GVHD *(Bone Marrow Transpl 45:662, 2010)*, but is not approved for this indication.
Candida spp.	SOT	Liver: Fluconazole 400 mg po q24h x 3 mos. High risk pts (re-transplants, dialysis, SBP)*(Transpl 75:2023, 2003)*. Fluconazole resistance *(Liver Transpl 12:850, 2006)*.
	HCT	Fluconazole 400 mg po or iv once daily from day 0 to engraftment of when ANC consistently >1000, or Posaconazole 200 mg po tid approved for high-risk patients (e.g., with GVHD or prolonged neutropenia), or Micafungin 50 mg iv once daily.
Coccidioides immitis	Any	Fluconazole 200-400 mg po q24h *(Transpl Inf Dis 5:3, 2003; Am J Transpl 6:340. 2006)*. See *COID 21:45, 2008* for approach at one center in endemic area; e.g., for positive serology without evidence of active infection, Fluconazole 400 mg q24h for first year post-transplant, then 200 mg q24h thereafter.
Pneumocystis jiroveci	SOT	TMP-SMX: 1 single-strength tab po q24h or 1 double-strength tab po once daily for 3 to 7 days per week. Duration: kidney: 6 mo to 1 year *(Amer J Transpl 9 (suppl 3): S59, 2009)*; heart, lung, liver: ≥ 1 year to life-long *(Amer J Transpl 4 (suppl 10): 135, 2004)*.
	HCT	TMP-SMX: 1 single-strength tab po q24h or 1 double-strength tab po once daily or once a day for 3 days per week, from engraftment to ≥ 6 mo post transplant.
Toxoplasma gondii	SOT	TMP-SMX (1 SS tab po q24h or 1 DS tab po once daily) x 3-7 days/wk for 6 mos post-transplant. *(See Clin Micro Infect 14:1089, 2008)*.
	HCT	TMP-SMX: 1 single-strength tab po q24h or 1 double-strength tab po once daily or once a day for 3 days per week, from engraftment to ≥ 6 mo post transplant for seropositive allogeneic transplant recipients.
Trypanosoma cruzi	Heart	May be transmitted from organs or transfusions *(CID 48:1534, 2009)*. Inspect peripheral blood of suspected cases for parasites *(MMWR 55:798, 2006)*. Risk of reactivation during immunosuppression is variable *(JAMA 298:2171,2007; JAMA 299:1134, 2008; J Cardiac Fail 15:249, 2009)*. If known Chagas disease in donor or recipient, contact CDC for treatment options *(phone 770-488-7775 or in emergency 770-488-7100)*.

TABLE 16 – PEDIATRIC DOSAGES OF SELECTED ANTIBACTERIAL AGENTS*

[Adapted from: (1) Nelson's Pocket Book of Pediatric Antimicrobial Therapy 2009, J. Bradley & J. Nelson, eds., American Academy of Pediatrics, 2009.

DRUG	DOSES IN MG PER KG PER DAY OR MG PER KG AT FREQUENCY INDICATED[1]				
	BODY WEIGHT <2000 gm		BODY WEIGHT >2000 gm		>28 DAYS OLD
	0–7 days	8–28 days	0–7 days	8–28 days	
Aminoglycosides, IV or IM (check levels; some dose by gestational age + wks of life; *see Nelson's Pocket Book, p. 25)*					
Amikacin	7.5 q18–24h	7.5 q12h	10 q12h	10 q12h	10 q8h
Gent/tobra	2.5 q18–24h	2.5 q12h	2.5 q12h	2.5 q12h	2.5 q8h
Aztreonam, IV	30 q12h	30 q8h	30 q8h	30 q6h	30 q6h
Cephalosporins					
Cefaclor					20–40 div tid
Cefadroxil					30 div bid (max 2 gm per day)
Cefazolin	25 q12h	25 q12h	25 q12h	25 q8h	25 q8h
Cefdinir					7 q12h or 14 q24h
Cefepime	30 q12h	30 q12h	30 q12h	30 q12h	150 div q8h
Cefixime					8 as q24h or div bid
Cefotaxime	50 q12h	50 q8h	50 q12h	50 q8h	50 q8h (75 q6h for meningitis)
Cefoxitin			20 q12h		80–160 div q6h
Cefpodoxime					10 div bid (max 400 mg per day)
Cefprozil					15–30 div bid (max 1 gm per day)
Ceftazidime	50 q12h	50 q8h	50 q12h	50 q8h	50 q8h
Ceftibuten					4.5 bid
Ceftizoxime					33–66 q8h
Ceftriaxone	25 q24h	50 q24h	25 q24h	50 q24h	50 q24h (meningitis 100)
Cefuroxime IV	50 q12h	50 q8h	50 q8h	50 q8h	50 q8h (80 q8h for meningitis)
po					10–15 bid (max 1 gm per day)
Cephalexin					25–50 div q6h (max 4 gm per day)
Loracarbef					15–30 div bid (max 0.8 gm per day)
Chloramphenicol IV	25 q24h	25 q24h	25 q24h	15 q12h	12.5–25 q6h (max 2–4 gm per day)
Clindamycin IV	5 q12h	5 q8h	5 q8h	5 q6h	7.5 q6h
po					
Ciprofloxacin[2] po					20–30 div bid (max 1.5 gm per day)
Ertapenem IV	No data	No data	No data	No data	15 q12h (max. 1g/day)
Imipenem[3] IV			25 q12h	25 q8h	15–25 q6h (max 2–4 gm per day)
Linezolid	10 q12h	10 q8h	10 q8h	10 q8h	10 q8h to age 12
Macrolides					
Erythro IV & po	10 q12h	10 q8h	10 q12h	13 q8h	10 q6h
Azithro po/IV	5 q24h	10 q24h	5 q24h	10 q24h	10 q24h
Clarithro po					7.5 q12h (max. 1 gm per day)
Meropenem IV	20 q12h	20 q8h	20 q12h	20 q8h	60–120 div q8h (120 for meningitis)
Metro IV & po	7.5 q24h	7.5 q12h	7.5 q12h	15 q12h	7.5 q6h
Penicillins					
Ampicillin	50 q12h	50 q8h	50 q8h	50 q6h	50 q6h
AMP-sulbactam					100–300 div q6h
Amoxicillin po				30 div bid	25–50 div tid
Amox-Clav po			30 div bid	30 div bid	45 or 90 (AM/CL-HD) div bid if over 12wks
Dicloxacillin					12–25 div q6h
Mezlocillin	75 q12h	75 q8h	75 q12h	75 q8h	75 q6h
Nafcillin, oxacillin IV	25 q12h	25 q8h	25 q8h	37 q6h	37 q6h (to max. 8–12 gm per day)
Piperacillin, PIP-tazo IV	50 q12h	100 q12h	100 q12h	100 q8h	100 q6h
Ticarcillin, TC/CL IV	75 q12h	75 q8h	75 q8h	75 q6h	75 q6h
Tinidazole					> Age 3: 50 mg/kg for 1 dose
Penicillin G, U/kg IV	50,000 q12h	75,000 q8h	50,000 q8h	50,000 q6h	50,000 units/kg per day
Penicillin V					25–50 mg per kg per day div q6–8h
Rifampin IV, po	10 q24h	10 q24h	10 q24h	10 q24h	10 q24h
Sulfisoxazole po					120–150 mg/kg per day div q4–6h
TMP-SMX po, IV; UTI: 8–12 TMP component div bid; Pneumocystis: 20 TMP component div q6h					
Tetracycline po (age 8 or older)					25–50 div q6h (>7yr old)
Doxycycline po, IV (age 8 or older)					2–4 div bid to max of 200 (>7yr old)
Vancomycin IV	12.5 q12h	15 q12h	18 q12h	22 q12h	40 div q6–8h [some start with 15 mg/kg IV q6h (normal renal function)]; 60 for meningitis.

[1] May need higher doses in patients with meningitis: *see CID 39:1267, 2004.*
[2] With exception of cystic fibrosis, anthrax, and complicated UTI, not approved for use under age 18.
[3] Not recommended in children with CNS infections due to risk of seizures.
* *See page 2 for abbreviations*

TABLE 17A – DOSAGE OF ANTIMICROBIAL DRUGS IN ADULT PATIENTS WITH RENAL IMPAIRMENT

- For listing of drugs with NO need for adjustment for renal failure, *see Table 17B.*
- Adjustments for renal failure are based on an estimate of creatinine clearance (CrCl) which reflects the glomerular filtration rate.
- **Different methods for calculating estimated CrCl are suggested for non-obese and obese patients.**
    - Calculations for ideal body weight (IBW) in kg:
        - *Men:* 50 kg plus 2.3 kg/inch over 60 inches height.
        - *Women:* 45 kg plus 2.3 kg/inch over 60 inches height.
    - Obese is defined as 20% over ideal body weight or body mass index (BMI) >30

- Calculations of estimated CrCl *(References, see (NEJM 354:2473, 2006 (non-obese), AJM 84:1053, 1988 (obese))*
    - **Non-obese patient**—
        - Calculate ideal body weight (IBW) in kg (as above)
        - Use the following formula to determine estimated CrCl

$$\frac{\text{(140 minus age)(IBW in kg)}}{\text{72 x serum creatinine}} = \text{CrCl in mL/min for men. Multiply answer by 0.85 for women (estimated)}$$

    - **Obese patient**—
        - Weight ≥20% over IBW or BMI >30
        - Use the following formulas to determine estimated CrCl

$$\frac{\text{(137 minus age) x ((0.285 x wt in kg) + (12.1 x ht in meters}^2\text{))}}{\text{51 x serum creatinine}} = \text{CrCl (obese male)}$$

$$\frac{\text{(146 minus age) x ((0.287 x wt in kg) + (9.74 x ht in meters}^2\text{))}}{\text{60 x serum creatinine}} = \text{CrCl (obese female)}$$

- If estimated CrCl ≥90 mL/min, *see Tables 10C and 10D for dosing.*
- What weight should be used to calculate dosage on a mg/kg basis?
    - If less than 20% over IBW, use the patient's actual weight for all drugs.
    - **For obese patients** (≥20% over IBW or BMI >30).
        - **Aminoglycosides:** (IBW plus 0.4(actual weight minus IBW) = adjusted weight.
        - **Vancomycin:** actual body weight whether non-obese or obese.
        - **All other drugs:** insufficient data *(Pharmacotherapy 27:1081, 2007).*

- For slow extended daily dialysis (SLEDD) over 6-12 hours, adjust does as for CRRT. For details, *see CID 49:433, 2009.*
- General reference: Drug Prescribing in Renal Failure, 5th ed., Aronoff, et al. (eds)*(Amer College Physicians, 2007 and drug package inserts).*

TABLE 17A (2)

ANTIMICROBIAL	HALF-LIFE (NORMAL/ ESRD) hr	DOSE FOR NORMAL RENAL FUNCTION	METHOD (*see footer*)	ADJUSTMENT FOR RENAL FAILURE Estimated creatinine clearance (CrCl), mL/min			HEMODIALYSIS, CAPD	COMMENTS & DOSAGE FOR CRRT
				>50–90	10–50	<10		
ANTIBACTERIAL ANTIBIOTICS								
Aminoglycoside Antibiotics: Traditional multiple daily doses—adjustment for renal disease								
Amikacin	1.4–2.3/17–150	7.5 mg per kg q12h or 15 mg per kg once daily (see below)	I	7.5 mg/kg q12h	7.5 mg/kg q24h **Same dose for CRRT**	7.5 mg/kg q48h	HEMO: ½ of normal renal function dose AD CAPD: 15–20 mg lost per L dialysate per day (see *Comment*)	**High flux hemodialysis** membranes lead to unpredictable aminoglycoside clearance, measure post-dialysis drug levels for efficacy and toxicity. With **CAPD**, pharmacokinetics highly variable—**check serum levels**. Usual method for CAPD: 2 liters of dialysis fluid placed qid or 8 liters per day (give 8Lx20 mg lost per L = 160 mg of amikacin supplement IV per day)
Gentamicin, Tobramycin	2–3/20–60	1.7 mg per kg q8h. Once daily dosing below	I	100% q8h	100% of q12-24h **Same dose for CRRT** *See Comment for SLEDD dose*	100% of q48h	HEMO: ½ of normal renal function dose AD CAPD: 3–4 mg lost per L dialysate per day	
Netilmicin[NUS]	2–3/35–72	2 mg per kg q8h. Once daily dosing below	I	100% q8h	100% of q12-24h **Same dose for CRRT**	100% of q48h	HEMO: ½ of normal renal function dose AD CAPD: 3–4 mg lost per L dialysate per day	Adjust dosing weight for obesity: [ideal body weight + 0.4 (actual body weight – ideal body weight)] (*CID 25:112, 1997*).
Streptomycin	2–3/30–80	15 mg per kg (max. of 1 gm) q24h. Once daily dosing below	I	q24h	q24–72h **Same dose for CRRT**	q72–96h	HEMO: ½ of normal renal function dose AD CAPD: 20–40 mg lost per L dialysate per day	**Gent SLEDD dose** in critically ill: 6 mg/kg IV q48h starting 30 min before start of SLEDD (daily SLEDD; q48h Gent)(*AAC54:3635, 2010*).

ONCE-DAILY AMINOGLYCOSIDE THERAPY: ADJUSTMENT IN RENAL INSUFFICIENCY *(see Table 10D for OD dosing/normal renal function)*

Creatinine Clearance (mL per min.)	>80	60–80	40–60	30–40	20–30	10–20	<10–0
Drug	Dose q24h (mg per kg)				Dose q48h (mg per kg)		Dose q72h and AD
Gentamicin/Tobramycin	5.1	4	3.5	2.5	4	3	2
Amikacin/kanamycin/streptomycin	15	12	7.5	4	7.5	4	3
Isepamicin[NUS]	8	8	8	8 q48h	8	8 q72h	8 q96h
Netilmicin[NUS]	6.5	5	4	2	3	2.5	2

ANTIMICROBIAL	HALF-LIFE (NORMAL/ ESRD) hr	DOSE FOR NORMAL RENAL FUNCTION	METHOD	>50–90	10–50	<10	HEMODIALYSIS, CAPD	COMMENTS & DOSAGE FOR CRRT
Carbapenem Antibiotics								
Doripenem	1/18	500 mg IV q8h	D&I	500 mg IV q8h	**≥30 – ≤50:** 250 mg IV q8h **>10 – <30:** 250 mg IV q12h	No data	No data	
Ertapenem	4/>4	1 gm q24h	D	1 gm q24h	0.5 gm q24h (CrCl <30)	0.5 gm q24h	HEMO: Dose as for CrCl <10; if dosed <6 hrs prior to HD, give 150 mg supplement AD	
Imipenem (*see Comment*)	1/4	0.5 gm q6h	D&I	250–500 mg q6–8h	250 mg q6–12h **Dose for CRRT: 0.5–1 gm bid** (*AAC 49:2421, 2005*)	125–250 mg q12h	HEMO: Dose AD CAPD: Dose for CrCl <10	↑ potential for seizures if recommended doses exceeded in pts with CrCl <20 mL per min. See pkg insert, esp. for pts <70 kg
Meropenem	1/6–8	1 gm q8h	D&I	1 gm q8h	1 gm q12h **Same dose for CRRT**	0.5 gm q24h	HEMO: Dose AD CAPD: Dose for CrCl <10	

Abbreviation Key: Adjustment Method: **D** = dose adjustment, **I** = interval adjustment; **CAPD** = continuous ambulatory peritoneal dialysis; **CRRT** = continuous renal replacement therapy; **HEMO** = hemodialysis; **AD** = after dialysis; **"Supplement"** or **"Extra"** is to replace drug lost during dialysis – additional drug beyond continuation of regimen for CrCl < 10 ml/min.

TABLE 17A (3)

ANTIMICROBIAL	HALF-LIFE (NORMAL/ ESRD) hr	DOSE FOR NORMAL RENAL FUNCTION	METHOD *(see footer)*	ADJUSTMENT FOR RENAL FAILURE Estimated creatinine clearance (CrCl), mL/min			HEMODIALYSIS, CAPD	COMMENTS & DOSAGE FOR CRRT
				>50–90	**10–50**	**<10**		
ANTIBACTERIAL ANTIBIOTICS *(continued)*								
Cephalosporin Antibiotics: DATA ON SELECTED **PARENTERAL** CEPHALOSPORINS								
Cefazolin	1.9/40–70	1 gm q8h	I	q8h	q12h **Same dose for CRRT**	q24–48h	HEMO: Extra 0.5–1 gm AD CAPD: 0.5 gm q12h	
Cefepime	2.2/18	2 gm q8h (max. dose)	D&I	2 gm q8h	2 gm q12–24h **Same dose for CRRT**	1 gm q24h	HEMO: Extra 1 gm AD CAPD: 1–2 gm q48h	
Cefotaxime, Ceftizoxime	1.7/15–35	2 gm q8h	I	q8–12h	q12–24h **Same dose for CRRT**	q24h	HEMO: Extra 1 gm AD CAPD: 0.5–1 gm q24h	Active metabolite of cefotaxime in ESRD. ↓ dose further for hepatic & renal failure.
Cefotetan	3.5/13–25	1–2 gm q12h	D	100%	1-2 gm q24h **Same dose for CRRT**	1-2 gm q48h	HEMO: Extra 1 gm AD CAPD: 1 gm q24h	CRRT dose: 750 mg q12h
Cefoxitin	0.8/13–23	2 gm q8h	I	q8h	q8–12h **Same dose for CRRT**	q24–48h	HEMO: Extra 1 gm AD CAPD: 1 gm q24h	May falsely increase serum creatinine by interference with assay.
Ceftaroline	1.6/–	600 mg IV q12h	D	600 mg q12h	30-50: 400 mg q12h 15-30: 300 mg q12h	< 15: 200 mg q12h	HEMO: 200 mg q12h	1-hr infusion for all doses
Ceftazidime	1.2/13–25	2 gm q8h	I	q8–12h	Q12–24h **Same dose for CRRT**	q24-48h	HEMO: Extra 1 gm AD CAPD: 0.5 gm q24h	Since 1/2 dose is dialyzed, post-dialysis dose is max. of 3 gm.
Ceftobiprole	2.9–3.3/21	500 mg IV q8-12h	I	500 mg IV q8-12h	**≥30 & ≤50:** 500 mg q12h over 2 hrs **≥10 & <30:** 250 mg q12h over 2 hrs	No data	No data	
Cefuroxime sodium	1.2/17	0.75–1.5 gm q8h	I	q8h	q8–12h **Same dose for CRRT**	q24h	HEMO: Dose AD CAPD: Dose for CrCl <10	
Fluoroquinolone Antibiotics								
Ciprofloxacin	3-6/6–9	500–750 mg po (or 400 mg IV) q12h	D	100%	50–75% CRRT 400 mg IV q24h	50%	HEMO: 250 mg po or 200 mg IV q12h CAPD: 250 mg po or 200 mg IV q8h	
Gatifloxacin[NUS]	7–14/11-40	400 mg po/IV q24h	D	400 mg q24h	400 mg, then 200 mg q24h Same dose for CRRT	400 mg, then 200 mg q24h	HEMO: 200 mg q24h AD CAPD: 200 mg q24h	
Gemifloxacin	7/>7	320 mg po q24h	D	320 mg q24h	160 mg q24h	160 mg q24h	HEMO: 160 mg q24h AD CAPD: 160 mg q24h	
Levofloxacin	6–8/76	750 mg q24h IV, PO	D&I	750 mg q24h	**20-49:** 750 q48h	**<20:** 750 mg once, then 500 mg q48h	HEMO/CAPD: Dose for CrCl <20	CRRT 750 mg once, then 500 mg q48h, although not FDA-approved.
Ofloxacin	7/28-37	200-400 mg q12h	D	200-400 mg q12h	200-400 mg q24h **Same dose for CRRT**	200 mg q24h	HEMO: Dose for CrCl <10, AD CAPD: 300 mg q24h	
Macrolide Antibiotics								
Clarithromycin	5–7/22	0.5–1 gm q12h	D	100%	75%	50–75%	HEMO: Dose AD CAPD: None	CRRT as for CrCl 10-50
Erythromycin	1.4/5–6	250–500 mg q6h	D	100%	100%	50–75%	HEMO/CAPD/CRRT: None	Ototoxicity with high doses in ESRD

Abbreviation Key: Adjustment Method: **D** = dose adjustment, **I** = interval adjustment; **CAPD** = continuous ambulatory peritoneal dialysis; **CRRT** = continuous renal replacement therapy; **HEMO** = hemodialysis; **AD** = after dialysis; **"Supplement"** or **"Extra"** is to replace drug lost during dialysis – additional drug beyond continuation of regimen for CrCl < 10 ml/min.

TABLE 17A (4)

ANTIMICROBIAL	HALF-LIFE (NORMAL/ ESRD) hr	DOSE FOR NORMAL RENAL FUNCTION	METHOD (see footer)	ADJUSTMENT FOR RENAL FAILURE Estimated creatinine clearance (CrCl), mL/min			HEMODIALYSIS, CAPD	COMMENTS & DOSAGE FOR CRRT
				>50–90	10–50	<10		
ANTIBACTERIAL ANTIBIOTICS *(continued)*								
Miscellaneous Antibacterial Antibiotics								
Colistin base	<6/≥48	2.5-5 mg/kg/day div q12h	D & I	Serum Cr 1.3-1.5: 2.5-3.8 mg/kg/day div q12h	Serum Cr: 1.6-2.5: 2.5 mg/kg q24h **Same dose for CRRT**	Serum Cr 2.6-4: 1.5 mg/kg q36h	HEMO: 1.5 mg/kg	*LnID 6:589, 2006*
Daptomycin	9.4/30	4–6 mg per kg per day	I	4–6 mg per kg per day	CrCl <30, 4–6 mg per kg q48h		HEMO & CAPD: 6 mg per kg q48h (after dialysis if possible)	
Linezolid	5-6/6-8	600 mg po/IV q12h	None	600 mg q12h	600 mg q12h **Same dose for CRRT**	600 mg q12h AD	HEMO: As for CrCl <10 CAPD & CRRT: No dose adjustment	Accumulation of 2 metabolites—risk unknown *(JAC 56:172, 2005)*
Metronidazole	6–14/7–21	7.5 mg per kg q6h	D	100%	100% **Same dose for CRRT**	50%	HEMO: Dose as for CrCl <10 AD CAPD: Dose for CrCl <10	
Nitrofurantoin	0.5/1	50–100 mg	D	100%	Avoid	Avoid	Not applicable	
Polymyxin B	6/≥ 48h	15,000-25,000 units/kg/day div q12h	D	15,000-25,000 units/kg/day div q12h	50-100% of normal dose div q12h	15% of normal dose div q12h	HEMO/CAPD: No data	
Sulfamethoxazole (SMX)	10/20–50	1 gm q8h	I	q12h	q18h Same dose for CAVH	q24h	HEMO: Extra 1 gm AD CAPD: 1 gm q24h	
Teicoplanin[NUS]	45/62–230	6 mg per kg per day	I	q24h	q48h **Same dose for CRRT**	q72h	HEMO: Dose for CrCl <10 CAPD: Dose for CrCl <10	
Telithromycin	10/15	800 mg q24h	D	800 mg q24h	600 mg q24h (<30 mL per min.)	600 mg q24h	HEMO: 600 mg AD CAPD: No data	If CrCl <30, reduce dose to 600 mg once daily. If both liver and renal failure, dose is 400 mg once daily
Telavancin	7-8/17.9	10 mg/kg q24h	D&I	10 mg/kg q24h	**30-50:** 7.5 mg/kg q24h	**<30:** 10 mg/kg q48h	No data	No data
Temocillin		1-2 gm q12h	I	1-2 gm q12h	1-2 gm q24h	1 gm q48h	HEMO: 1 gm q48h AD CAPD: 1 gm q48h	
Trimethoprim (TMP)	11/20–49	100–200 mg q12h	I	q12h	**>30:** q12h **10-30:** q18h **Same dose for CRRT**	q24h	HEMO: Dose AD CAPD: q24h	CRRT dose: q18h
Trimethoprim-sulfamethoxazole-DS (Doses based on TMP component)								
Treatment (based on TMP component)	*As for TMP*	5–20 mg/kg/day divided q6-12h	D	5–20 mg/kg/d divided q6-12h	**30–50:** 5–7.5 mg/kg q8h (same dose for CRRT) **10–29:** 5–10 mg/kg q12h	Not recommended; but if used: 5–10 mg/kg per dose q24h	Not recommended; but if used: 5–10 mg/kg q24h	
TMP-SMX Prophylaxis	*As for TMP*	1 tab po q24h or 3 times per week	No change	100%	100%	100%		

Abbreviation Key: Adjustment Method: **D** = dose adjustment **I** = interval adjustment; **CAPD** = continuous ambulatory peritoneal dialysis; **CRRT** = continuous renal replacement therapy; **HEMO** = hemodialysis; **AD** = after dialysis; **"Supplement"** or **"Extra"** is to replace drug lost during dialysis – additional drug beyond continuation of regimen for CrCl < 10 ml/min.

TABLE 17A (5)

ANTIMICROBIAL	HALF-LIFE (NORMAL/ ESRD) hr	DOSE FOR NORMAL RENAL FUNCTION	METHOD *(see footer)*	ADJUSTMENT FOR RENAL FAILURE Estimated creatinine clearance (CrCl), mL/min			HEMODIALYSIS, CAPD	COMMENTS & DOSAGE FOR CRRT
				>50–90	10–50	<10		
ANTIBACTERIAL ANTIBIOTICS *(continued)*								
Vancomycin[1]	6/200–250	1 gm q12h	D&I	1 gm q12h	1 gm q24–96h	1 gm q4–7 days	HEMO/CAPD: Dose for CrCl <10	CAVH/CVVH: 500 mg q24–48h. New hemodialysis membranes ↑ clear. of vanco; **check levels**
Penicillins								
Amoxicillin Ampicillin	1/5–20 1/7–20	250–500 mg q8h 250 mg–2 gm q6h	I I	q8h q6h	q8–12h q6–12h	q24h q12–24h	HEMO: Dose AD CAPD: 250 mg q12h	IV amoxicillin not available in the U.S. CRRT: dose for CrCl 10-50
Amoxicillin/ Clavulanate[2]	1.3 AM/1 5–20/4	500/125 mg q8h *(see Comments)*	D&I	500/125 mg q8h	250–500 mg AM component q12h	250–500 mg AM component q24h	HEMO: As for CrCl <10; extra dose after dialysis	**If CrCl ≤30 per mL, do not use 875/125 or 1000/62.5 AM/CL**
Amoxicillin ext. rel. tabs	1.5/?	775 mg once daily		Once daily	CrCl <30, no data, avoid usage			
Ampicillin (AM/ Sulbactam(SB)	1 (AM)/1 (SB) 9 (AM)/10 (SB)	2 gm AM + 1 gm SB q6h	I	q6h	q8–12h	q24h	HEMO: Dose AD CAPD: 2 gm AM/1 gm SB q24h	CRRT dose: 1.5 AM/0.75 SB q12h
Aztreonam	2/6–8	2 gm q8h	D	100%	50–75% **Same dose for CRRT**	25%	HEMO: Extra 0.5 gm AD CAPD: Dose for CrCl <10	Technically is a β-lactam antibiotic.
Penicillin G	0.5/6–20	0.5–4 million U q4h	D	100%	75% **Same dose for CRRT**	20–50%	HEMO: Dose AD CAPD: Dose for CrCl <10	1.7 mEq potassium per million units. ↑s potential of seizure. 10 million units per day max. dose in ESRD.
Piperacillin	1/3.3–5.1	3–4 gm q4–6h	I	q4–6h	q6–8h **Same dose for CRRT**	q8h	HEMO: 2 gm q8h plus 1 gm extra AD CAPD: Dose for CrCl <10	1.9 mEq sodium per gm
Pip (P)/Tazo(T)	0.71-1.2 (both)/2-6	3.375 – 4.5 gm q6-8h	D&I	100%	2.25 gm q6h **<20**: q8h **Same dose for CRRT**	2.25 gm q8h	HEMO: Dose for CrCl <10 + 0.75 gm AD CAPD: 4.5 gm q12h; CRRT: 2.25 gm q6h	
Ticarcillin	1.2/13	3 gm q4h	D&I	1–2 gm q4h	1–2 gm q8h **Same dose for CRRT**	1–2 gm q12h	HEMO: Extra 3.0 gm AD CAPD: Dose for CrCl <10	5.2 mEq sodium per gm
Ticarcillin/ Clavulanate[2]	1.2/11-16	3.1 gm q4h	D&I	3.1 gm q4h	3.1 gm q8-12h **Same dose for CRRT**	2 gm q12h	HEMO: Extra 3.1 gm AD CAPD: 3.1 gm q12h	*See footnote*[2]
Tetracycline Antibiotics								
Tetracycline	6–10/57–108	250–500 mg qid	I	q8–12h	q12–24h **Same dose for CRRT**	q24h	HEMO/CAPD/CAVH: None	Avoid in ESRD
ANTIFUNGAL ANTIBIOTICS								
Amphotericin B & Lipid-based ampho B	24h-15 days//unchanged	Non-lipid: 0.4–1 mg/kg/day ABLC: 5 mg/kg/day LAB: 3–5 mg/kg/day	I	q24h	q24h **Same dose for CRRT**	q24h	HEMO/CAPD/CRRT: No dose adjustment	For ampho B, toxicity lessened by saline loading; risk amplified by concomitant cyclosporine A, aminoglycosides, or pentamidine

[1] If renal failure, use EMIT assay to measure levels; levels overestimated by RIA or fluorescent immunoassay.

[2] Clavulanate cleared by liver, not kidney. Hence as dose of combination decreased, a deficiency of clavulanate may occur *(JAMA 285:386, 2001)*.

Abbreviation Key: Adjustment Method: **D** = dose adjustment, **I** = interval adjustment; **CAPD** = continuous ambulatory peritoneal dialysis; **CRRT** = continuous renal replacement therapy; **HEMO** = hemodialysis; **AD** = after dialysis; **"Supplement"** or **"Extra"** is to replace drug lost during dialysis – additional drug beyond continuation of regimen for CrCl < 10 ml/min.

TABLE 17A (6)

ANTIMICROBIAL	HALF-LIFE (NORMAL/ ESRD) hr	DOSE FOR NORMAL RENAL FUNCTION	METHOD (see footer)	ADJUSTMENT FOR RENAL FAILURE Estimated creatinine clearance (CrCl), mL/min			HEMODIALYSIS, CAPD	COMMENTS & DOSAGE FOR CRRT
				>50–90	10–50	<10		
ANTIFUNGAL ANTIBIOTICS *(continued)*								
Fluconazole	37/100	100–400 mg q24h	D	100%	50%	50%	HEMO: 100% of recommended dose AD CAPD: Dose for CrCl <10	CRRT: 200-400 mg q24h
Flucytosine	3–6/75–200	37.5 mg per kg q6h	I	q12h	q12–24h **Same dose for CRRT**	q24h	HEMO: Dose AD CAPD: 0.5–1 gm q24h	Goal is peak serum level >25 mcg per mL and <100 mcg per mL
Itraconazole, po soln	21/25	100–200 mg q12h	D	100%	100% **Same dose for CRRT**	50%	HEMO/CAPD: oral solution: 100 mg q12-24h	
Itraconazole, IV	21/25	200 mg IV q12h	–	200 mg IV bid	Do not use IV itra if CrCl <30 due to accumulation of carrier: cyclodextrin			
Terbinafine	36–200/?	250 mg po per day	–	q24h	Use has not been studied. Recommend avoidance of drug.			
Voriconazole, IV	Non-linear kinetics	6 mg per kg IV q12h times 2, then 4 mg per kg q12h	–	No change	If CrCl <50 mL per min., accum. of IV vehicle (cyclodextrin). Switch to po or DC **For CRRT:** 4 mg/kg po q12h			
ANTIPARASITIC ANTIBIOTICS								
Pentamidine	3-12/73-18	4 mg per kg per day	I	q24h	q24h **Same dose for CRRT**	q24–36h	HEMO: As for CrCl <10 plus 0.75 g AD. CAPD: Dose for CrCl<10	
Quinine	5–16/5–16	650 mg q8h	I	650 mg q8h	650 mg q8–12h **Same dose for CRRT**	650 mg q24h	HEMO: Dose AD CAPD: Dose for CrCl <10	Marked tissue accumulation
ANTITUBERCULOUS ANTIBIOTICS *(Excellent review: Nephron 64:169, 1993)*								
Ethambutol	4/7–15	15–25 mg per kg q24h	I	q24h	q24–36h **Same dose for CRRT**	q48h	HEMO: Dose AD CAPD: Dose for CrCl <10	25 mg per kg 4–6 hr prior to 3 times per wk dialysis. Streptomycin instead of ethambutol in renal failure.
Ethionamide	2.1/?	250–500 mg q12h	D	100%	100%	50%	HEMO/CAPD/CRRT: No dosage adjustment	
Isoniazid	0.7–4/8–17	5 mg per kg per day (max. 300 mg)	D	100%	100% **Same dose for CRRT**	100%	HEMO: Dose AD CAPD/: Dose for CrCl <10	
Pyrazinamide	9/26	25 mg per kg q24h (max. dose 2.5 gm q24h)	D	100%	100% **Same dose for CRRT**	12–25 mg per kg q24h	HEMO: 40 mg/kg 24 hrs before each 3x/week dialysis CAPD: No reduction;	
Rifampin	1.5–5/1.8–11	600 mg per day	D	600 mg q24h	300–600 mg q24h **Same dose for CRRT**	300–600 mg q24h	HEMO: No adjustment CAPD/: Dose for CrCl <10	Biologically active metabolite
ANTIVIRAL AGENTS For ANTIRETROVIRALS *See CID 40:1559, 2005*								
Acyclovir, IV	2-4/20	5–12.4 mg per kg q8h	D&I	100% q8h	100% q12–24h	50% q24h	HEMO: Dose AD CAPD: Dose for CrCl <10	Rapid IV infusion can cause ↑ Cr. CRRT dose: 5-10 mg/kg q24h
Adefovir	7.5/15	10 mg po q24h	I	10 mg q24h	10 mg q48–72h[3]	10 mg q72h[3]	HEMO: 10 mg q week AD	CAPD: No data; CRRT: Dose ?
Amantadine	12/500	100 mg po bid	I	q12h	q24-48h	q 7 days	HEMO/CAPD: Dose for CrCl<10/	CRRT: Dose for CrCl 10-50

[3] Ref: *Transplantation 80:1086, 2005*

Abbreviation Key: Adjustment Method: **D** = dose adjustment, **I** = interval adjustment; **CAPD** = continuous ambulatory peritoneal dialysis; **CRRT** = continuous renal replacement therapy; **HEMO** = hemodialysis; **AD** = after dialysis; **"Supplement"** or **"Extra"** is to replace drug lost during dialysis – additional drug beyond continuation of regimen for CrCl < 10 ml/min.

TABLE 17A (7)

ANTIMICROBIAL	HALF-LIFE (NORMAL/ ESRD) hr	DOSE FOR NORMAL RENAL FUNCTION	METHOD *(see footer)*	ADJUSTMENT FOR RENAL FAILURE Estimated creatinine clearance (CrCl), mL/min >50–90	10–50	<10	HEMODIALYSIS, CAPD	COMMENTS & DOSAGE FOR CRRT
ANTIVIRAL AGENTS For ANTIRETROVIRALS *(continued)*								
Atripla	See each drug	200 mg emtricitabine + 300 mg tenofovir + 600 mg efavirenz	I	Do not use if CrCl <50				
Cidofovir: **Complicated dosing—*see package insert***								
Induction	2.5/unknown	5 mg per kg once per wk for 2 wks	–	5 mg per kg once per wk	Contraindicated in pts with CrCl ≤ 55 ml/min.			Major toxicity is renal. No efficacy, safety, or pharmacokinetic data in pts with moderate/severe renal disease.
Maintenance	2.5/unknown	5 mg per kg q2wks	–	5 mg per kg q2wks	Contraindicated in pts with CrCl ≤ 55 ml/min.			
Didanosine tablets[4]	0.6–1.6/4.5	125–200 mg q12h buffered tabs	D	200 mg q12h	200 mg q24h	<60 kg: 150 mg q24h >60 kg: 100 mg q24h	HEMO: Dose AD CAPD/CRRT: Dose for CrCl <10	Based on incomplete data. Data are estimates.
		400 mg q24h enteric-coated tabs	D	400 mg q24h	125–200 mg q24h	**Do not use EC tabs**	HEMO/CAPD: Dose for CrCl <10	**If <60 kg & CrCl <10 mL per min, do not use EC tabs**
Emtricitabine (CAPS)	10/>10	200 mg q24h	I	200 mg q24h	**30–49:** 200 mg q48h **10–29:** 200 mg q72h	200 mg q96h	HEMO: Dose for CrCl <10	*See package insert for oral solution.*
Emtricitabine + Tenofovir	See each drug	200-300 mg q24h	I	No change	**30–50:** 1 tab q48h	**CrCl <30:** Do not use		
Entecavir	128–149/?	0.5 mg q24h	D	0.5 mg q24h	0.15–0.25 mg q24h	0.05 mg q24h	HEMO/CAPD: 0.05 mg q24h	Give after dialysis on dialysis days
Famciclovir	2.3–3/10–22	500 mg q8h	D&I	500 mg q8h	500 mg q12–24h	250 mg q24h	HEMO: Dose AD CAPD: No data	CRRT: Not applicable

ANTIMICROBIAL	HALF-LIFE (NORMAL/ ESRD) hr	CrCl (mL/min per kg body weight—only for Foscarnet)	>1.4	>1-1.4	>0.8-1	>0.6-0.8	>0.5-0.6	>0.4-0.5	<0.4	COMMENTS
Foscarnet (CMV dosage). Dosage adjustment based on est. CrCl divided by wt (kg)	Normal half-life (T½) 3 hrs with terminal T½ of 18-88 hrs. T½ very long with ESRD	Induction: 60 mg/kg IV q8h x 2-3 wks	60 q8h	45 q8h	50 q12h	40 q12h	60 q24h	50 q24h	Do not use	*See package insert for further details*
		Maintenance: 90-120 mg/kg/day IV	120 q24h	90 q24h	65 q24h	105 q48h	80 q8h	65 q48h	Do not use	

ANTIMICROBIAL	HALF-LIFE (NORMAL/ ESRD) hr	DOSE FOR NORMAL RENAL FUNCTION	METHOD	>50–90	10–50	<10	HEMODIALYSIS, CAPD	COMMENTS & DOSAGE FOR CRRT
Ganciclovir	3.6/30 IV:	Induction 5 mg per kg q12h IV	D&I	5 mg per kg q12h	1.25–2.5 mg per kg q24h	1.25 mg per kg 3 times per wk	HEMO: Dose AD CAPD: Dose for CrCl <10	
		Maintenance 5 mg per kg q24h IV	D&I	2.5–5.0 mg per kg q24h	0.6–1.25 mg per kg q24h	0.625 mg per kg 3 times per wk	HEMO: 0.6 mg per kg AD CAPD: Dose for CrCl <10	
	po:	1 gm tid po	D&I	0.5–1 gm tid	0.5–1 gm q24h	0.5 gm 3 times per week	HEMO: 0.5 gm AD	

[4] Ref: for NRTIs and NNRTIs: *Kidney International 60:821, 2001*

Abbreviation Key: Adjustment Method: **D** = dose adjustment, **I** = interval adjustment; **CAPD** = continuous ambulatory peritoneal dialysis; **CRRT** = continuous renal replacement therapy; **HEMO** = hemodialysis; **AD** = after dialysis; **"Supplement"** or **"Extra"** is to replace drug lost during dialysis – additional drug beyond continuation of regimen for CrCl < 10 ml/min.

TABLE 17A (8)

ANTIMICROBIAL	HALF-LIFE (NORMAL/ ESRD) hr	DOSE FOR NORMAL RENAL FUNCTION	METHOD (see footer)	ADJUSTMENT FOR RENAL FAILURE Estimated creatinine clearance (CrCl), mL/min			HEMODIALYSIS, CAPD	COMMENTS & DOSAGE FOR CRRT
				>50–90	10–50	<10		
ANTIVIRAL AGENTS For ANTIRETROVIRALS *(continued)*								
Maraviroc	14–18/No data	300 mg bid		300 mg bid				Risk of side effects increased if concomitant CYP3A inhibitor
Lamivudine[5]	5–7/15–35	300 mg po q24h	D&I	300 mg po q24h	50–150 mg q24h	25–50 mg q24h	HEMO: Dose AD; CAPD: Dose for CrCl<10. CRRT: 100 mg 1st days, then 50 mg/day.	
Oseltamivir, therapy	6-10/>20	75 mg po bid – treatment	I	75 mg q12h	**30-50:** 75 mg bid **<30:** 75 mg once daily	No data	HEMO: 30 mg non-dialysis days[6]; CAPD: 30 mg once per week	Dose for prophylaxis if CrCl <30: 75 mg once daily CRRT: 75 mg po bid
Peramivir		600 mg once daily	P&I	600 mg q24h	**31-49:** 150 mg q24h **10-30:** 100 mg q24h	100 mg (single dose) then 15 mg q24h	HEMO: 100 mg (single dose) then 100 mg 2 hrs AD (dialysis days only)	CRRT: *http://www.cdc.gov/h1n1flu/eva/peramivir.htm*
Ribavirin	Use with caution in patients with creatinine clearance <50 mL per min.							
Rimantadine	13–65/Prolonged	100 mg bid po	I	100 mg bid	100 mg q24h–bid	100 mg q24h	HEMO/CAPD: No data	Use with caution, little data
Stavudine, po[5]	1–1.4/5.5–8	30–40 mg q12h	D&I	100%	50% q12–24h	≥60 kg: 20 mg per day <60 kg: 15 mg per day	HEMO: Dose as for CrCl <10 AD CAPD: No data CRRT: Full dose	
Telbivudine	40-49/No data	600 mg po daily	I	600 mg q24h	**30-49:** 600 mg q48H **<30:** 600 mg q72h	600 mg q96h	HEMO: As for CrCl <10 AD	
Tenofovir, po	17/?	300 mg q24h		300 mg q24h	**30-49:** 300 mg q48h **10-29:** 300 mg q72-96h	No data	HEMO: 300 mg q7d or after 12 hrs of HEMO.[7]	
Valacyclovir	2.5–3.3/14	1 gm q8h	D&I	1 gm q8h	1 gm q12–24h **Same dose for CRRT**	0.5 gm q24h	HEMO: Dose AD CAPD: Dose for CrCl <10	CAVH dose: As for CrCl 10–50
Valganciclovir	4/67	900 mg po bid	D&I	900 mg po bid	450 mg q24h to 450 mg every other day	DO NOT USE	See package insert	
Zalcitabine[5]	2/>8	0.75 mg q8h	D&I	0.75 mg q8h	0.75 mg q12h **Same dose for CRRT**	0.75 mg q24h	HEMO: Dose AD CAPD: No data	CRRT dose: As for CrCl 10–50
Zidovudine[5]	1.1–1.4/1.4–3	300 mg q12h	D&I	300 mg q12h	300 mg q12h **Same dose for CRRT**	100 mg q8h	HEMO: Dose for CrCl <10 AD CAPD: Dose for CrCl <10	

[5] Ref. for NRTIs and NNRTIs: *Kidney International 60:821, 2001*

[6] HEMO wt-based dose adjustments for children age >1 yr (dose after each HEMO): ≤15 kg: 7.5 mg; 16-23 kg: 10 mg; 24–40 kg: 15 mg; > 40 kg: 30 mg *(CID 50:127, 2010)*.

[7] Acute renal failure and Fanconi syndrome reported.

Abbreviation Key: Adjustment Method: **D** = dose adjustment, **I** = interval adjustment; **CAPD** = continuous ambulatory peritoneal dialysis; **CRRT** = continuous renal replacement therapy; **HEMO** = hemodialysis; **AD** = after dialysis; **"Supplement"** or **"Extra"** is to replace drug lost during dialysis – additional drug beyond continuation of regimen for CrCl < 10 ml/min.

TABLE 17B – NO DOSAGE ADJUSTMENT WITH RENAL INSUFFICIENCY BY CATEGORY*

Antibacterials		Antifungals	Anti-TBc	Antivirals	
Azithromycin	Metronidazole	Anidulafungin	Rifabutin	Abacavir	Lopinavir
Ceftriaxone	Minocycline	Caspofungin	Rifapentine	Atazanavir	Nelfinavir
Chloramphenicol	Moxifloxacin	Itraconazole oral solution		Darunavir	Nevirapine
Ciprofloxacin XL	Nafcillin	Ketoconazole		Delavirdine	Raltegravir
Clindamycin	Pyrimethamine	Micafungin		Efavirenz	Ribavirin
Doxycycline	Rifaximin	Voriconazole, **po only**		Enfuvirtide[1]	Saquinavir
Linezolid	Tigecycline			Fosamprenavir	Tipranavir
				Indinavir	

[1] Enfuvirtide: Not studied in patients with CrCl <35 mL/min. DO NOT USE

TABLE 18 – ANTIMICROBIALS AND HEPATIC DISEASE: DOSAGE ADJUSTMENT*

The following alphabetical list indicates antibacterials excreted/metabolized by the liver **wherein a dosage adjustment may be indicated** in the presence of hepatic disease. Space precludes details; consult the PDR or package inserts for details. List is **not** all-inclusive:

Antibacterials		Antifungals	Antivirals[§]	
Ceftriaxone	Nafcillin	Caspofungin	Abacavir	Indinavir
Chloramphenicol	Rifabutin	Itraconazole	Atazanavir	Lopinavir/ritonavir
Clindamycin	Rifampin	Voriconazole	Darunavir	Nelfinavir
Fusidic acid	Synercid**		Delavirdine	Nevirapine
Isoniazid	Telithromycin[++]		Efavirenz	Rimantadine
Metronidazole	Tigecycline		Enfuvirtide	Ritonavir
	Tinidazole		Fosamprenavir	

[§] Ref. on antiretrovirals: *CID 40:174, 2005* ** Quinupristin/dalfopristin [++] Telithro: reduce dose in renal & hepatic failure

TABLE 19 – TREATMENT OF CAPD PERITONITIS IN ADULTS*

(Periton Dial Intl 20:396, 2000 & 29:5, 2009)[2]

EMPIRIC Intraperitoneal Therapy:[3] Culture Results Pending

Drug		Residual Urine Output	
		<100 mL per day	>100 mL per day
Cefazolin +	Can mix in same bag	1 gm per bag, q24h	20 mg per kg BW per bag, q24h
Ceftazidime		1 gm per bag, q24h	20 mg per kg BW per bag, q24h

Drug Doses for SPECIFIC Intraperitoneal Therapy—Culture Results Known. NOTE: Few po drugs indicated

Drug	Intermittent Dosing (once per day)		Continuous Dosing (per liter exchange)	
	Anuric	Non-Anuric	Anuric	Non-Anuric
Gentamicin	0.6 mg per kg	↑ dose 25%	MD 8 mg	↑ MD by 25%
Cefazolin	15 mg per kg	20 mg per kg	LD 500 mg, MD 125 mg	LD 500 mg, ↑ MD 25%
Ceftazidime	1000–1500 mg	ND	LD 250 mg, MD 125 mg	ND
Ampicillin	250–500 mg po bid	ND	250–500 mg po bid	ND
Ciprofloxacin	500 mg po bid	ND	LD 50 mg, MD 25 mg	ND
Vancomycin	15–30 mg per kg q5–7 days	↑ dose 25%	MD 30–50 mg per L	↑ MD 25%
Metronidazole	250 mg po bid	ND	250 mg po bid	ND
Amphotericin B	NA	NA	MD 1.5 mg	NA
Fluconazole	200 mg q24h	ND	200 mg q24h	ND
Itraconazole	100 mg q12h	100 mg q12h	100 mg q12h	100 mg q12h
Amp-sulbactam	2 gm q12h	ND	LD 1 gm, MD 100 mg	ND
TMP-SMX	320/1600 mg po q1–2 days	ND	LD 320/1600 mg po, MD 80/400 mg po q24h	ND

CAPD = continuous ambulatory peritoneal dialysis

[1] Ref. for NRTIs and NNRTIs: *Kidney International 60:821, 2001*
[2] **All doses IP unless indicated otherwise.**
LD = loading dose, **MD** = maintenance dose, **ND** = no data; **NA** = not applicable—dose as normal renal function.
Anuric = <100 mL per day, **non-anuric** = >100 mL per day
[3] **Does not provide treatment for MRSA.** If Gram-positive cocci on Gram stain, include vancomycin.

* *See page 2 for other abbreviations*

TABLE 20A – ANTI-TETANUS PROPHYLAXIS, WOUND CLASSIFICATION, IMMUNIZATION

WOUND CLASSIFICATION

Clinical Features	Tetanus Prone	Non-Tetanus Prone
Age of wound	> 6 hours	≤ 6 hours
Configuration	Stellate, avulsion	Linear
Depth	> 1 cm	≤ 1 cm
Mechanism of injury	Missile, crush, burn, frostbite	Sharp surface (glass, knife)
Devitalized tissue	Present	Absent
Contaminants (dirt, saliva, etc.)	Present	Absent

(From ACS Bull. 69:22,23, 1984, No. 10)

IMMUNIZATION SCHEDULE

History of Tetanus Immunization	Dirty, Tetanus-Prone Wound		Clean, Non-Tetanus Prone Wound	
	Td[1,2]	**TIG**	**Td**	**TIG**
Unknown or < 3 doses	Yes	Yes	Yes	No
3 or more doses	No[3]	No	No[4]	No

See Footnotes

[From MMWR 39:37, 1990; MMWR 46(SS-2):15, 1997]

---

[1] Td = Tetanus & diphtheria toxoids adsorbed (adult) - TIG = Tetanus immune globulin (human)

[2] Yes if wound >24 hr old. For children <7 yrs, DPT (DT if pertussis vaccine contraindicated); For persons ≥7 yrs, Td preferred to tetanus toxoid alone.

[3] Yes if >5 years since last booster.

[4] Yes if >10 years since last booster.

TABLE 20B – RABIES POST-EXPOSURE PROPHYLAXIS

All wounds should be cleaned immediately & thoroughly with soap & water. This has been shown to protect 90% of experimental animals![5]

Post-Exposure Prophylaxis Guide, United States, 2000
(CID 30:4, 2000; NEJM 351:2626, 2004; MMWR 57: RR-3, 2008).

Animal Type	Evaluation & Disposition of Animal	Recommendations for Prophylaxis
Dogs, cats, ferrets	Healthy & available for 10-day observation	Don't start unless animal develops sx, then immediately begin HRIG + HDCV or RVA
	Rabid or suspected rabid	Immediate vaccination
	Unknown (escaped)	Consult public health officials
Skunks, raccoons, bats,* foxes, coyotes, most carnivores	Regard as rabid	Immediate vaccination
Livestock, rodents, rabbits; includes hares, squirrels, hamsters, guinea pigs, gerbils, chipmunks, rats, mice, woodchucks		Almost never require anti-rabies rx. Consult public health officials.

* Most recent cases of human rabies in U.S. due to contact (not bites) with silver-haired bats or rarely big brown bats but risk of acquiring rabies from non-contact bat exposure is exceedingly low *(CID 48:1493, 2009)*. For more detail, *see CID 30:4, 2000; JAVMA 219:1687, 2001; CID 37:96, 2003 (travel medicine advisory); Ln 363:959, 2004; EID 11:1921, 2005; MMWR 55 (RR-5), 2006.*

Post-Exposure Rabies Immunization Schedule

IF NOT PREVIOUSLY VACCINATED

Treatment	Regimen[6]
Local wound cleaning	**All post-exposure treatment should begin with immediate, thorough cleaning of all wounds with soap & water.**
Human rabies immune globulin (HRIG)	20 units per kg body weight given once on day 0. If anatomically feasible, the full dose should be infiltrated around the wound(s), the rest should be administered IM in the gluteal area. HRIG should **not** be administered in the **same syringe**, **or** into the **same anatomical site** as vaccine, or more than 7 days after the initiation of vaccine. Because HRIG may partially suppress active production of antibody, no more than the recommended dose should be given.[7]
Vaccine	Human diploid cell vaccine (HDCV), rabies vaccine adsorbed (RVA), or purified chick embryo cell vaccine (PCECV) 1 mL **IM (deltoid area[8])**, one each days 0, 3, 7, 14[9].

IF PREVIOUSLY VACCINATED[10]

Treatment	Regimen[6]
Local wound cleaning	All post-exposure treatment should begin with immediate, thorough cleaning of all wounds with soap **&** water.
HRIG	HRIG should **not** be administered
Vaccine	HDCV, RVA or PCEC, 1 mL **IM (deltoid area[4])**, one each on days 0 & 3

CORRECT VACCINE ADMINISTRATION SITES

Age Group	Administration Site
Children & adults	**DELTOID[8]** only (**NEVER** in gluteus)
Infants & young children	Outer aspect of thigh (anterolateral thigh) may be used (**NEVER** in gluteus)

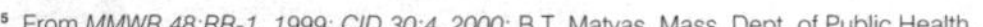

[5] From *MMWR 48:RR-1, 1999; CID 30:4, 2000;* B.T. Matyas, Mass. Dept. of Public Health.

[6] These regimens are applicable for all age groups, including children.

[7] In most reported post-exposure treatment failures, only identified deficiency was failure to infiltrate wound(s) with HRIG *(CID 22:228, 1996)*. However, several failures reported from SE Asia in patients in whom WHO protocol followed *(CID 28:143, 1999)*.

[8] The **deltoid** area is the **only** acceptable site of vaccination for adults & older children. For infants & young children, outer aspect of the thigh (anterolateral thigh) may be used. Vaccine should **NEVER** be administered in gluteal area.

[9] Note that this is a change from previous recommendation of 5 doses (days 0, 3, 7, 14 & 28) based on new data & recommendations from ACIP. Note that the number of doses for persons with altered immunocompetence remains unchanged (5 doses on days 0, 3, 7, 14 & 28) and recommendations for pre-exposure prophylaxis remain 3 doses administered on days 0, 7 and 21 or 28 *(MMWR 59 (RR-2), 2010)*.

[10] Any person with a history of pre-exposure vaccination with HDCV, RVA, PCECV; prior post-exposure prophylaxis with HDCV, RVA, PCEC; or previous vaccination with any other type of rabies vaccine & a documented history of antibody response to the prior vaccination.

TABLE 21 SELECTED DIRECTORY OF RESOURCES

ORGANIZATION	PHONE/FAX	WEBSITE(S)
ANTIPARASITIC DRUGS & PARASITOLOGY INFORMATION *(CID 37:694, 2003)*		
CDC Drug Line	Weekdays: 404-639-3670 Evenings, weekends, holidays: 404-639-2888	http://www.cdc.gov/ncidod/srp/drugs/drug-service.html
DPDx: Lab ID of parasites		www.dpd.cdc.gov/dpdx/default.htm
Gorgas Course Tropical Medicine		http://info.dom.uab.edu/gorgas
Malaria	daytime: 770-488-7788 other: 770-488-7100	www.cdc.gov/malaria
Expert Compound. Pharm.	800-247-9767/818-787-7256	www.uniquerx.com
World Health Organization (WHO)		www.who.int
Parasites & Health		www.dpd.cdc.gov/dpdx/HTML/Para_Health.htm
BIOTERRORISM		
Centers for Disease Control & Prevention	770-488-7100	www.bt.cdc.gov
Infectious Diseases Society of America	703-299-0200	www.idsociety.org
Johns Hopkins Center Civilian Biodefense		www.jhsph.edu
Center for Biosecurity of the Univ. of Pittsburgh Med. Center		www.upmc-biosecurity.org
US Army Medical Research Institute of Inf. Dis.		www.usamriid.army.mil
HEPATITIS B		
Hepatitis B Foundation		www.hepb.org
HEPATITIS C *(CID 35:754, 2002)*		
CDC		www.cdc.gov/ncidod/diseases/hepatitis/C
Individual		http://hepatitis-central.com
Medscape		www.medscape.com
HIV		
General		
HIV InSite		http://hivinsite.ucsf.edu
Johns Hopkins AIDS Service		www.hopkins-aids.edu
Drug Interactions		
Johns Hopkins AIDS Service		www.hopkins-aids.edu
Liverpool HIV Pharm. Group		www.hiv-druginteractions.org
Other		http://AIDS.medscape.com
Prophylaxis/Treatment of Opportunistic Infections; HIV Treatment		www.aidsinfo.nih.gov
IMMUNIZATIONS *(CID 36:355, 2003)*		
CDC, Natl. Immunization Program	404-639-8200	www.cdc.gov/vaccines/
FDA, Vaccine Adverse Events	800-822-7967	www.fda.gov/cber/vaers/vaers.htm
National Network Immunization Info.	877-341-6644	www.immunizationinfo.org
Influenza vaccine, CDC	404-639-8200	www.cdc.gov/vaccines/
Institute for Vaccine Safety		www.vaccinesafety.edu
OCCUPATIONAL EXPOSURE, BLOOD-BORNE PATHOGENS (HIV, HEPATITIS B & C)		
National Clinicians' Post-Exposure Hotline	888-448-4911	www.ucsf.edu/hivcntr
Q-T$_c$ INTERVAL PROLONGATION BY DRUGS		www.qtdrugs.org
SEXUALLY TRANSMITTED DISEASES		www.cdc.gov/std/treatment/TOC2002TG.htm Slides: http://www.phac-aspc.gc.ca/slm-maa/slides/index.html
TRAVELERS' INFO: Immunizations, Malaria Prophylaxis, More		
Amer. Soc. Trop. Med. & Hyg.		www.astmh.org
CDC, general	877-394-8747/888-232-3299	http://wwwn.cdc.gov/travel/default.asp
CDC, Malaria:		www.cdc.gov/malaria
Prophylaxis		http://wwwn.cdc.gov/travel/default.asp
Treatment	770-488-7788	www.who.int/health_topics/malaria
MD Travel Health		www.mdtravelhealth.com
Pan American Health Organization		www.paho.org
World Health Organization (WHO)		www.who.int/home-page
VACCINE & IMMUNIZATION RESOURCES *(CID 36:355, 2003)*		
American Academy of Pediatrics		www.cispimmunize.org
CDC, National Immunization Program		www.cdc.gov/vaccines/
National Network for Immunization Information		www.immunizationinfo.org

TABLE 22A – ANTI-INFECTIVE DRUG-DRUG INTERACTIONS

Importance: ± = theory/anecdotal; + = of probable importance; ++ = of definite importance
To check for interactions between more than 2 drugs, *see: http://www.drugs.com/drug_interactions.html and http://www.healthline.com/druginteractions*

ANTI-INFECTIVE AGENT (A)	OTHER DRUG (B)	EFFECT	IMPORT
Amantadine (Symmetrel)	Alcohol	↑ CNS effects	+
	Anticholinergic and anti-Parkinson agents (ex. Artane, scopolamine)	↑ effect of B: dry mouth, ataxia, blurred vision, slurred speech, toxic psychosis	+
	Trimethoprim	↑ levels of A & B	+
	Digoxin	↑ levels of B	±
Aminoglycosides—parenteral (amikacin, gentamicin, kanamycin, netilmicin, sisomicin, streptomycin, tobramycin)	Amphotericin B	↑ nephrotoxicity	++
	Cis platinum (Platinol)	↑ nephro & ototoxicity	+
	Cyclosporine	↑ nephrotoxicity	+
	Neuromuscular blocking agents	↑ apnea or respiratory paralysis	+
	Loop diuretics (e.g., furosemide)	↑ ototoxicity	++
	NSAIDs	↑ nephrotoxicity	+
	Non-polarizing muscle relaxants	↑ apnea	+
	Radiographic contrast	↑ nephrotoxicity	+
	Vancomycin	↑ nephrotoxicity	+
Aminoglycosides—oral (kanamycin, neomycin)	**Oral anticoagulants (dicumarol, phenindione, warfarin)**	↑ prothrombin time	+
Amphotericin B and ampho B lipid formulations	Antineoplastic drugs	↑ nephrotoxicity risk	+
	Digitalis	↑ toxicity of B if K^+ ↓	+
	Nephrotoxic drugs: aminoglycosides, cidofovir, cyclosporine, foscarnet, pentamidine	↑ nephrotoxicity of A	++
Ampicillin, amoxicillin	Allopurinol	↑ frequency of rash	++
Artemether-lumefantrine	CYP3A inhibitors: amiodarone, atazanavir, itraconazole, ritonavir, voriconazole	↑ levels of A; ↑ QTc interval	++
	CYP2D6 substrates: flecainide, imipramine, amitriptyline	↑ levels of B; ↑ QTc interval	++
Fosamprenavir	Antiretrovirals—*see Table 22B*		
	Contraceptives, oral	↓ levels of A & B; use other contraception	++
	Lovastatin/simvastatin	**↑ levels of B—avoid**	++
	Rifabutin	↑ levels of B (↓ dose by 50–75%)	++
	Rifampin	**↓ levels of A—avoid**	++
Atazanavir	*See protease inhibitors and Table 22B*		
Atovaquone	Rifampin (perhaps rifabutin)	↓ serum levels of A; ↑ levels of B	+
	Metoclopramide	↓ levels of A	+
	Tetracycline	↓ levels of A	++

Azole Antifungal Agents [***Flu*** = fluconazole; ***Itr*** = itraconazole; ***Ket*** = ketoconazole; ***Posa*** = posaconazole ***Vor*** = voriconazole; **+** = occurs; ***blank space*** = either studied & no interaction OR no data found (may be in pharm. co. databases)]

Flu	Itr	Ket	Posa	Vor	OTHER DRUG (B)	EFFECT	IMPORT
+	+				Amitriptyline	↑ levels of B	+
+	+	+		+	Calcium channel blockers	↑ levels of B	++
	+			+	Carbamazepine (vori contraindicated)	↓ levels of A	++
+	+	+	+	+	Cyclosporine	↑ levels of B, ↑ risk of nephrotoxicity	+
	+	+			Didanosine	↓ absorption of A	+
	+	+	+	+	Efavirenz	↓ levels of A, ↑ levels of B	++ **(avoid)**
	+	+	+		H_2 blockers, antacids, sucralfate	↓ absorption of A	+
+	+	+	+	+	Hydantoins (phenytoin, Dilantin)	↑ levels of B, ↓ levels of A	++
	+	+			Isoniazid	↓ levels of A	+
	+			+	Lovastatin/simvastatin	Rhabdomyolysis reported; ↑ levels of B	++
				+	Methadone	↑ levels of B	+
+	+	+	+	+	Midazolam/triazolam, po	↑ levels of B	++
+	+	+		+	Oral anticoagulants	↑ effect of B	++
+	+			+	Oral hypoglycemics	↑ levels of B	++
			+	+	Pimozide	↑ levels of B—**avoid**	++
	+	+		+	Protease inhibitors	↑ levels of B	++
	+	+	+	+	Proton pump inhibitors	↓ levels of A, ↑ levels of B	++
+	+	+	+	+	Rifampin/rifabutin (vori contraindicated)	↑ levels of B, ↓ serum levels of A	++
			+	+	Sirolimus (vori and posa contraindicated)	↑ levels of B	++
+		+	+	+	Tacrolimus	↑ levels of B with toxicity	++
+		+			Theophyllines	↑ levels of B	+
		+			Trazodone	↑ levels of B	++
+					Zidovudine	↑ levels of B	+

TABLE 22A (2)

ANTI-INFECTIVE AGENT (A)	OTHER DRUG (B)	EFFECT	IMPORT
Azole Antifungal Agents *(continued)*			
Caspofungin	Cyclosporine	↑ levels of A	++
	Tacrolimus	↓ levels of B	++
	Carbamazepine, dexamethasone, efavirenz, nevirapine, phenytoin, rifamycin	↓ levels of A; ↑ dose of caspofungin to 70 mg/d	++
Cephalosporins with methyl-tetrathiozolethiol side-chain	Oral anticoagulants (dicumarol, warfarin), heparin, thrombolytic agents, platelet aggregation inhibitors	↑ effects of B, bleeding	+
Chloramphenicol	Hydantoins	↑ toxicity of B, nystagmus, ataxia	++
	Iron salts, Vitamin B12	↓ response to B	++
	Protease inhibitors—HIV	↑ levels of A & B	++
Clindamycin (Cleocin)	Kaolin	↓ absorption of A	++
	Muscle relaxants, e.g., atracurium, baclofen, diazepam	↑ frequency/duration of respiratory paralysis	++
	St John's wort	↓ levels of A	++
Cycloserine	Ethanol	↑ frequency of seizures	+
	INH, ethionamide	↑ frequency of drowsiness/dizziness	+
Dapsone	Didanosine	↓ absorption of A	+
	Oral contraceptives	↓ effectiveness of B	+
	Pyrimethamine	↑ in marrow toxicity	+
	Rifampin/Rifabutin	↓ serum levels of A	+
	Trimethoprim	↑ levels of A & B (methemoglobinemia)	+
	Zidovudine	May ↑ marrow toxicity	+
Daptomycin	HMG-CoA inhibitors (statins)	DC statin while on dapto	++
Delavirdine (Rescriptor)	*See Non-nucleoside reverse transcriptase inhibitors (NNRTIs) and Table 22B*		
Didanosine (ddI) (Videx)	Allopurinol	↑ levels of A—**AVOID**	++
	Cisplatin, dapsone, INH, metronidazole, nitrofurantoin, stavudine, vincristine, zalcitabine	↑ risk of peripheral neuropathy	+
	Ethanol, lamivudine, pentamidine	↑ risk of pancreatitis	+
	Fluoroquinolones	↓ absorption 2° to chelation	+
	Drugs that need low pH for absorption: dapsone, indinavir, itra/ketoconazole, pyrimethamine, rifampin, trimethoprim	↓ absorption	+
	Methadone	↓ levels of A	++
	Ribavirin	↑ levels ddI metabolite—**avoid**	++
	Tenofovir	↑ levels of A **(reduce dose of A)**	++
Doripenem	Probenecid	↑ levels of A	++
	Valproic acid	↓ levels of B	++
Doxycycline	Aluminum, bismuth, iron, Mg^{++}	↓ absorption of A	+
	Barbiturates, hydantoins	↓ serum t/2 of A	+
	Carbamazepine (Tegretol)	↓ serum t/2 of A	+
	Digoxin	↑ serum levels of B	+
	Warfarin	↑ activity of B	++
Efavirenz (Sustiva)	*See non-nucleoside reverse transcriptase inhibitors (NNRTIs) and Table 22B*		
Ertapenem (Invanz)	Probenecid	↑ levels of A	++
	Valproic acid	↓ levels of B	++
Ethambutol (Myambutol)	Aluminum salts (includes didanosine buffer)	↓ absorption of A & B	+
Etravirine	***See non-nucleoside reverse transcriptase inhibitors (NNRTIs) and Table 22B***		

Fluoroquinolones (***Cipro*** = ciprofloxacin; ***Gati*** = gatifloxacin; ***Gemi*** = gemifloxacin; ***Levo*** = levofloxacin; ***Moxi*** = moxifloxacin; ***Oflox*** = ofloxacin)

Cipro	Gati	Gemi	Levo	Moxi	Oflox	***NOTE: Blank space*** *= either studied and no interaction OR no data found (pharm. co. may have data)*	EFFECT	IMPORT
	+		+	+		**Antiarrhythmics (procainamide, amiodarone)**	↑ Q-T interval (torsade)	++
+	+		+	+	+	Insulin, oral hypoglycemics	↑ & ↓ blood sugar	++
+						Caffeine	↑ levels of B	+
+					+	Cimetidine	↑ levels of A	+
+					+	Cyclosporine	↑ levels of B	±
+	+		+	+	+	Didanosine	↓ absorption of A	++
+	+	+	+	+	+	**Cations: Al+++, Ca++, Fe++, Mg++, Zn++ (antacids, vitamins, dairy products), citrate/citric acid**	↓ absorption of A (some variability between drugs)	++
+						Methadone	↑ levels of B	++
+			+		+	**NSAIDs**	↑ risk CNS stimulation/seizures	++
+						Phenytoin	↑ or ↓ levels of B	+
+	+	+			+	Probenecid	↓ renal clearance of A	+
+						Rasagiline	↑ levels of B	++

TABLE 22A (3)

ANTI-INFECTIVE AGENT (A)	OTHER DRUG (B)	EFFECT	IMPORT
Fluoroquinolones *(continued)*			

Cipro	Gati	Gemi	Levo	Moxi	Oflox	***NOTE: Blank space*** = either studied and no interaction OR no data found (pharm. co. may have data)		
				+		Rifampin	↓ levels of A *(CID 45:1001, 2007)*	++
+	+	+	+		+	**Sucralfate**	**↓ absorption of A**	++
+						Theophylline	↑ levels of B	++
+						Thyroid hormone	↓ levels of B	++
+						Tizanidine	↑ levels of B	++
+			+	+	+	Warfarin	↑ prothrombin time	+

ANTI-INFECTIVE AGENT (A)	OTHER DRUG (B)	EFFECT	IMPORT
Ganciclovir (Cytovene) & **Valganciclovir** (Valcyte)	Imipenem	↑ risk of seizures reported	+
	Probenecid	↑ levels of A	+
	Zidovudine	↓ levels of A, ↑ levels of B	+
Gentamicin	*See Aminoglycosides—parenteral*		
Imipenem & Meropenem	BCG	↓ effectiveness of B – avoid combination	++
	Divalproex	↓ levels of B	++
	Ganciclovir	↑ seizure risk	++
	Probenecid	↑ levels of A	++
	Valproic acid	↓ levels of B	++
Indinavir	*See protease inhibitors and Table 22B*		
Isoniazid	**Alcohol, rifampin**	**↑ risk of hepatic injury**	++
	Aluminum salts	↓ absorption (take fasting)	++
	Carbamazepine, phenytoin	↑ levels of B with nausea, vomiting, nystagmus, ataxia	++
	Itraconazole, ketoconazole	↓ levels of B	+
	Oral hypoglycemics	↓ effects of B	+
Lamivudine	Zalcitabine	**Mutual interference—do not combine**	++
Linezolid (Zyvox)	Adrenergic agents	Risk of hypertension	++
	Aged, fermented, pickled or smoked foods —↑ tyramine	Risk of hypertension	+
	Rasagiline (MAO inhibitor)	Risk of serotonin syndrome	+
	Rifampin	↓ levels of A	++
	Serotonergic drugs (SSRIs)	Risk of serotonin syndrome	++
Lopinavir	*See protease inhibitors*		

Macrolides [***Ery*** = erythromycin; ***Azi*** = azithromycin; ***Clr*** = clarithromycin; **+** = occurs; ***blank space*** = either studied and no interaction OR no data (pharm. co. may have data)]

Ery	Azi	Clr	OTHER DRUG (B)	EFFECT	IMPORT
+		+	Carbamazepine	↑ serum levels of B, nystagmus, nausea, vomiting, ataxia	**++ (avoid w/ erythro)**
+		+	Cimetidine, **ritonavir**	↑ levels of B	+
+			Clozapine	↑ serum levels of B, CNS toxicity	+
		+	**Colchicine**	**↑ levels of B (potent, fatal)**	**++(avoid)**
+			Corticosteroids	↑ effects of B	+
+	+	+	Cyclosporine	↑ serum levels of B with toxicity	+
+	+	+	Digoxin, digitoxin	↑ serum levels of B (10% of cases)	+
		+	Efavirenz	↓ levels of A	++
+		+	Ergot alkaloids	↑ levels of B	++
+		+	Lovastatin/simvastatin	↑ levels of B; rhabdomyolysis	++
+			Midazolam, triazolam	↑ levels of B, ↑ sedative effects	+
+		+	Phenytoin	↑ levels of B	+
+	+	+	Pimozide	**↑ Q-T interval**	++
+		+	Rifampin, rifabutin	↓ levels of A	+
+		+	Tacrolimus	↑ levels of B	++
+		+	Theophylline	↑ serum levels of B with nausea, vomiting, seizures, apnea	++
+		+	Valproic acid	↑ levels of B	+
+		+	Warfarin	May ↑ prothrombin time	+
		+	Zidovudine	↓ levels of B	+

ANTI-INFECTIVE AGENT (A)	OTHER DRUG (B)	EFFECT	IMPORT
Maraviroc	Clarithromycin	↑ serum levels of A	++
	Delavirdine	↑ levels of A	++
	Itraconazole/ketoconazole	↑ levels of A	++
	Nefazodone	↑ levels of A	++
	Protease Inhibitors (not tipranavir/ritonavir)	↑ levels of A	++
	Anticonvulsants: carbamazepine, phenobarbital, phenytoin	↓ levels of A	++
	Efavirenz	↓ levels of A	++
	Rifampin	↓ levels of A	++

TABLE 22A (4)

ANTI-INFECTIVE AGENT (A)	OTHER DRUG (B)	EFFECT	IMPORT
Macrolides *(continued)*			
Mefloquine	ß-adrenergic blockers, calcium channel blockers, quinidine, quinine	↑ arrhythmias	+
	Divalproex, valproic acid	↓ level of B with seizures	++
	Halofantrine	Q-T prolongation	++ **(avoid)**
Meropenem	*See Imipenem*		
Methenamine mandelate or hippurate	Acetazolamide, sodium bicarbonate, thiazide diuretics	↓ antibacterial effect 2° to ↑ urine pH	++
Metronidazole Tinidazole	**Alcohol**	Disulfiram-like reaction	+
	Cyclosporin	↑ levels of B	++
	Disulfiram (Antabuse)	Acute toxic psychosis	+
	Lithium	↑ levels of B	++
	Oral anticoagulants	↑ anticoagulant effect	++
	Phenobarbital, hydantoins	↑ levels of B	++
Micafungin	Nifedipine	↑ levels of B	+
	Sirolimus	↑ levels of B	+
Nelfinavir	*See protease inhibitors and Table 22B*		
Nevirapine (Viramune)	*See non-nucleoside reverse transcriptase inhibitors (NNRTIs) and Table 22B*		
Nitrofurantoin	Antacids	↓ absorption of A	+

Non-nucleoside reverse transcriptase inhibitors (NNRTIs): For interactions with protease inhibitors, *see Table 22B*.
Del = delavirdine; ***Efa*** = efavirenz; ***Etr*** = etravirine; ***Nev*** = nevirapine

Del	Efa	Etr	Nev	Co-administration contraindicated *(See package insert)*:		
+		+		Anticonvulsants: carbamazepine, phenobarbital, phenytoin		++
+		+		Antimycobacterials: rifabutin, rifampin		++
+				Antipsychotics: pimozide		++
+	+	+		Benzodiazepines: alprazolam, midazolam, triazolam		++
+	+			Ergotamine		++
+	+	+		HMG-CoA inhibitors (statins): lovastatin, simvastatin, atorvastatin, pravastatin		++
+		+		St. John's wort		++
				Dose change needed:		
+				Amphetamines	↑ levels of B—**caution**	++
+		+	+	Antiarrhythmics: amiodarone, lidocaine, others	↓ or ↑ levels of B—**caution**	++
+	+	+	+	Anticonvulsants: carbamazepine, phenobarbital, phenytoin	↓ levels of A and/or B	++
+	+	+	+	Antifungals: itraconazole, ketoconazole, voriconazole, posaconazole	Potential ↓ levels of B, ↑ levels of A	++ **(avoid)**
+			+	Antirejection drugs: cyclosporine, rapamycin, sirolimus, tacrolimus	↑ levels of B	++
+			+	Calcium channel blockers	↑ levels of B	++
+		+	+	Clarithromycin	↑ levels of B metabolite, ↑ levels of A	++
+		+	+	Cyclosporine	↑ levels of B	++
+		+		Dexamethasone	↓ levels of A	++
+	+	+	+	Sildenafil, vardenafil, tadalafil	↑ levels of B	++
+			+	Fentanyl, methadone	↑ levels of B	++
+				Gastric acid suppression: antacids, H-2 blockers, proton pump inhibitors	↓ levels of A	++
	+	+	+	Methadone, fentanyl	↓ levels of B	++
	+		+	Oral contraceptives	↑ or ↓ levels of B	++
+	+	+	+	Protease inhibitors—*see Table 22B*		
+	+	+	+	**Rifabutin, rifampin**	↑ or ↓ levels of rifabutin; ↓ levels of A—**caution**	++
+	+	+	+	St. John's wort	↓ levels of B	++
+		+	+	Warfarin	↑ levels of B	++

ANTI-INFECTIVE AGENT (A)	OTHER DRUG (B)	EFFECT	IMPORT
Pentamidine, IV	Amphotericin B	↑ risk of nephrotoxicity	+
	Pancreatitis-assoc drugs, eg, alcohol, valproic acid	↑ risk of pancreatitis	+
Piperacillin	Cefoxitin	Antagonism vs pseudomonas	++
Pip-tazo	Methotrexate	↑ levels of B	++
Polymyxin B	Curare paralytics	Avoid: neuromuscular blockade	++
Polymyxin E (Colistin)	Curare paralytics	Avoid: neuromuscular blockade	++
	Aminoglycosides, Ampho B, Vanco	↑ nephrotoxicity risk	++
Primaquine	Chloroquine, dapsone, INH, probenecid, quinine, sulfonamides, TMP/SMX, others	**↑ risk of hemolysis in G6PD-deficient patients**	++

TABLE 22A (5)

Protease Inhibitors—Anti-HIV Drugs. (***Atazan*** = atazanavir; ***Darun*** = darunavir; ***Fosampren*** = fosamprenavir; ***Indin*** = *indinavir;* ***Lopin*** = lopinavir; ***Nelfin*** = nelfinavir ; ***Saquin*** = saquinavir; ***Tipran*** = tipranavir). For interactions with antiretrovirals, *see Table 22B* ***Only a partial list—check package insert***

Also see http://aidsinfo.nih.gov
To check for interactions between more than 2 drugs, see: http://www.drugs.com/drug_interactions.html and http://www.healthline.com/druginteractions

ANTI-INFECTIVE AGENT (A)	Atazan	Darun	Fosampren	Indin	Lopin	Nelfin	Saquin	Tipran	OTHER DRUG (B)	EFFECT	IMPORT
									Analgesics:		
								+	1. Alfentanil, fentanyl, hydrocodone, tramadol	↑ levels of B	+
		+			+		+	+	2. Codeine, hydromorphone, morphine, methadone	↓ levels of B *(JAIDS 41:563, 2006)*	+
	+	+	+	+	+	+		+	**Anti-arrhythmics: amiodarone, lidocaine, mexiletine, flecainide**	↑ levels of B; **do not co-administer or use caution *(See package insert)***	++
		+		+	+	+	+		**Anticonvulsants: carbamazepine, clonazepam, phenobarbital**	↓ levels of A, ↑ levels of B	++
	+		+	+				+	Antidepressants, all tricyclic	↑ levels of B	++
	+	+						+	Antidepressants, all other	↑ levels of B; do not use pimozide	++
		+							Antidepressants: SSRIs	↓ levels of B - avoid	++
								+	Antihistamines	**Do not use**	++
	+	+	+	+	+	+		+	**Benzodiazepines, e.g., diazepam, midazolam, triazolam**	**↑ levels of B—do not use**	++
	+	+	+	+	+	+	+	+	Calcium channel blockers (all)	↑ levels of B	++
	+	+			+	+	+	+	Clarithro, erythro	↑ levels of B if renal impairment	+
	+	+			+	+		+	Contraceptives, oral	↓ levels of A & B	++
		+	+		+		+		Corticosteroids: prednisone, dexa-methasone	↓ levels of A, ↑ levels of B	+
	+	+	+	+	+	+	+	+	Cyclosporine	↑ levels of B, monitor levels	+
							+		Digoxin	↑ levels of B	++
	+	+	+	+	+	+	+	+	Ergot derivatives	**↑ levels of B—do not use**	++
			+	+		+	+		Erythromycin, clarithromycin	↑ levels of A & B	+
				+		+	+		Grapefruit juice (>200 mL/day)	↓ indinavir & ↑ saquinavir levels	++
	+	+	+	+	+	+	+		H2 receptor antagonists	↓ levels of A	++
	+	+	+	+	+	+	+	+	**HMG-CoA reductase inhibitors (statins): lovastatin, simvastatin**	**↑ levels of B—do not use**	++
	+								Irinotecan	**↑ levels of B—do not use**	++
		+	+	+	+	+	+	+	Ketoconazole, itraconazole, ? vori.	↑ levels of A, ↑ levels of B	+
		+	+	+	+	+	+	+	Posaconazole	↑ levels of A, no effect on B	++
					+			+	Metronidazole	Poss. disulfiram reaction, alcohol	+
					+				Phenytoin *(JAIDS 36:1034, 2004)*	↑ levels of A & B	++
	+	+	+	+	+	+	+	+	**Pimozide**	**↑ levels of B—do not use**	++
	+	+		+	+	+	+		Proton pump inhibitors	↓ levels of A	++
	+	+	+	+	+	+	+	+	Rifampin, rifabutin	↓ levels of A, ↑ levels of B **(avoid)**	++ **(avoid)**
	+	+	+	+	+	+	+	+	Sildenafil (Viagra), tadalafil, vardenafil	Varies, some ↑ & some ↓ levels of B	++
	+	+	+	+	+	+	+	+	**St. John's wort**	**↓ levels of A—do not use**	++
	+	+	+	+	+	+	+	+	**Sirolimus, tracrolimus**	**↑ levels of B**	++
	+								Tenofovir	↓ levels of A—add ritonavir	++
		+		+	+				Theophylline	↓ levels of B	+
	+		+		+			+	Warfarin	↑ levels of B	+
Pyrazinamide									INH, rifampin	May ↑ risk of hepatotoxicity	±
Pyrimethamine									Lorazepam	↑ risk of hepatotoxicity	+
									Sulfonamides, TMP/SMX	↑ risk of marrow suppression	+
									Zidovudine	↑ risk of marrow suppression	+
Quinine									Digoxin	↑ digoxin levels; ↑ toxicity	++
									Mefloquine	↑ arrhythmias	+
									Oral anticoagulants	↑ prothrombin time	++
Quinupristin- dalfopristin (Synercid)									Anti-HIV drugs: NNRTIs & PIs	↑ levels of B	++
									Antineoplastic: vincristine, docetaxel, paclitaxel	↑ levels of B	++
									Calcium channel blockers	↑ levels of B	++
									Carbamazepine	↑ levels of B	++
									Cyclosporine, tacrolimus	↑ levels of B	++
									Lidocaine	↑ levels of B	++
									Methylprednisolone	↑ levels of B	++
									Midazolam, diazepam	↑ levels of B	++
									Statins	↑ levels of B	++

TABLE 22A (6)

ANTI-INFECTIVE AGENT (A)	OTHER DRUG (B)	EFFECT	IMPORT
Protease Inhibitors—Anti-HIV Drugs *(continued)*			
Raltegravir	**Rifampin**	**↓ levels of A**	++
Ribavirin	Didanosine	↑ levels of B → toxicity—**avoid**	++
	Stavudine	↓ levels of B	++
	Zidovudine	↓ levels of B	++
Rifamycins (rifampin, rifabutin)	Al OH, ketoconazole, PZA	↓ levels of A	+
Ref.: *ArIM 162:985, 2002*	Atovaquone	↑ levels of A, ↓ levels of B	+
The following is a partial list of drugs with rifampin-induced ↑ metabolism and hence lower than anticipated serum levels: ACE inhibitors, dapsone, diazepam, digoxin, diltiazem, doxycycline, fluconazole, fluvastatin, haloperidol, moxifloxacin, nifedipine, progestins, triazolam, tricyclics, voriconazole, zidovudine *(Clin Pharmocokinet 42:819, 2003).*	Beta adrenergic blockers (metoprolol, propranolol)	↓ effect of B	+
	Caspofungin	↓ levels of B—increase dose	++
	Clarithromycin	↑ levels of A, ↓ levels of B	++
	Corticosteroids	↑ replacement requirement of B	++
	Cyclosporine	↓ effect of B	++
	Delavirdine	**↑ levels of A, ↓ levels of B—avoid**	++
	Digoxin	↓ levels of B	++
	Disopyramide	↓ levels of B	++
	Fluconazole	↑ levels of A	+
	Amprenavir, indinavir, nelfinavir, ritonavir	↑ levels of A (↓ dose of A), ↓ levels of B	++
	INH	Converts INH to toxic hydrazine	++
	Itraconazole, ketoconazole	↓ levels of B, ↑ levels of A	++
	Linezolid	↓ levels of B	++
	Methadone	↓ serum levels (withdrawal)	+
	Nevirapine	**↓ levels of B—avoid**	++
	Oral anticoagulants	Suboptimal anticoagulation	++
	Oral contraceptives	↓ effectiveness; spotting, pregnancy	+
	Phenytoin	↓ levels of B	+
	Protease inhibitors	**↓ levels of A, ↑ levels of B—CAUTION**	++
	Quinidine	↓ effect of B	+
	Raltegravir	↓ levels of B	++
	Sulfonylureas	↓ hypoglycemic effect	+
	Tacrolimus	**↓ levels of B**	++
	Theophylline	↑ levels of B	+
	TMP/SMX	↓ levels of A	+
	Tocainide	↓ effect of B	+
Rimantadine	*See Amantadine*		
Ritonavir	*See protease inhibitors and Table 22B*		
Saquinavir	*See protease inhibitors and Table 22B*		
Stavudine	Dapsone, INH	May ↑ risk of peripheral neuropathy	±
	Ribavirin	↓ levels of A—**avoid**	++
	Zidovudine	Mutual interference—do not combine	++
Sulfonamides	Beta blockers	↑ levels of B	++
	Cyclosporine	↓ cyclosporine levels	+
	Methotrexate	↑ antifolate activity	+
	Oral anticoagulants	↑ prothrombin time; bleeding	+
	Phenobarbital, rifampin	↓ levels of A	+
	Phenytoin	↑ levels of B; nystagmus, ataxia	+
	Sulfonylureas	↑ hypoglycemic effect	+
Telithromycin (Ketek)	Carbamazine	↓ levels of A	++
	Digoxin	↑ levels of B—do digoxin levels	++
	Ergot alkaloids	**↑ levels of B—avoid**	++
	Itraconazole; ketoconazole	↑ levels of A; no dose change	+
	Metoprolol	↑ levels of B	++
	Midazolam	↑ levels of B	++
	Oral anticoagulants	↑ prothrombin time	+
	Phenobarbital, phenytoin	↓ levels of A	++
	Pimozide	**↑ levels of B; QT prolongation—AVOID**	++
	Rifampin	**↓ levels of A—avoid**	++
	Simvastatin & other "statins"	↑ levels of B (↑ risk of myopathy)	++
	Sotalol	↓ levels of B	++
	Theophylline	↑ levels of B	++
Tenofovir	Atazanavir	↓ levels of B—add ritonavir	++
	Didanosine (ddI)	**↑ levels of B (reduce dose)**	++

TABLE 22A (7)

ANTI-INFECTIVE AGENT (A)	OTHER DRUG (B)	EFFECT	IMPORT
Protease Inhibitors—Anti-HIV Drugs *(continued)*			
Terbinafine	Cimetidine	↑ levels of A	+
	Phenobarbital, rifampin	↓ levels of A	+
Tetracyclines	*See Doxycycline, plus:*		
	Atovaquone	↓ levels of B	+
	Digoxin	↑ toxicity of B (may persist several months—up to 10% pts)	++
	Methoxyflurane	↑ toxicity; polyuria, renal failure	+
	Sucralfate	↓ absorption of A (separate by ≥2 hrs)	+
Thiabendazole	Theophyllines	↑ serum theophylline, nausea	+
Tigecycline	Oral contraceptives	↓ levels of B	++
Tinidazole (Tindamax)	*See Metronidazole—similar entity, expect similar interactions*		
Tobramycin	*See Aminoglycosides*		
Trimethoprim	Amantadine, dapsone, digoxin, methotrexate, procainamide, zidovudine	↑ serum levels of B	++
	Potassium-sparing diuretics	↑ serum K^+	++
	Repaglinide	↑ levels of B (hypoglycemia)	++
	Thiazide diuretics	↓ serum Na^+	+
Trimethoprim-Sulfameth-oxazole	Ace inhibitors	↑ serum K+	++
	Amantadine	↑ levels of B (toxicity)	++
	Azathioprine	Reports of leukopenia	+
	Cyclosporine	↓ levels of B, ↑ serum creatinine	+
	Loperamide	↑ levels of B	+
	Methotrexate	Enhanced marrow suppression	++
	Oral contraceptives, pimozide, and 6-mercaptopurine	↓ effect of B	+
	Phenytoin	↑ levels of B	+
	Rifampin	↑ levels of B	+
	Warfarin	↑ activity of B	+
Valganciclovir (Valcyte)	*See Ganciclovir*		
Vancomycin	Aminoglycosides	↑ frequency of nephrotoxicity	++
Zalcitabine (ddC) (HIVID)	Valproic acid, pentamidine (IV), alcohol, lamivudine	↑ pancreatitis risk	+
	Cisplatin, INH, metronidazole, vincristine, nitrofurantoin, d4T, dapsone	↑ risk of peripheral neuropathy	+
Zidovudine (ZDV) (Retrovir)	Atovaquone, fluconazole, methadone	↑ levels of A	+
	Clarithromycin	↓ levels of A	±
	Indomethacin	↑ levels of ZDV toxic metabolite	+
	Nelfinavir	↓ levels of A	++
	Probenecid, TMP/SMX	↑ levels of A	+
	Rifampin/rifabutin	↓ levels of A	++
	Stavudine	**Interference—DO NOT COMBINE!**	++
	Valproic Acid	↑ levels of A	++

TABLE 22B – DRUG-DRUG INTERACTIONS BETWEEN NON-NUCLEOSIDE REVERSE TRANSCRIPTASE INHIBITORS (NNRTIS) AND PROTEASE INHIBITORS
(Adapted from Guidelines for the Use of Antiretroviral Agents in HIV-Infected Adults & Adolescents; see *www.aidsinfo.nih.gov*)

NAME (Abbreviation, Trade Name)	Atazanavir (ATV, Reyataz)	DARUNAVIR (DRV, Prezista)	Fosamprenavir (FOS-APV, Lexiva)	Indinavir (IDV, Crixivan)	Lopinavir/Ritonavir (LP/R, Kaletra)	Nelfinavir (NFV, Viracept)	Saquinavir (SQV, Invirase)	Tipranavir (TPV)
Delavirdine (DLV, Rescriptor)	No data	No data	**Co-administration not recommended**	IDV levels ↑ 40%. Dose: IDV 600 mg q8h, DLV standard	Expect LP levels to ↑. No dose data	NFV levels ↑ 2X; DLV levels ↓ 50%. Dose: No data	SQV levels ↑ 5X. Dose: SQV 800 mg q8h, DLV standard	No data
Efavirenz (EFZ, Sustiva)	ATV AUC ↓ 74%. Dose: EFZ standard; ATA/RTV 300/100 mg q24h with food	Standard doses of both drugs	FOS-APV levels ↓. Dose: EFZ standard; FOS-APV 1400 mg + RTV 300 mg q24h or 700 mg FOS-APV + 100 mg RTV q12h	Levels: IDV ↓ 31%. Dose: IDV 1000 mg q8h. EFZ standard	Level of LP ↓ 40%. Dose: LP/R 533/133 mg q12h, EFZ standard	Standard doses	Level: SQV ↓ 62%. Dose: SQV 400 mg + RTV 400 mg q12h	No dose change necessary
Etravirine (ETR, Intelence)	↑ ATV & ↑ ETR levels.	Standard doses of both drugs	↑ levels of FOS-APV.	↓ level of IDV.	↑ levels of ETR, ↓ **levels of LP/R.**	↑ levels of NFV.	↓ ETR levels 33%; SQV/R no change. Standard dose of both drugs.	↓ levels of ETR, ↑ levels of TPV & RTV. **Avoid combination.**
Nevirapine (NVP, Viramune)	Avoid combination. ATZ increases NVP concentrations > 25%; NVP decreases ATZ AUC by 42%	Standard doses of both drugs	Use with caution. NVP AUC increased 14% (700/100 Fos/rit; NVP AUC inc 29% (Fos 1400 mg BID).	IDV levels ↓ 28%. Dose: IDV 1000 mg q8h or combine with RTV; NVP standard	LP levels ↓ 53%. Dose: LP/R 533/133 mg q12h; NVP standard	Standard doses	Dose: SQV + RTV 400/400 mg, both q12h	**Standard doses**

TABLE 23 – LIST OF GENERIC AND COMMON TRADE NAMES

GENERIC NAME: TRADE NAMES

Abacavir: Ziagen
Abacavir + Lamivudine: Epzicom
Abacavir + Lamivudine+Zidovudine: Trizivir
Acyclovir: Zovirax
Adefovir: Hepsera
Albendazole: Albenza
Amantadine: Symmetrel
Amikacin: Amikin
Amoxicillin: Amoxil, Polymox
Amoxicillin extended release: Moxatag
Amox./clav.: Augmentin, Augmentin ES-600; Augmentin XR
Amphotericin B: Fungizone
Ampho B-liposomal: AmBisome
Ampho B-lipid complex: Abelcet
Ampicillin: Omnipen, Polycillin
Ampicillin/sulbactam: Unasyn
Artemether-Lumefantrine: Coartem
Atazanavir: Reyataz
Atovaquone: Mepron
Atovaquone + proguanil: Malarone
Azithromycin: Zithromax
Azithromycin ER: Zmax
Aztreonam: Azactam, Cayston
Caspofungin: Cancidas
Cefaclor: Ceclor, Ceclor CD
Cefadroxil: Duricef
Cefazolin: Ancef, Kefzol
Cefdinir: Omnicef
Cefditoren pivoxil: Spectracef
Cefepime: Maxipime
Cefixime[NUS]: Suprax
Cefoperazone-sulbactam: Sulperazon[NUS]
Cefotaxime: Claforan
Cefotetan: Cefotan
Cefoxitin: Mefoxin
Cefpodoxime proxetil: Vantin
Cefprozil: Cefzil
Ceftaroline: Teflaro
Ceftazidime: Fortaz, Tazicef, Tazidime
Ceftibuten: Cedax
Ceftizoxime: Cefizox
Ceftobiprole: Zeftera
Ceftriaxone: Rocephin
Cefuroxime: Zinacef, Ceftin
Cephalexin: Keflex
Cephradine: Anspor, Velosef
Chloroquine: Aralen
Cidofovir: Vistide
Ciprofloxacin: Cipro, Cipro XR
Clarithromycin: Biaxin, Biaxin XL
Clindamycin: Cleocin
Clofazimine: Lamprene
Clotrimazole: Lotrimin, Mycelex
Cloxacillin: Tegopen
Colistimethate: Coly-Mycin M
Cycloserine: Seromycin
Daptomycin: Cubicin
Darunavir: Prezista

Delavirdine: Rescriptor
Dicloxacillin: Dynapen
Didanosine: Videx
Diethylcarbamazine: Hetrazan
Diloxanide furoate: Furamide
Doripenem: Doribax
Doxycycline: Vibramycin

GENERIC NAME: TRADE NAMES

Drotrecogin alfa: Xigris
Efavirenz: Sustiva
Efavirenz/Emtricitabine/Tenofovir: Atripla
Emtricitabine: Emtriva
Emtricitabine + tenofovir: Truvada
Enfuvirtide (T-20): Fuzeon
Entecavir: Baraclude
Ertapenem: Invanz
Etravirine: Intelence
Erythromycin(s): Ilotycin
Ethyl succinate: Pediamycin
Glucoheptonate: Erythrocin
Estolate: Ilosone
Erythro/sulfisoxazole: Pediazole
Ethambutol: Myambutol
Ethionamide: Trecator
Famciclovir: Famvir
Fluconazole: Diflucan
Flucytosine: Ancobon
Fosamprenavir: Lexiva
Foscarnet: Foscavir
Fosfomycin: Monurol
Ganciclovir: Cytovene
Gatifloxacin: Tequin
Gemifloxacin: Factive
Gentamicin: Garamycin
Griseofulvin: Fulvicin
Halofantrine: Halfan
Idoxuridine: Dendrid, Stoxil
INH + RIF: Rifamate
INH + RIF + PZA: Rifater
Interferon alfa: Intron A
Interferon, pegylated: PEG-Intron, Pegasys
Interferon + ribavirin: Rebetron
Imipenem + cilastatin: Primaxin, Tienam
Imiquimod: Aldara
Indinavir: Crixivan
Itraconazole: Sporanox
Iodoquinol: Yodoxin
Ivermectin: Stromectol
Kanamycin: Kantrex
Ketoconazole: Nizoral
Lamivudine: Epivir, Epivir-HBV
Lamivudine + abacavir: Epzicom
Levofloxacin: Levaquin
Linezolid: Zyvox
Lomefloxacin: Maxaquin
Lopinavir/ritonavir: Kaletra
Loracarbef: Lorabid
Mafenide: Sulfamylon
Maraviroc: Selzentry
Mebendazole: Vermox
Mefloquine: Lariam
Meropenem: Merrem
Mesalamine: Asacol, Pentasa
Methenamine: Hiprex, Mandelamine
Metronidazole: Flagyl
Micafungin: Mycamine
Minocycline: Minocin
Moxifloxacin: Avelox
Mupirocin: Bactroban
Nafcillin: Unipen
Nelfinavir: Viracept
Nevirapine: Viramune
Nitazoxanide: Alinia
Nitrofurantoin: Macrobid, Macrodantin

GENERIC NAME: TRADE NAMES

Nystatin: Mycostatin
Ofloxacin: Floxin
Oseltamivir: Tamiflu
Oxacillin: Prostaphlin
Palivizumab: Synagis
Paromomycin: Humatin
Pentamidine: NebuPent, Pentam 300
Piperacillin: Pipracil
Piperacillin/tazobactam: Zosyn, Tazocin
Piperazine: Antepar
Podophyllotoxin: Condylox
Polymyxin B: Poly-Rx
Posaconazole: Noxafil
Praziquantel: Biltricide
Primaquine: Primachine
Proguanil: Paludrine
Pyrantel pamoate: Antiminth
Pyrimethamine: Daraprim
Pyrimethamine/sulfadoxine: Fansidar
Quinupristin/dalfopristin: Synercid
Raltegravir: Isentress
Retapamulin: Altabax
Ribavirin: Virazole, Rebetol
Rifabutin: Mycobutin
Rifampin: Rifadin, Rimactane
Rifapentine: Priftin
Rifaximin: Xifaxan
Rimantadine: Flumadine
Ritonavir: Norvir
Saquinavir: Invirase
Spectinomycin: Trobicin
Stavudine: Zerit
Stibogluconate: Pentostam
Silver sulfadiazine: Silvadene
Sulfamethoxazole: Gantanol
Sulfasalazine: Azulfidine
Sulfisoxazole: Gantrisin
Telbivudine : Tyzeka
Telavancin: Vibativ
Telithromycin: Ketek
Temocillin: Negaban, Temopen
Tenofovir: Viread
Terbinafine: Lamisil
Thalidomide: Thalomid Thiabendazole: Mintezol
Ticarcillin: Ticar
Tigecycline: Tygacil
Tinidazole: Tindamax
Tipranavir: Aptivus
Tobramycin: Nebcin
Tretinoin: Retin A
Trifluridine: Viroptic
Trimethoprim: Primsol
Trimethoprim/sulfamethoxazole: Bactrim, Septra
Valacyclovir: Valtrex
Valganciclovir: Valcyte
Vancomycin: Vancocin
Voriconazole: Vfend
Zalcitabine: HIVID
Zanamivir: Relenza
Zidovudine (ZDV): Retrovir
Zidovudine + 3TC: Combivir
Zidovudine + 3TC + abacavir: Trizivir

TABLE 23 (2)
LIST OF COMMON TRADE AND GENERIC NAMES

TRADE NAME: GENERIC NAME
Abelcet: Ampho B-lipid complex
Albenza: Albendazole
Aldara: Imiquimod
Alinia: Nitazoxanide
Altabax: Retapamulin
AmBisome: Ampho B-liposomal
Amikin: Amikacin
Amoxil: Amoxicillin
Ancef: Cefazolin
Ancobon: Flucytosine
Anspor: Cephradine
Antepar: Piperazine
Antiminth: Pyrantel pamoate
Aptivus: Tipranavir
Aralen: Chloroquine
Asacol: Mesalamine
Atripla: Efavirenz/emtricitabine/tenofovir Augmentin, Augmentin ES-600
Augmentin XR: Amox./clav.
Avelox: Moxifloxacin
Azactam: Aztreonam
Azulfidine: Sulfasalazine
Bactroban: Mupirocin
Bactrim: Trimethoprim/sulfamethoxazole
Baraclude: Entecavir
Biaxin, Biaxin XL: Clarithromycin
Biltricide: Praziquantel
Cancidas: Caspofungin
Cayston: Aztreonam (inhaled)
Ceclor, Ceclor CD: Cefaclor
Cedax: Ceftibuten
Cefizox: Ceftizoxime
Cefotan: Cefotetan
Ceftin: Cefuroxime axetil
Cefzil: Cefprozil
Cipro, Cipro XR: Ciprofloxacin & extended release
Claforan: Cefotaxime
Coartem: Artemether-Lumefantrine
Coly-Mycin M: Colistimethate
Combivir: ZDV + 3TC
Crixivan: Indinavir
Cubicin: Daptomycin
Cytovene: Ganciclovir
Daraprim: Pyrimethamine
Diflucan: Fluconazole
Doribax: Doripenem
Duricef: Cefadroxil
Dynapen: Dicloxacillin
Emtriva: Emtricitabine
Epivir, Epivir-HBV: Lamivudine
Epzicom: Lamivudine + abacavir
Factive: Gemifloxacin
Famvir: Famciclovir
Fansidar: Pyrimethamine + sulfadoxine
Flagyl: Metronidazole
Floxin: Ofloxacin
Flumadine: Rimantadine
Foscavir: Foscarnet
Fortaz: Ceftazidime
Fulvicin: Griseofulvin
Fungizone: Amphotericin B
Furadantin: Nitrofurantoin
Fuzeon: Enfuvirtide (T-20)
Gantanol: Sulfamethoxazole
Gantrisin: Sulfisoxazole
Garamycin: Gentamicin
Halfan: Halofantrine
Hepsera: Adefovir
Herplex: Idoxuridine
Hiprex: Methenamine hippurate
HIVID: Zalcitabine
Humatin: Paromomycin
Ilosone: Erythromycin estolate
Ilotycin: Erythromycin
Intelence: Etravirine
Intron A: Interferon alfa
Invanz: Ertapenem
Invirase: Saquinavir
Isentress: Raltegravir
Kantrex: Kanamycin
Kalotra: Lopinavir/ritonavir
Keflex: Cephalexin
Ketek: Telithromycin
Lamisil: Terbinafine
Lamprene: Clofazimine
Lariam: Mefloquine
Levaquin: Levofloxacin
Lexiva: Fosamprenavir
Lorabid: Loracarbef
Macrodantin, Macrobid: Nitrofurantoin
Malarone: Atovaquone + proguanil
Mandelamine: Methenamine mandel.
Maxaquin: Lomefloxacin
Maxipime: Cefepime
Mefoxin: Cefoxitin
Mepron: Atovaquone
Merrem: Meropenem
Minocin: Minocycline
Mintezol: Thiabendazole
Monocid: Cefonicid
Monurol: Fosfomycin
Moxatag: Amoxicillin extended release
Myambutol: Ethambutol
Mycamine: Micafungin
Mycobutin: Rifabutin
Mycostatin: Nystatin
Nafcil: Nafcillin
Nebcin: Tobramycin
NebuPent: Pentamidine
Nizoral: Ketoconazole
Norvir: Ritonavir
Noxafil: Posaconazole
Omnicef: Cefdinir
Omnipen: Ampicillin
Pediamycin: Erythro. ethyl succinate
Pediazole: Erythro. ethyl succinate + sulfisoxazole
Pegasys, PEG-Intron: Interferon, pegylated
Pentam 300: Pentamidine
Pentasa: Mesalamine
Pipracil: Piperacillin
Polycillin: Ampicillin
Polymox: Amoxicillin
Poly-Rx: Polymyxin B
Prezista: Darunavir
Priftin: Rifapentine
Primaxin: Imipenem + cilastatin
Primsol: Trimethoprim
Prostaphlin: Oxacillin
Rebetol: Ribavirin
Rebetron: Interferon + ribavirin
Relenza: Zanamivir
Rescriptor: Delavirdine
Retin A: TretinoinRetrovir: Zidovudine (ZDV)
Reyataz: Atazanavir
Rifadin: Rifampin
Rifamate: INH + RIF
Rifater: INH + RIF + PZA
Rimactane: Rifampin
Rocephin: Ceftriaxone
Selzentry: Maraviroc
Septra: Trimethoprim/sulfa
Seromycin: Cycloserine
Silvadene: Silver sulfadiazine
Spectracef: Cefditoren pivoxil
Sporanox: Itraconazole
Stoxil: Idoxuridine
Stromectol: Ivermectin
Sulfamylon: Mafenide
Sulperazon[NUS]: Cefoperazone-sulbactam
Suprax: Cefixime[NUS]
Sustiva: Efavirenz
Symmetrel: Amantadine
Synagis: Palivizumab
Synercid: Quinupristin/dalfopristin
Tamiflu: Oseltamivir
Tazicef: Ceftazidime
Teflaro: Ceftaroline
Tegopen: Cloxacillin
Tequin: Gatifloxacin
Thalomid: Thalidomide
Ticar: Ticarcillin
Tienam: Imipenem
Timentin: Ticarcillin-clavulanic acid
Tinactin: Tolnaftate
Tindamax: Tinidazole
Trecator SC: Ethionamide
Trizivir: Abacavir + ZDV + 3TC
Trobicin: Spectinomycin
Truvada: Emtricitabine + tenofovir
Tygacil: Tigecycline
Tyzeka: Telbivudine
Unasyn: Ampicillin/sulbactam
Unipen: Nafcillin
Valcyte: Valganciclovir
Valtrex: Valacyclovir
Vancocin: Vancomycin
Vantin: Cefpodoxime proxetil
Velosef: Cephradine
Vermox: Mebendazole
Vfend: Voriconazole
Vibativ: Telavancin
Vibramycin: Doxycycline
Videx: Didanosine
Viracept: Nelfinavir
Viramune: Nevirapine
Virazole: Ribavirin
Viread: Tenofovir
Vistide: Cidofovir
Xifaxan: Rifaximin
Xigris: Drotrecogin alfa
Yodoxin: Iodoquinol
Zerit: Stavudine
Zeftera: Ceftobiprole
Ziagen: Abacavir
Zinacef: Cefuroxime
Zithromax: Azithromycin
Zmax: Azithromycin ER
Zovirax: Acyclovir
Zosyn: Piperacillin/tazobactam
Zyvox: Linezolid

INDEX OF MAJOR ENTITIES

PAGES (page numbers bold if major focus)

Bold numbers indicate major considerations. Antibiotic selection often depends on modifying circumstances and alternative agents.

PAGES (page numbers bold if major focus)

PAGES (page numbers bold if major focus)

PAGES (page numbers bold if major focus)

N

PAGES (page numbers bold if major focus)

O

P

PAGES (page numbers bold if major focus)

PAGES (page numbers bold if major focus)

PAGES (page numbers bold if major focus)